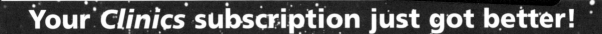
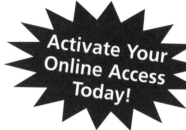
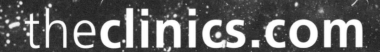

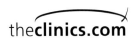

MAGNETIC RESONANCE IMAGING CLINICS
of North America

Abdominal MR Imaging

DIEGO R. MARTIN, MD, PhD
Guest Editor

May 2005 • Volume 13 • Number 2

SAUNDERS

An Imprint of Elsevier, Inc.
PHILADELPHIA   LONDON   TORONTO   MONTREAL   SYDNEY   TOKYO

W.B. SAUNDERS COMPANY
A Divison of Elsevier Inc.

Elsevier, Inc. • 1600 John F. Kennedy Boulevard • Suite 1800 • Philadelphia, Pennsylvania 19103-2899

http://www.theclinics.com

MRI CLINICS OF NORTH AMERICA   **Volume 13, Number 2**
May 2005   **ISSN 1064-9689**
Editor: Barton Dudlick   **ISBN 1-4160-2731-9**

Reprints: For copies of 100 or more, of articles in this publication, please contact the Commercial Re-prints Department, Elsevier Inc., 360 Park Avenue South, New York, New York 10010-1710. Tel. (212) 633-3813 Fax: (212) 462-1935 email: reprints@elsevier.com.

The ideas and opinions expressed in *Magnetic Resonance Imaging Clinics of North America* do not neces-sarily reflect those of the Publisher. The Publisher does not assume any responsibility for any injury and/or damage to persons or property arising out of or related to any use of the material contained in this periodical. The reader is advised to check the appropriate medical literature and the product in-formation currently provided by the manufacturer of each drug to be administered to verify the dosage, the method and duration of administration, or contraindications. It is the responsibility of the treating physician or other health care professional, relying on independent experience and knowledge of the patient, to determine drug dosages and the best treatment for the patient. Mention of any product in this issue should not be construed as endorsement by the contributors, editors, or the Publisher of the product or manufacturers' claims.

Magnetic Resonance Imaging Clinics of North America (ISSN 1064-9689) is published quarterly by the W.B. Saunders Company. Corporate and editorial offices: Elsevier, Inc., 1600 John F. Kennedy Boule-vard, Suite 1800, Philadelphia, PA 19103-2899. Accounting and circulation offices: 6277 Sea Harbor Drive, Orlando, FL 32887-4800. Periodicals postage paid at Orlando, FL 32862, and additional mailing offices. Subscription prices are $190.00 per year (US individuals), $290.00 per year (US institutions), $95.00 (US students and residents), $214.00 per year (Canadian individuals), $352.00 per year (Canadian institutions), $255.00 per year (foreign individuals), and $352.00 per year (foreign institutions). To re-ceive student and resident rate, orders must be accompanied by name of affiliated institution, date of term, and the *signature* of program/residency coordinator on institution letter-head. Orders will be billed at individual rate until proof of status is received. Foreign air speed delivery is included in all *Clinics* subscription prices. All prices are subject to change without notice. POSTMASTER: Send address changes to *Magnetic Resonance Imaging Clinics of North America*, W.B. Saunders Company, Periodicals Fulfillment, Orlando, FL 32887-4800. **Customer Service: 1-800-654-2452 (US). From outside of the US, call 1-407-345-4000. E-mail: hhspcs@harcourt.com.**

Magnetic Resonance Imaging Clinics of North America is covered in the *RSNA Index of Imaging Literature, Index Medicus, MEDLINE,* and *EMBASE/Excerpta Medica.*

Printed in the United States of America.

GUEST EDITOR

DIEGO R. MARTIN, MD, PhD, Professor and Director of MRI, Department of Radiology, Emory University School of Medicine, Atlanta, Georgia

CONTRIBUTORS

WALEED AJAJ, MD, Department of Diagnostic and Interventional Radiology and Neuroradiology, University Hospital Essen, Essen, Germany

N. CEM BALCI, MD, Associate Professor of Radiology, Department of Radiology, University of Kocaeli, Derince, Kocaeli, Turkey

MICHELLE BRADBURY, MD, PhD, Department of Radiology, Memorial Sloan Kettering Cancer Center, New York, New York

MICHÈLE A. BROWN, MD, Assistant Professor, Department of Radiology, UCSD Medical Center, San Diego, California

RAMAN DANRAD, MD, Department of Radiology, Emory University School of Medicine, Atlanta, Georgia

JAN DE BECKER, PhD, Clinical Scientist, Philips Medical Systems, Best, The Netherlands

J. PAUL FINN, MD, Professor of Radiology, Department of Radiological Sciences, David Geffen School of Medicine, University of California Los Angeles, Los Angeles, California

HARRY T. FRIEL, MS, Clinical Scientist, Philips Medical Systems, Highland Heights, Ohio

SAMANTHA L. HELLER, MD, PhD, Department of Radiology, New York University Medical Center, New York, New York

HEDVIG HRICAK, MD, PhD, Department of Radiology, Memorial Sloan Kettering Cancer Center, New York, New York

SHAHID M. HUSSAIN, MD, Head, Section of Abdominal Imaging, Department of Radiology, Erasmus University Medical Center, Rotterdam, The Netherlands

W. BRIAN HYSLOP, MD, PhD, Department of Radiology, University of North Carolina, Chapel Hill, North Carolina

CHRISTIANE A. KUEHLE, MD, Department of Diagnostic and Interventional Radiology and Neuroradiology, University Hospital Essen, Essen, Germany

ANDREA LAGHI, MD, Researcher, Department of Radiological Sciences, University of Rome "La Sapienza," Latina, Italy

GERHARD LAUB, PhD, Siemens Medical Solutions, Los Angeles, California

THOMAS C. LAUENSTEIN, MD, Department of Diagnostic and Interventional Radiology and Neuroradiology, University Hospital Essen, Essen, Germany

VIVIAN S. LEE, MD, PhD, Professor and Vice-Chair of Research, Department of Radiology, New York University Medical Center, New York, New York

DIEGO R. MARTIN, MD, PhD, Professor and Director of MRI, Department of Radiology, Emory University School of Medicine, Atlanta, Georgia

KAMBIZ NAEL, MD, Department of Radiological Sciences, David Geffen School of Medicine, University of California Los Angeles, Los Angeles, California

ERTAN PAMUKLAR, MD, Department of Radiology, University of North Carolina, Chapel Hill, North Carolina

PASQUALE PAOLANTONIO, MD, Fellow, Department of Radiological Sciences, University of Rome "La Sapienza," Rome, Italy

ROBERTO PASSARIELLO, MD, Professor and Chairman, Department of Radiological Sciences, University of Rome "La Sapienza," Rome, Italy

RICHARD C. SEMELKA, MD, Professor of Radiology; Director of MR Services; and Vice Chairman of Clinical Research, Department of Radiology, University of North Carolina, Chapel Hill, North Carolina

CLAUDE B. SIRLIN, MD, Assistant Professor, Department of Radiology, UCSD Medical Center, San Diego, California

CONTENTS

article also introduces concepts and the specific alteration of sequence parameters for optimization of abdominal–pelvic imaging at 3 Tesla.

MR imaging features of liver masses are described on current state-of-the-art MR imaging sequences. Liver masses are divided into solid and nonsolid lesions. The description of nonsolid masses includes cysts, biliary hamartomas, and hemangiomas. The description of solid lesions includes metastases to the liver and primary liver lesions (such as focal nodular hyperplasia, hepatocellular adenomas, and hepatocellular carcinomas). Finally, MR imaging is compared with other modalities.

This article discusses MR imaging sequences that are used for the evaluation of diffuse liver diseases, including processes that lead to abnormal lipid metabolization, iron deposition disease, and perfusion abnormalities.

MR imaging is an established technique for the diagnosis of a spectrum of biliary and gallbladder pathologies. It continues to improve with the advent of technologic advances, which include new contrast agents and new sequences that are capable of improving upon the contrast resolution and signal-to-noise that are afforded by conventional MR imaging. This article reviews conventional and more recent MR imaging approaches to diseases of the gallbladder and biliary system.

MR imaging is a valuable tool in the assessment of the full spectrum of pancreatic diseases. MR imaging is effective as a problem-solving modality because, in the majority of cases, it distinguishes chronic pancreatitis from the normal pancreas and chronic pancreatitis with focal enlargement from pancreatic cancer.

MR imaging, using modern equipment and a rigorous technical approach, is able to offer detailed morphologic information and functional data on the small bowel. Technical requirements include a high magnetic field and fast imaging. An adequate small bowel distension is mandatory for an accurate study and is obtained by using an oral contrast agent ("MR follow-through") or a naso-jejunal catheter ("MR enteroclysis"). A major clinical indication is the evaluation of patients who have suspected inflammatory bowel disease, in particular, Crohn's disease. The absence of ionizing radiation, considering the young age of most of the patients and the frequency of the examinations, is an important advantage over other techniques (radiograph and CT enteroclysis).

FORTHCOMING ISSUES

RECENT ISSUES

THE CLINICS ARE NOW AVAILABLE ONLINE!

Access your subscription at:
www.theclinics.com

GOAL STATEMENT

The goal of *Magnetic Resonance Imaging Clinics of North America* is to keep practicing radiologists and radiology residents up to date with current clinical practice in radiology by providing timely articles reviewing the state of the art in patient care.

ACCREDITATION

The *Magnetic Resonance Imaging Clinics of North America* is planned and implemented in accordance with the Essential Areas and Policies of the Accreditation Council for Continuing Medical Education (ACCME) through the joint sponsorship of the University of Virginia School of Medicine and Elsevier. The University of Virginia School of Medicine is accredited by the ACCME to provide continuing medical education for physicians.

The University of Virginia School of Medicine designates this educational activity for a maximum of 60 category 1 credits per year, 15 category 1 credits per issue, toward the AMA Physician's Recognition Award. Each physician should claim only those credits that he/she actually spent in the activity.

The American Medical Association has determined that physicians not licensed in the US who participate in this CME activity are eligible for AMA PRA category 1 credit.

Category 1 credit can be earned by reading the text material, taking the CME examination online at http://www.theclinics.com/home/cme, and completing the evaluation. After taking the test, you will be required to review any and all incorrect answers. Following completion of the test and evaluation, your credit will be awarded and you may print your certificate.

FACULTY DISCLOSURE

As a provider accredited by the Accreditation Council for Continuing Medical Education (ACCME), the Office of Continuing Medical Education of the University of Virginia School of Medicine must ensure balance, independence, objectivity, and scientific rigor in all its individually sponsored or jointly sponsored educational activities. All authors/editors participating in a sponsored activity are expected to disclose to the readers any significant financial interest or other relationship (1) with the manufacturer(s) of any commercial product(s) and/or provider(s) of commercial services discussed in an educational presentation and (2) with any commercial supporters of the activity (significant financial interest or other relationship can include such things as grants or research support, employee, consultant, stock holder, member of speakers bureau, etc.) The intent of this disclosure is not to prevent authors/editors with a significant financial or other relationship from writing an article, but rather to provide readers with information on which they can make their own judgments. It remains for the readers to determine whether the author's/editor's interest or relationships may influence the article with regard to exposition or conclusion.

The authors/editors listed below have identified no professional or financial affiliations related to their presentation:
N. Cem Balci, MD; Michelle Bradbury, MD, PhD; Michèle A. Brown, MD; Barton Dudlick, Acquisitions Editor; Harry T. Friel, MS; Hedvig Hricak, MD, PhD; Shahid M. Hussain, MD; Christiane A. Kuehle, MD; Andrea Laghi, MD; Thomas C. Lauenstein, MD; Diego R. Martin, MD, PhD; Kambiz Nael, MD; Ertan Pamuklar, MD; Pasquale Paolantonio, MD; Roberto Passariello, MD; Richard C. Semelka, MD; and Claude B. Sirlin, MD.

The author listed below has identified the following professional or financial affiliation related to his presentation:
Gerhard Laub, PhD, is a Siemens Medical Solutions, Inc. employee.
J. Paul Finn, MD, has received research support from Siemens Medical Solutions, Inc.

Disclosure of Discussion of non-FDA approved uses for pharmaceutical products and/or medical devices: The University of Virginia School of Medicine, as an ACCME provider, requires that all authors identify and disclose any "off label" uses for pharmaceutical and medical device products. The University of Virginia School of Medicine recommends that each physician fully review all the available data on new products or procedures prior to instituting them with patients.

All authors who provided disclosures will not be discussing off-label uses except the following:
J. Paul Finn, MD, Gerhard Laub, PhD, and Kambiz Nael, MD, will discuss the use of gadodiamide.

The authors listed below have not provided disclosure or off-label information:
Waleed Ajaj, MD; Raman Danrad, MD; Jan De Becker, PhD; Samantha L. Heller, MD, PhD; W. Brian Hyslop, MD, PhD; and Vivian S. Lee, MD, PhD.

TO ENROLL

To enroll in the *Magnetic Resonance Imaging Clinics of North America* Continuing Medical Education program, call customer service at 1-800-654-2452 or visit us online at http://www.theclinics.com/home/cme. The CME program is available to subscribers for an additional fee of $165.00.

Magn Reson Imaging Clin N Am
13 (2005) xi–xii

MAGNETIC
RESONANCE
IMAGING CLINICS
of North America

Preface

Abdominal MR Imaging

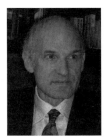

Diego R. Martin, MD, PhD
Guest Editor

Diagnostic cross-sectional imagers should agree on certain principles with regard to future directions. The ultimate goals for our techniques should include the ability to safely and non-invasively make specific and accurate diagnoses of tissue pathology in living functional tissue and to replace the need for extracting tissue specimens for the purpose of histopathology that have been considered historically to represent a diagnostic gold standard. Clinical diagnostic MR imaging of the abdomen and pelvis has been shown to provide an imaging technology that may be optimal for diagnostic sensitivity and specificity for a wide range of applications compared with ultrasound or CT. Although MR imaging historically has been perceived as being more complex and less accessible than CT, there has been strong incentive to continue to pursue MR development to minimize the need for CT with associated ionizing radiation, to avoid the use of iodinated contrast agents with potentially greater health risks compared with MR contrast agents, and to exploit MR capabilities for tissues characterization, both morphologically and functionally.

One of the major themes to which I would like to draw the attention of the reader of this issue of the *Magnetic Resonance Imaging Clinics of North America* is that MR imaging provides more information about the tissues beyond morphology. This information is based on the capacity to generate contrast from tissues based on the composition of intracellular and extracellular molecular elements, and it is this information that facilitates diagnostic conclusions about tumors and assessment of diffuse diseases of organ systems, such as hepatitis, hemochromatosis, or abnormal intracellular lipid accumulation. The use of intravenously administered contrast agents is critically important for both CT and MR imaging of tissue diseases; however, here again, there are clear benefits of MR imaging: one major factor being that following the injected contrast, as it perfuses through the tissues, requires repeated imaging with adequate temporal resolution, and this can be achieved by way of MR imaging without any concern for accumulation of radiation dosages.

Another major theme is that MR imaging is in a period of rapid development. Much of the earlier work on MR imaging concentrated on understanding the appearance of various diseases using different sequences and establishing the fundamental methodology. These fundamental methodologic principles are discussed in the article on imaging development at 3 Tesla. The concepts guiding future development are discussed in the articles on future perspectives, molecular imaging, and contrast agents. These articles discuss the fundamental concepts addressing the technical development of MR systems and of new methods for generating contrast from the tissues, including new contrast agents, and aspects of MR that inherently generate information that is based on the molecular and cellular composition and structure of tissues, such as spectroscopy.

Rather than being an exhaustive review of all organ systems, a selection of important MR imaging applications were chosen, including liver, bile ducts and gallbladder, pancreas, and the female pelvis (the kidney and male pelvis having being discussed in detail in recent issues of the *Magnetic Resonance Imaging Clinics of North America*). Imaging of the small and large bowel are recent applications that are becoming well established in selected centers. MR angiography is widely used, but the use and approach to imaging at a higher 3 Tesla field strength warranted specific discussion, particularly given the increasing number of higher field strength systems being introduced into imaging centers in North America and indeed globally.

Finally, this issue should contribute to establishing the utilization of MR imaging for routine evaluation of most of the important diseases affecting the soft tissues within the abdomen and pelvis. It is my impression that, unfortunately, the utility of MR imaging still exceeds the utilization in most imaging centers. There may be many reasons for this discrepancy, with the need for further education and dissemination of knowledge of these applications representing one contributing factor. It is my sincere hope that the articles in this issue of the *Magnetic Resonance Imaging Clinics of North America* may have a positive impact on increasing the general desire and comfort level for exploiting abdominal MR imaging tools for common applications.

Diego R. Martin, MD, PhD
Department of Radiology
Emory University Hospital
1364 Clifton Road NE
Atlanta, GA 30322, USA

E-mail address: diego_martin@emoryhealthcare.org

ELSEVIER
SAUNDERS

Magn Reson Imaging Clin N Am
13 (2005) 211–224

MAGNETIC
RESONANCE
IMAGING CLINICS
of North America

Future Horizons in MR Imaging

W. Brian Hyslop, MD, PhD[a], N. Cem Balci, MD[b],
Richard C. Semelka, MD[a],*

[a]Department of Radiology, University of North Carolina, 101 Manning Drive, CB #7510,
Chapel Hill, NC 27599-7510, USA
[b]Department of Radiology, University of Kocaeli, Derince, Kocaeli, Turkey

Body MR imaging continues to experience rapid growth in the type and number of studies performed. Given the rapid pace of technologic innovation in body MR imaging and the subsequent development of clinical applications, long-range predictions are difficult to make. By reviewing the current state-of-the-art in selected topics in body MR imaging, it is reasonable to project their potential for novel clinical or research applications in the near future.

We divide the field of body MR imaging into five areas of development: contrast agents, molecular imaging, technologic advances, image processing, and screening. Contrast agents and molecular imaging applications are distinguished by morphologic versus metabolic imaging, although overlap exists. Technologic advances include the continued development of an already well-established parallel imaging technology and experience with newer high-field systems. Image processing includes examples from volume segmentation techniques that aid in quantification and classification of images and image registration or fusion techniques. This article concludes with a discussion of screening MR imaging and its potential in comparison to that of CT.

Contrast agents

Contrast agents in nonpulmonary body MR imaging can be classified as extracellular, liver-specific, reticuloendothelial system (RES)-specific, and intravascular agents. The most commonly used agents are extracellular agents comprised of Gd-chelates [1]. They are usually injected into the circulation at a concentration of 0.1 MMOL/kg at a flow rate of 2 to3 mL/s for body imaging; potentially higher flow rates are used for MR angiographic studies. Optimization of scanning for liver imaging with an extracellular contrast agent typically uses three successive postcontrast T1-weighted liver scans [2]. The first scan is timed to occur 15 to 20 seconds after the initiation of contrast injection to best image the liver during the arterial-dominant phase. This images the early enhancement pattern of a lesion to aid in characterization and optimizes detection of hypervascular lesions. The optimal timing exhibits contrast in hepatic arteries and portal veins without contrast in the hepatic veins. The second scan (portal venous phase) is delayed 45 to 75 seconds after the initiation of contrast injection. This typically allows time for the initial scan to be completed in a breath hold and permits a brief rest period before a second breath hold. The portal venous phase optimizes the detection of hypovascular metastases and can be used to evaluate the contrast washout pattern, which is a useful discriminating feature. A delayed scan can be obtained 90 seconds to 5 minutes after contrast injection in the interstitial phase of liver enhancement and aids in evaluating persistent enhancement of hemangiomata, washout characteristics of liver lesions, or delayed enhancement in tumors such as cholangiocarcinoma.

Liver-specific contrast agents may be classified as hepatocyte specific [3] or RES specific. Agents

---

* Corresponding author.

 E-mail address: richsem@med.unc.edu
(R.C. Semelka).

1064-9689/05/$ - see front matter © 2005 Elsevier Inc. All rights reserved.
doi:10.1016/j.mric.2005.03.011

that are of greatest clinical interest combine perfusional information with tissue-specific properties. Two contrast agents that have achieved clinical use that combine the properties of a non-specific gadolinium-based contrast agent with that of a hepatocyte-specific agent are gadobenate dimeglumine (Gd-BOPTA multihance, Bracco, Milan, [+]) and Gd-EOB-DTPA. Gd-BOPTA distributes to the extracellular fluid space but is selectively taken up by functioning hepatocytes and excreted into the bile [4]. It is mainly eliminated by the kidneys and has a biliary excretion rate of 3% to 5% [5]. The hepatobiliary contrast enhancement is prominent 1 to 2 hours postinjection. In a trial comparing Gd-BOPTA and gadopentetate dimeglumine, the dynamic postcontrast images were comparable in efficacy, whereas on delayed images, Gd-BOPTA was rated as superior in terms of showing additional information over non-enhanced scans [3,6]. Fig. 1 demonstrates an arterial-dominant and hepatic parenchymal phase image of a hypervascular tumor. The relatively long delay between initial injection and hepatocyte-specific imaging is more cumbersome when compared with imaging solely with an extracellular contrast agent. Gd-BOPTA has been clinically available for use in Europe for a number of years and has recently received FDA approval. A recent supplement to the *Journal of European Radiology* was devoted to the uses of this agent [7].

Gd-EOB-DTPA (Primovist, Schering, Berlin, Germany) is another paramagnetic hepatobiliary contrast agent. In contrast to Gd-BOPTA, fecal excretion by way of biliary fluid accounts for 50% of the excreted dose. Because of the high biliary excretion fraction, this agent may be used to obtain T1-weighted MR cholangiographic images of the biliary system [8]. Hepatobiliary contrast enhancement reaches a maximum at 10 to 20 minutes postinjection, with a 2-hour plateau phase. A phase III clinical trial demonstrated the highest liver-to-lesion contrast 20 to 45 minutes after injection [9]. This same clinical trial demonstrated a frequency of correctly detected lesions of 77%, 81%, and 87% for biphasic CT, non-enhanced MR imaging, and Gd-EOB-DTPA-enhanced MR imaging, respectively [9]. Because of the shorter delay between initial contrast injection and subsequent hepatobiliary-specific imaging, this agent results in a shorter total time to study a given patient. Primovist was approved for clinical use in Europe in 2005.

Superparamagnetic iron oxide particles

Iron oxide particles are used extensively in clinical and molecular imaging [10]. Ultrasmall superparamagnetic iron oxide (USPIO) agents may have potentially important future applications because they permit combined early perfusion and late RES-specific uptake or are taken up in lymph nodes. Their longer circulatory half-life has led to targeted imaging of macrophages in lymph nodes and bone marrow. In lymph nodes containing metastases, the USPIO concentration is reduced, leading to relative hyperintensity (ie, no enhancement) in a metastasis-containing node. This results in improved sensitivity for the detection of nodal metastasis in nodes that are normal by size criteria. Nearing completion of their clinical trials, USPIO products such as Combidex have been used to assess metastatic disease in multiple types of cancer, including head and neck cancers [11], breast cancer [12], and pelvic malignancies (eg, prostate [13] and rectal

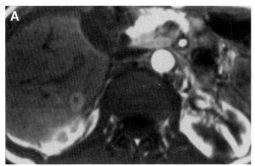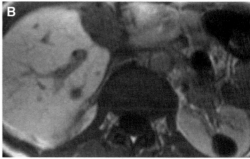

Fig. 1. (*A*) Dynamic and (*B*) delayed hepatic parenchymal enhancement using Gd-BOPTA. (*A*) A hypervascular neuroendocrine tumor on arterial-dominant imaging. (*B*) The mass becomes hypointense to the liver during parenchymal imaging.

cancer [14]). Head and neck and pelvic imaging may be particularly well suited for USPIO imaging because respiratory motion has less of an effect on the high-resolution imaging needed to distinguish between normal and abnormal lymph nodes. Fig. 2 demonstrates an application of USPIOs in the detection of metastatic lymph nodes in a patient with prostate cancer. In a prospective study using 216 histopathologically proven lymph nodes imaged in vivo in 36 patients with genitourinary malignancy, semiautomated assessment of lymph nodes using a T2* >17.3 milliseconds (corresponding to contrast excluded from the lymph node) and pixel variance in intranodal intensity beyond a certain threshold resulted in an accuracy of 98.6% in distinguishing between normal and malignant lymphadenopathy [15]. The ability to noninvasively detect nodal metastases aids in surgical and radiation planning, in the selection of patients for neo-adjuvant chemotherapy before surgery, in the evaluation of the nodal location within the body without need for multimodality image fusion techniques (such as with CT-PET), and in the reduction in the use of more invasive lymphangiographic or endoscopic techniques [15].

Intravascular contrast agents

The relatively short half-life of extracellular Gd-based contrast agents in blood requires rapid dynamic imaging of the vasculature prior to decrease in S/N. This has led to research on intravascular contrast agents that, by prolonging their intravascular half-life, allows imaging of the vasculature over a longer time period with

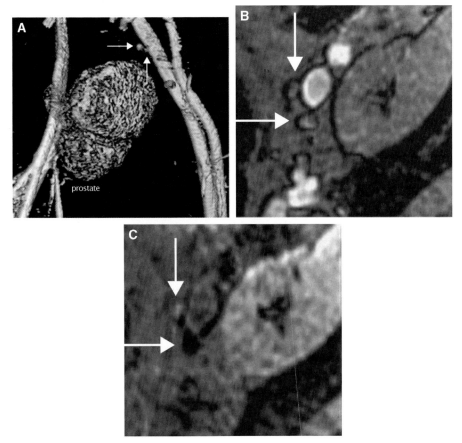

Fig. 2. (A) A 3D reconstruction of the prostate, iliac vessels, and metastatic (*thick arrow*) and normal (*thin arrow*) lymph nodes. (B) Conventional MR imaging shows the signal intensity is isointense between the two nodes. (C) USPIO-enhanced lymph node shows that the signal in the normal node is decreased (*thick arrow*) but remains elevated in the metastatic node (*thin arrow*). (Courtesy of M.G. Harisinghani, Boston, MA.)

a corresponding increase in S/N. Strategies to prolong the intravascular half-life include the chelation of paramagnetic ions to macromolecules and the use of USPIO agents. Human pilot studies have been done for USPIO agents [16,17], and Gd bound to human serum album (Gadofosveset or MS-325) has undergone phase III clinical trials [18]. No intravascular agent has received FDA approval.

Pulmonary imaging

A novel type of contrast is the use of hyper-polarized 3-He or 129-Xe to evaluate the pulmonary airspaces [19]. The technical requirements (gas supply, laser optical pumping technology, and rf hardware that can be tuned to the Larmor frequency of the hyperpolarized gas) limit this work to research applications. An estimated 500 to 1000 human subjects have been imaged. Optimization of imaging protocols continues for static ventilation imaging, dynamic ventilation imaging with a frame refreshment rate of 10 milliseconds or less [20], diffusion imaging to indirectly assess the underlying pulmonary parenchymal architecture, and regional oxygen tension measurement [19]. The latter is obtained by using the paramagnetic properties of oxygen to obtain a volumetric distribution of 3-He relaxation times over the pulmonary parenchyma, inferring the regional oxygen uptake by monitoring the change in 3-He relaxation times over time and thus obtaining a noninvasive ventilation/perfusion map at higher resolution than conventional scintigraphic imaging [21].

A novel application for the first FDA-approved MR imaging contrast agent is that of aerosolized Gd-DTPA for use in ventilatory static imaging [22]. A human pilot study demonstrated a 37% improvement in S/N of the pulmonary parenchyma when using a T1-weighted turbo spin-echo pulse sequence. Although there is much less experience with human subjects, the relative ease of implementation may make this an attractive alternative for pulmonary imaging.

Molecular imaging

The imaging of targeted molecules or cells can be defined as molecular or cellular imaging, respectively [10]. Applications might include the imaging of a labeled molecule or the target of that molecule (ie, a receptor or cellular target). For both types of imaging, the relatively low relaxivity of gadolinium chelates and the toxicity of free Gd

make iron oxide particles the preferred agent for many cellular imaging studies. The clinical application of USPIOs described in the previous section is an example of targeted cellular imaging to macrophages for the purpose of imaging the lymph nodes.

Molecular imaging using MR imaging with iron-labeled and Gd-labeled antibodies and peptides has been demonstrated in several model systems [10]. For example, magnetically labeled monoclonal antibodies have been used for visualization of myocardial infarction [23] and lung cancer [24]. Cholecystokinin- and secretin-linked particles have aided in the MR visualization of their respective pancreatic receptors [25,26]. Contrast enhancement of apoptotic tumor cells treated with chemotherapeutics was demonstrated in an in vivo animal model for conjugated iron oxide-C2 domain synaptotagmin I [27]. Polymerized nanoparticles with chelated Gd have been successfully targeted to angiogenic vessels in a rabbit carcinoma model and imaged with MR imaging [28].

In experimental studies, imaging of monocyte/macrophage activity in small animals has been applied to such diverse areas as experimental autoimmune encephalomyelitis [29], renal injury [30], graft rejection [31,32], and atherosclerotic plaque [33]. The last example was developed into a prospective preliminary trial that demonstrated USPIOs in macrophages in predominantly ruptured and rupture-prone human atherosclerotic lesions in carotid endarterectomy specimens with resultant decrease in signal intensity on T2-weighted imaging, suggesting a role for differentiating between high- and low-risk plaques [34].

The ability to image stem cells and progenitor cells is of interest because the viability of stem-cell transplantation in the clinical setting depends on their prolonged survival and their ability to migrate from the initial site of injection. The labeling of nonphagocytic cells with magnetic particulate agents has been achieved using a number of techniques [10]. Techniques for cellular labeling include linking magnetic particles to the HIV tat peptide [35], monoclonal antibodies that internalize the magnetic particles within the cell, and magnetodendrimers [36]. A mixture of commercially available transfection agents and SPIOs may be attractive because of the commercial availability of both components. Transfection agents are used to permit entry of the USPIO into the cell through the formation of endosomes. Labeled mesenchymal stem cells have been used to follow the fate of such cells after intramyocardial injection [37]. Dendritic cells, T cells, and endothelial progenitors are other targeted cells for which magnetic labeling has been performed.

As recently reviewed by Danthi [38], smart activatable agents have been designed for MR imaging and MR relaxometry. In one model system, a contrast agent (a Gd-bound chelator with one coordination site blocked by a galactopyranose residue) became activated when cells expressing the gene for β-galactosidase cleaved the residue from the contrast agent [39]. With non-imaging techniques such as MR relaxometry, magnetic nanoparticles coated with antiviral antibodies have been used as a sensitive assay for the detection of as few as five viral particles in 10 μL of 25% protein solution, which represents an improvement over PCR methods and current ELISA assays [40]. Magnetic nanoparticles have been used to detect enzymatic activity and to assay DNA and proteins at the femtomolar level in unpurified samples [41], thus demonstrating their potential sensitivity for MR imaging microscopy applications.

In summary, cellular labeling with SPIO and USPIO agents is well established in clinical imaging. Molecular and cellular imaging via MR imaging and MR relaxometry is a powerful tool to study gene expression and targeted cell migration and serve as a sensitive assay for viral and enzymatic activity. For further information, the interested reader is directed to a recent issue of *Academic Radiology* devoted to the topic of molecular imaging [42].

Technology

Parallel imaging

Parallel imaging simultaneously acquires data from an array of rf coils over an imaging volume. With calibration of the rf sensitivity profiles from individual elements of the rf array, this information can be used in conjunction with a decreased number of gradient phase-encoding steps to reduce the amount of time required to obtain an imaging data set or to increase the imaging resolution within a given time duration (eg, breath hold) if the resolution is not already signal-to-noise limited.

Techniques for parallel imaging fall into two classes [43]. SMASH [44] (SiMultaneous Acquisition of Spatial Harmonics) and its successors (such as GRAPPA [45]) explicitly calculate missing k-space lines before Fourier transformation of the data to recover an image. SENSE [46] (SENSitivity-Encoded) MR imaging and its successors (such as mSENSE [modified SENSE] or tSENSE [temporal SENSE]) use an alternative approach that reconstructs an image with a reduced field-of-view (FOV) for each of the individual coil elements and combines these individual images into a single full FOV image by using knowledge of the spatial distribution of rf coil sensitivities. GRAPPA and mSENSE acquire additional data in the center of k-space to auto calibrate the sensitivity profile of the rf coils. Both classes of parallel imaging are vendor supported.

Parallel imaging can be used for a variety of purposes in body MR imaging [47]. For example, data acquisition within a single breath hold plays a significant role in state-of-the-art abdominal imaging. For a patient who can hold his breath without difficulty, the acceleration in imaging from parallel techniques may be used to acquire more data during the breath hold, resulting in improved image resolution. Alternatively, if a patient has difficulty holding his breath, parallel imaging can be used to shorten scan times with comparable resolution, assuming the resolution is not signal-to-noise limited. For fast scans with long echo trains, there is intrinsic image filtering and loss of resolution due to the acquisition of multiple lines of k-space during a single TR. Parallel imaging may be used in this situation to reduce the length of the echo train resulting in a decrease in low-pass filtering and associated image blurring.

Clinical applications of parallel imaging in body MR imaging

Examples of parallel imaging applications to body MR imaging include dynamic liver, renal, and cardiac imaging. Fig. 3 shows an example of parallel imaging applied to decrease the breath hold time for a T1-weighted spoiled gradient echo scan of the liver from 21 to 13 seconds using an acceleration factor of 2.

MR imaging has the potential to perform a high-resolution, morphologic, and functional evaluation of the kidneys in a single setting [48,49]. The functional evaluation relies on measuring the time-dependent cortical and medullary enhancement of the kidneys with subsequent modeling to calculate the glomerular filtration rate or differential renal function. Such measurements benefit

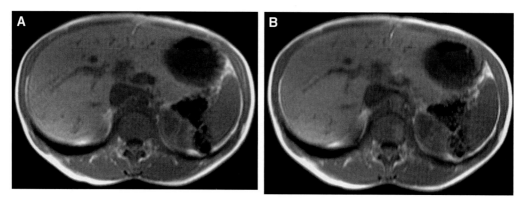

Fig. 3. T1-weighted spoiled gradient echo axial image of the liver without (*A*) and with (*B*) parallel imaging. The total scan time for the liver decreased from 21 to 13 seconds with an R of two.

from the improved temporal resolution of parallel imaging.

High temporal resolution is important in cardiac cine imaging to evaluate global cardiac function and wall motion abnormalities and in first-pass perfusion imaging to evaluate for ische- mia. Theoretical [50] and experimental [51] anal- ysis of cine true FISP imaging with steady-state free precession suggested a temporal resolution of 40 to 50 ms/cine frame was needed for accurate assessment of global cardiac function at a heart rate of 60 bpm. Using a GRAPPA technique with acceleration factor of 2, a single breath-hold real- time cine MR technique was used to obtain 9 to 11 short axis cine images from base to apex with a temporal resolution of 48 milliseconds [52]. Although obtained at lower spatial resolution, the resultant assessment of stroke volume and ejection fraction was not significantly different from the relatively high spatial resolution tech- nique single-slice/breath hold technique using multiple breath holds. Using a GRAPPA tech- nique, the difference in scan time was approxi- mately 20 seconds versus 10 minutes after accounting for the multiple breath holds and a recovery time.

Fig. 4 demonstrates two cine frames from a real-time SSFP pulse sequence using TSENSE [53]. Adaptive TSENSE combines temporally in- terleaved k-space lines to obtain coil sensitivity maps directly from the acquired data without additionally sampled central k-space lines. It can be used with any dynamic imaging technique that acquires data repeatedly over time, including cine and first-pass perfusion imaging. Despite the volunteer's free breathing during the study, the

cine images do not show significant breathing or flow artifacts.

High-field imaging systems

Several commercial vendors have produced clinical 3T imaging magnets, and prototype high-field imaging systems have been developed. The initial cost of a clinical high-field magnet and its associated higher-frequency rf electronics is greater than that of conventional 1.5T systems, as is the cost of cryogenics. Although the use of active shielding on many clinical 3T magnets lessens siting restrictions for the FDA 5 gauss exclusion zone, fringe fields (0.5 to 5 gauss) may extend well beyond that of the 1.5T counterpart. Consequently, careful consideration of the pros and cons of high-field body imaging is warranted given the increased cost of purchasing and main- taining such a unit.

The primary advantage of a 3T magnet is the increase in the strength of the MR signal due to the increased equilibrium magnetization and higher Larmor frequency [54]. This must be weighed against several potential disadvantages. Susceptibility variations within the patient (due, for example, to the presence of air or metallic clips) result in locoregional magnetic field distor- tions, which are proportional to the static mag- netic field and are thus worsened at higher fields. Increasing field strength results in a prolonged T1, which reduces the available signal in short TR sequences. Conversely, the reduction in T2 results in low-pass filtering and a loss in resolution for sequences with long readout trains. Although rf energy deposited in the patient scales theoretically with the square of the Larmor frequency at lower

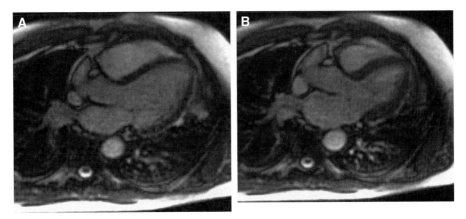

Fig. 4. Free-breathing self-gating TSENSE imaging of an inflow/outflow view of the heart in diastole (*A*) and systole (*B*).

frequencies, the measured increase in rf energy deposition in neuroimaging when going from 4T to 7T was only 60% as much as the theoretical prediction of a threefold increase [55]. Nonetheless, rapid imaging sequences at higher fields are more likely to exceed specific absorption rate (SAR) limits [56]. Finally, acoustic noise levels from gradient switching increase with static field strength and may pose additional constraints on rapid gradient-echo sequences.

As recently reviewed by Pruessman [56], there is significant synergism between high-field and parallel imaging. Many of the disadvantages in high-field imaging may be compensated for with the use of parallel imaging. For example, the problems of increased T2* effects in scans with long echo trains, increased SAR from high frequency rf, and increased acoustic noise levels due to rapid gradient switching may be corrected, at least in part, with the use of parallel imaging. Additionally, theoretical [57] and experimental work suggest that further increases in field strength beyond 3T result in additional benefits when parallel imaging is applied [58] because the local geometry factor g (which is inversely proportional to the acceleration factor) decreases with increasing field strength, thus allowing one to use a higher acceleration factor for a comparable SNR reduction when parallel imaging is used.

Figs. 5 and 6 provide clinical examples of 3T imaging. Fig. 5 demonstrates a pathology-proven insulinoma. Fig. 6 demonstrates a patient with pelvic prolapse. The additional S/N obtained with 3T imaging is put to advantage by using a high-resolution matrix (384 × 512) on T2-weighted imaging to image the asymmetric levator ani musculature.

Imaging at 3T requires optimization of the pulse sequence parameters normally used at 1.5T. Care must be given to steady-state free precession (SSFP) techniques used in cardiac imaging because they are sensitive to static field inhomogeneities that can lead to flow-related artifacts. The longer T1 associated with higher field strengths and the increased rf power deposition are other considerations that need to be addressed. With optimization of the sequence parameters (rf power, TR, and flip angle) and localized shimming and resonance frequency determination, high-quality SSFP cine images are obtained during short breath holds [59].

Image processing

With the explosion of three-dimensional (3D) data sets in MR imaging, the need for sophisticated image processing and visualization techniques has never been greater. Image processing techniques to facilitate feature extraction and computer-aided diagnosis, segmentation algorithms, and image registration algorithms within the same or across different imaging modalities are areas of active commercial and academic research. These techniques may aid in oncologic diagnosis, surgical or radiation planning, and cardiology [60].

Image registration techniques have been extensively validated in brain registration [61]. However, image registration techniques for different organ systems require independent verification of accuracy. Real-time MR image-ultrasound image fusion has been reported, with the goal of using a previously acquired MR image of the prostate

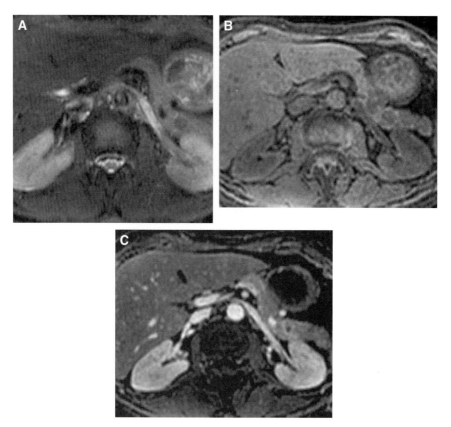

Fig. 5. (*A*) STIR image of the pancreatic tail at 3T demonstrating a hypointense mass. (*B*) Precontrast T1-weighted axial image demonstrating a hypointense pancreatic mass. (*C*) Contrast-enhanced axial T1-weighted image demonstrating rim enhancement of the mass. (Courtesy of D.R. Martin, MD, PhD, Emory University, Atlanta, GA.)

and fusing it with a transrectal ultrasound examination to facilitate biopsy localization [62]. CT/MR image fusion in radiation therapy planning to the prostate has been used as a supplement [63] and as an alternative [64] to CT-based treatment.

In liver imaging, segmentation and registration techniques may be used to aid in preoperative surgical planning, ablation procedures, or biopsy localization. Fig. 7 is a 3D segmentation of hepatic and portal venous anatomy extracted from a postcontrast 3D VIBE data set of the liver [65]. This patient was undergoing a preoperative liver transplant evaluation, and images such as these can be used to better evaluate for venous anomalies that might alter the surgical approach. Fig. 8 is an example of image registration of a 3D VIBE MR image of the liver with a 3D ultrasound of the liver. This technique could be used to facilitate biopsy or ablative treatment of a lesion that was seen by

MR imaging but that could not be visualized on ultrasound [66].

In 2000, the National Library of Medicine funded the creation of the Insight Toolkit (ITK), an open-source software environment to develop an application programming interface for multidimensional image processing. In 2004, the project produced its fifth release of ITK. Such open-software projects should aid in the dissemination of a well-tested core of software algorithms that may be used by the larger medical imaging community to process data [67].

Screening

The great majority of whole-body screening studies have used CT. Whole-body CT screening remains controversial. Arguments against it include the potential for increased cancer risk

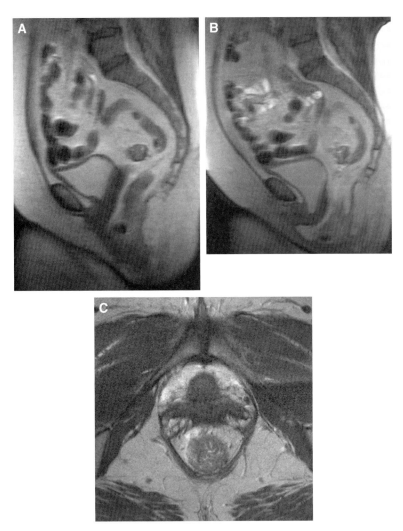

Fig. 6. (*A*) Pre- and (*B*) post-strain sagittal HASTE image demonstrates pelvic floor prolapse. (*C*) Axial high-resolution (384 × 512) T2-weighted turbo spin-echo image demonstrating asymmetry of the levator musculature. (Courtesy of D.R. Martin, MD, PhD, Emory University, Atlanta, GA.)

secondary to exposure to ionizing radiation [68], the risk of an allergic reaction or nephrotoxicity related to iodinated contrast if this is administered as part of the screening examination, medicolegal liability associated with "missed" findings on a noncontrast CT examination [69] or a contrast-related injury suffered by an asymptomatic patient undergoing a screening study performed with iodinated contrast, the morbidity and economic costs associated with evaluating indeterminate findings on a screening examination [70], the variability in diagnostic yield of noncontrast CT examinations between screening centers [71], and the economic cost of the screening examination.

Several of the arguments against CT screening are addressed with the use of MR imaging. Any risk of cancer induction secondary to ionizing radiation is removed. The safety profile of MR contrast agents is favorable when compared with that of iodinated contrast with CT [1]. The ability to perform multiple imaging sequences in a given region of the body without concern over the cumulative risk of ionizing radiation is an additional advantage of MR imaging. The resultant improved accuracy of MR imaging compared with CT for characterization of liver lesions [72] would be expected to result in fewer indeterminate findings in need of additional workup, but the

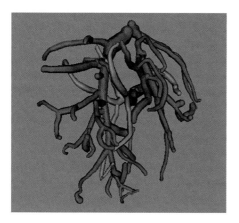

Fig. 7. Segmented hepatic and portal venous anatomy from a 3D MR image of the liver. (Courtesy of S. Aylward, PhD, Chapel Hill, NC.)

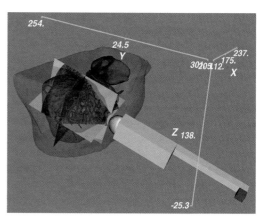

Fig. 8. Schematic demonstrating image registration of a 3D MR image and 3D ultrasound to aid in ultrasound-guided ablation of a liver mass. (Courtesy of S. Aylward, PhD, Chapel Hill, NC.)

cost/benefit ratio for screening MR imaging requires large-scale trials to prospectively evaluate.

Surveillance MR examinations are performed for patients at increased risk for a particular underlying malignancy. Liver MR imaging for patients with underlying liver disease at increased risk for hepatocellular carcinoma is an example [73]. Other targeted populations include breast MR imaging for patients with increased risk of breast cancer due to BRCA1/2 genetic susceptibility [74]. Because of its cost, MR imaging is not typically considered for use as a screening examination.

A dedicated MR screening protocol has been evaluated for virtual colonoscopy with MR imaging [75] using nontagged [76] and barium-based fecal tagging [77]. Although most polyps <5 mm were missed [75], such lesions statistically have a low likelihood of malignancy. Because the fecal tagging procedure does not require colonic cleansing, patient acceptance of the procedure might be improved when compared with colonoscopy.

Preliminary results of a whole-body MR imaging screening protocol performed on 298 subjects were recently reported [78]. The study was optimized for the detection of significant cerebrovascular or atherosclerotic disease, pulmonary nodules, cardiac imaging, and colonic polyps. The hour-long study incorporated pre- and post-contrast neuroimaging; whole-body MR angiography; HASTE imaging of the thorax, cine, and delayed hyperenhancement imaging of the heart; and MR colonography after a tap water enema. Two hundred ninety studies were diagnostic. Signs of cerebrovascular, peripheral vascular, or cardiovascular disease were seen in 21% of patients. Nine pulmonary nodules ranging in size from 3 to 7 mm were found. Cardiac imaging revealed myocardial infarction in one patient, reduced contractility in five patients, valvular abnormalities in 11 patients, and left ventricular hypertrophy in 17 patients. Virtual colonoscopy revealed 12 polyps confirmed by polypectomy. Incidental findings included one renal cell carcinoma.

With parallel imaging techniques, further reductions in scan time may be anticipated. An alternative MR imaging screening protocol developed at this institution uses pre- and postcontrast imaging of the abdomen coupled with postcontrast VIBE and HASTE imaging of the head, chest, and pelvis (Fig. 9). Such a study can be completed in 15 minutes using parallel imaging with an acceleration factor of two. Longitudinal studies in a research setting are required to determine the value of any of these screening protocols.

Summary

In this article, we defined the major areas of active research in clinical MR imaging. Further increases in the number of parallel coils within an imaging array and in advances in parallel imaging pulse sequences and postprocessing will lead to further reductions in imaging time analogous to the impact of multidetector CT on helical CT. The synergism between parallel and high-field imaging will aid the development of high-field imaging.

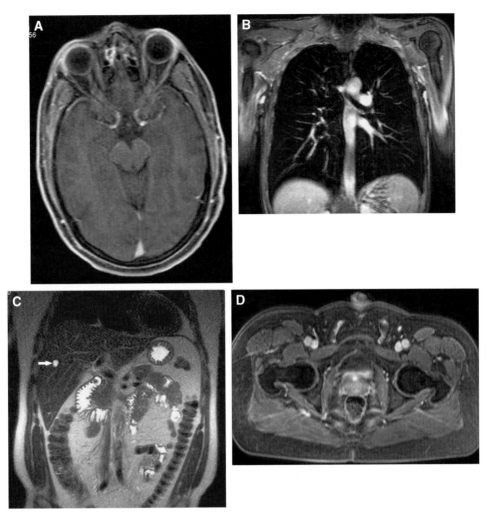

Fig. 9. Sample images from a single patient during a 15-minute prototype screening protocol. (*A*) Transverse T1-weighted fat-suppressed 3D gradient echo post-gadolinium image of the head. (*B*) Coronal T1-weighted fat-suppressed 3D gradient echo post-gadolinium image of the chest. (*C*) Coronal T2-weighted single-shot echo train spin-echo image of the abdomen. (*D*) Transverse T1-weighted fat-suppressed 3D gradient echo post-gadolinium image.

The combined dynamic and hepatic parenchymal enhancement of new contrast agents that have or may soon receive FDA approval will enable improved detection and characterization of liver lesions. The lymphotropic SPIO agents will remain an active area of clinical research to further assess their role in oncologic staging. Molecular imaging contrast research using magnetic particles and MR microscopy will continue to flourish. Screening examinations by MR imaging will remain an area of research for the short- and intermediate term, with the final outcome dependent more on socioeconomic costs than the underlying capability of achieving high-quality screening studies.

References

[1] Runge VM. Safety of magnetic resonance contrast agents. Top Magn Reson Imaging 2001;12:309–14.
[2] Semelka RC, Helmberger TK. Contrast agents for MR imaging of the liver. Radiology 2001;218:27–38.
[3] Reimer P, Schneider G, Schima W. Hepatobiliary contrast agents for contrast-enhanced MRI of the liver: properties, clinical development and applications. Eur Radiol 2004;14:559–78.

[4] Spinazzi A, Lorusso V, Pirovano G, et al. Safety, tolerance, biodistribution, and MR imaging enhancement of the liver with gadobenate dimeglumine: results of clinical pharmacologic and pilot imaging studies in nonpatient and patient volunteers. Acad Radiol 1999;6:282–91.

[5] de Haen C, Gozzini L. Soluble-type hepatobiliary contrast agents for MR imaging. J Magn Reson Imaging 1993;3:179–86.

[6] Kuwatsuru R, Kadoya M, Ohtoma K, et al. Comparison of gadobenate dimeglumine with gadopentetate dimeglumine for magnetic resonance imaging of liver tumors. Invest Radiol 2001;36:632–41.

[7] Proceedings of the Multihance (gadobenate dimeglumine) user group meeting. Eur Radiol 2004; 14(Suppl 7):1–88.

[8] Carlos RC, Branam JD, Dong Q, et al. Biliary imaging with Gd-EOB-DTPA: is a 20-minute delay sufficient? Acad Radiol 2002;9:1322–5.

[9] Huppertz A, Balzer T, Blakeborough A, et al. Improved detection of focal liver lesions in MRI: a multicenter comparison of Gd-EOB-DTPA with intraoperative findings. Radiology 2004;230: 266–75.

[10] Bulte JWM, Kraitchman DL. Iron oxide MR contrast agents for molecular and cellular imaging. NMR Biomed 2004;17:484–99.

[11] Anzai Y. Superparamagnetic iron oxide nanoparticles: nodal metastases and beyond. Top Magn Reson Imaging 2004;15:103–11.

[12] Michel SC, Keller TM, Frohlich JM, et al. Preoperative breast cancer staging: MR imaging of the axilla with ultrasmall superparamagnetic iron oxide enhancement. Radiology 2002;225:527–36.

[13] Harisinghani MG, Barentsz J, Hahn PF, et al. Noninvasive detection of clinically occult lymph-node metastases in prostate cancer. N Engl J Med 2003; 348:2491–9.

[14] Dow-Mu K, Brown G, Temple L, et al. Rectal cancer: mesorectal lymph nodes at MR imaging with USPIO versus histopathologic findings: initial observations. Radiology 2004;231:91–9.

[15] Harisinghani MG, Weissleder R. Sensitive, noninvasive detection of lymph node metastases. PloS Med 2004;1:e66.

[16] Tombach B, Reimer P, Bremer C, et al. First-pass and equilibrium-MRA of the aortoiliac region with a superparamagnetic iron oxide blood pool MR contrast agent (SH U 555 C): results of a human pilot study. NMR Biomed 2004;17:500–6.

[17] Aschauer M, Deutschmann HA, Stollberger R, et al. Value of a blood pool contrast agent in MR venography of the lower extremities and pelvis: preliminary results in 12 patients. Magn Reson Med 2003; 50:993–1002.

[18] Perreault P, Edelman MA, Baum RA, et al. MR angiography with gadofosveset trisodium for peripheral vascular disease: phase II trial. Radiology 2003;229:811–20.

[19] van Beek EJR, Wild JM, Kauczor HU, et al. Functional MRI of the lung using hyperpolarized 3-helium gas. J Magn Reson Imaging 2004;20: 540–54.

[20] Wild JM, Paley MNJ, Kasuboski L, et al. Dynamic radial projection MRI of inhaled hyperpolarization 3He. Magn Reson Med 2003;49:991–7.

[21] Deninger AJ, Eberle B, Bermuth J, et al. Assessment of a single-acquisition imaging sequence for oxygensensitive 3He-MRI. Magn Reson Med 2002;47: 105–14.

[22] Haage P, Karaagac S, Spuntrup E, et al. Feasibility of pulmonary ventilation visualization with aerosolized magnetic resonance contrast media. Invest Radiol 2005;40:85–8.

[23] Weissleder R, Lee AS, Khaw BA, et al. Polyclonal human immunoglobulin G labeled with polymeric iron oxide: antibody MR imaging. Radiology 1991;181:245–9.

[24] Remsen LG, McCormick CI, Roman-Goldstein S, et al. MR of carcinoma-specific monoclonal antibody conjugated to monocrystalline iron oxide nanoparticles: the potential for non-invasive diagnosis. AJNR Am J Neuroradiol 1996;17:411–8.

[25] Reimer P, Weissleder R, Shen T, et al. Pancreatic receptors: initial feasibility studies with a targeted contrast agent for MR imaging. Radiology 1994; 193:527–31.

[26] Shen TT, Bogdanov A Jr, Bogdanova A, et al. magnetically labelled secretin retains receptor affinity to pancreas acinar cells. Bioconjug Chem 1996;7: 311–6.

[27] Zhao M, Beauregard DA, Loizou L, et al. Noninvasive detection of apoptosis using magnetic resonance imaging and a target contrast agent. Nat Med 2001;7:1241–4.

[28] Sipkins DA, Cheresh DA, Kazerni MR, et al. Detection of tumor angiogenesis in vivo by αβ-targeted magnetic resonance imaging. Nat Med 1998;4: 623–6.

[29] Rausch M, Hiestand P, Baumann D, et al. MRI-based monitoring of inflammation and tissue damage in acute and chronic relapsing EAE. Magn Reson Med 2003;50:309–14.

[30] Jo SK, Hu X, Kobayashi H, et al. Detection of inflammation following renal ischemia by magnetic resonance imaging. Kidney Int 2003;64:43–51.

[31] Zhang Y, Dodd SJ, Hendrich KS, et al. Magnetic resonance imaging detection of rat renal transplant rejection by monitoring macrophage infiltration. Kidney Int 2000;58:1300–10.

[32] Kanno S, Wu YJ, Lee PC, et al. Macrophage accumulation associated with rat cardiac allograft rejection detected by magnetic resonance imaging with ultrasmall superparamagnetic iron oxide particles. Circulation 2001;104:934–8.

[33] Ruehm SG, Corot C, Vogt P, et al. Magnetic resonance imaging of atherosclerotic plaque with ultrasmall superparamagnetic particles of iron oxide in

hyperlipidemic rabbits. Circulation 2001;103:415–22.

[34] Kooi ME, Cappendijk VC, Cleutjens KBJM, et al. Accumulation of ultrasmall superparamagnetic particles of iron oxide in human atherosclerotic plaques can be detected by in vivo magnetic resonance imaging. Circulation 2001;103:415–22.

[35] Josephson L, Tung CH, Moore A, et al. High-efficiency intracellular magnetic labeling with novel superparamagnetic-Tat peptide conjugates. Bioconjug Chem 1999;10:186–91.

[36] Bulte JWM, Douglas T, Witwer B, et al. Magnetodendrimers allow endosomal magnetic labeling and in vivo tracking of stem cells. Nat Biotechnol 2001;19:1141–7.

[37] Kraitchman DL, Heldman AW, Atalar E, et al. In vivo magnetic resonance imaging of mesenchymal stem cells in myocardial infarction. Circulation 2003;229:838–46.

[38] Danthi SN, Pandit SD, Li KCP. A primer on molecular biology for imagers: VII. molecular imaging probes. Acad Radiol 2004;11:1047–54.

[39] Louie AY, Huber MM, Ahrens ET, et al. In vivo visualization of gene expression using magnetic resonance imaging. Nat Biotechnol 2000;18:321–5.

[40] Perez JM, Simeone FJ, Saeki Y, et al. Viral-induced self-assembly of magnetic nanoparticles allows the detection of viral particles in biological media. J Am Chem Soc 2003;125:10192–3.

[41] Perez JM, Josephson L, Weissleder R. Use of magnetic nanoparticles as nanosensors to probe for molecular interactions. ChemBioChem 2004;5:261–4.

[42] Li KCP. Molecular imaging. Acad Radiol 2004;11(Suppl 1):S1–108.

[43] Bammer R, Schoenberg SO. Current concepts and advances in clinical parallel magnetic resonance imaging. Top Magn Reson Imaging 2004;15:129–58.

[44] Sodickson DK, Manning WJ. Simultaneous acquisition of spatial harmonics (SMASH): fast imaging with radiofrequency coil arrays. Magn Reson Med 1997;38:591–603.

[45] Griswold MA, Jakob PM, Heidemann RM, et al. Generalized autocalibrating partially parallel acquisitions (GRAPPA). Magn Reson Med 2002;47:1202–10.

[46] Pruessman KP, Weiger M, Scheidegger MB. SENSE: sensitivity encoding for fast MRI. Magn Reson Med 1999;42:952–62.

[47] Margolis DJA, Bammer R, Chow LC. Parallel imaging of the abdomen. Top Magn Reson Imaging 2004;15:197–206.

[48] Huang AJ, Lee VS, Rusinek H. MR imaging of renal function. Radiol Clin North Am 2003;41:1001–17.

[49] Rohrschneider WK, Haufe S, Clorius JH, et al. MR to assess renal function in children. Eur Radiol 2003;13:1033–45.

[50] Setser RM, Fischer SE, Lorenz CH. Quantification of left ventricular function with magnetic resonance images acquired in real time. J Magn Reson Imaging 2000;12:430–8.

[51] Miller S, Simonetti OP, Carr J, et al. MR imaging of the heart with cine true fast imaging with steady-state precession: influence of spatial and temporal resolutions on left ventricular functional parameters. Radiology 2002;223:263–9.

[52] Wintersperger BJ, Nikolaou K, Dietrich O, et al. Single breathhold real-time cine MR imaging: improved temporal resolution using generalized autocalibrating partially parallel acquisition (GRAPPA) algorithm. Eur Radiol 2003;13:1931–6.

[53] Kellman P, Epstein FH, McVeigh ER. Adaptive sensitivity encoding incorporating temporal filtering (TSENSE). Magn Reson Med 2001;45:846–52.

[54] Norris DG. High field human imaging. J Magn Reson Imaging 2003;18:519–29.

[55] Vaughan JT, Garwood M, Collins CM, et al. RF power, homogeneity, and signal-to-noise comparison in head images. Magn Reson Med 2001;46:24–30.

[56] Pruessmann KP. Parallel imaging at high field strength: synergies and joint potential. Top Magn Reson Imaging 2004;15:237–44.

[57] Wiesinger F, Boesiger P, Pruessmann KP. Electrodynamics and ultimate SNR in parallel MR imaging. Magn Reson Med 2004;52:376–90.

[58] Wiesinger F, Van de Moortele P-F, Adriany G, et al. Parallel imaging performance as a function of field strength: an experimental investigation using electrodynamic scaling. Magn Reson Med 2004;52:953–64.

[59] Schar M, Kozerke S, Fischer SE, et al. Cardiac SSFP imaging at 3 Tesla. Magn Reson Med 2004;51:799–806.

[60] Slomka PJ. Software approach to merging molecular with anatomic information. J Nucl Med 2004;45:36S–45S.

[61] West J, Fitzpatrick JM, Wang MY, et al. Comparison and evaluation of retrospective intermodality brain image registration techniques. J Comput Assist Tomogr 1997;21:554–66.

[62] Kaplan I, Oldenburg NE, Meskell P, et al. Real time MRI-ultrasound image guided stereotactic prostate biopsy. Magn Reson Imaging 2002;20:295–9.

[63] McLaughlin PW, Narayana V, Meriowitz A, et al. Vessel-sparing prostate radiotherapy: dose limitation to critical erectile vascular structures (internal pudendal artery and corpus cavernosum) defined by MRI. Int J Radiat Oncol Biol Phys 2005;61:20–31.

[64] Chen L, Price RA, Nguyen TB, et al. Dosimetric evaluation of MRI-based treatment planning for prostate cancer. Phys Med Biol 2004;49:5157–70.

[65] Aylward SR, Jomier J, Weeks S, et al. Registration and analysis of vascular images. Int J Comp Vision 2003;55:123–8.

[66] Aylward SR, Jomier J, Guyon JP, et al. Intra-operative 3D ultrasound augmentation. In: Proceedings of the IEEE International Symposium on Biomedical Imaging. Washington (DC): IEEE; 2002. p. 421–4.

[67] Yoo TS, Ackerman MJ. Open source software for medical image processing and visualization. Comm ACM 2005;48:55–9.

[68] de González AB, Darby S. Risk of cancer from diagnostic x-rays: estimates for the UK and 14 other countries. Lancet 2004;363:345–51.

[69] Berlin L. Medicolegal and ethical issues in radiologic screening. Radiol Clin North Am 2004;42:779–88.

[70] Casarella WJ. A patient's viewpoint on current controversy: letter to the editor. Radiology 2002;224:927.

[71] Berland LL, Berland NW. Whole-body computed tomography screening. Radiol Clin North Am 2004;42:699–710.

[72] Semelka RC, Martin D, Balci C, et al. Focal liver lesions: comparison of dual-phase CT and multisequence multiplanar MR imaging including dynamic gadolinium enhancement. J Magn Reson Imaging 2001;13:397–401.

[73] Hussain SM, Semelka RC, Mitchell DG. MR imaging of hepatocellular carcinoma. Magn Reson Imaging Clin North Am 2002;10:31–52.

[74] Kriege M, Brekelmans CT, Boetes C, et al. Efficacy of MRI and mammography for breast-cancer screening in women with a familial or genetic predisposition. N Engl J Med 2004;351:427–37.

[75] Luboldt W, Bauerfeind P, Wildermuth S, et al. Colonic masses: detection with MR colonography. Radiology 2000;216:383–8.

[76] Lauenstein TC, Holtmann G, Schoenfelder D, et al. MR colonography without bowel cleansing: a new strategy to improve patient acceptance. AJR 2001; 177:823–7.

[77] Lauenstein TC, Goehde SC, Ruehm SG, et al. MR-colonography with barium-based fecal tagging: initial clinical experience. Radiology 2002; 223:248–54.

[78] Goehde SC, Hunold P, Vogt FM, et al. Full-body cardiovascular and tumor MRI for early detection of disease: feasibility and initial experience in 298 subjects. AJR 2005;184:598–611.

ELSEVIER
SAUNDERS

Magn Reson Imaging Clin N Am
13 (2005) 225–240

MAGNETIC
RESONANCE
IMAGING CLINICS
of North America

Molecular MR Imaging in Oncology

Michelle Bradbury, MD, PhD*, Hedvig Hricak, MD, PhD

Department of Radiology, Memorial Sloan Kettering Cancer Center, 1275 York Avenue, New York, NY 10021, USA

The translation of molecular biology into clinical practice is the future of medicine, including oncology. The genomics and proteomics (and now metabolomics) revolution has made the incorporation of molecular medicine into clinical practice inevitable, with molecular imaging playing an essential role in this transformation. Imaging plays, and will continue to play, a pivotal role in preclinical and clinical cancer detection, staging, targeted therapy, monitoring treatment response, and treatment follow-up. The continued role of imaging, in part, will be predicated on the ability to image tumor biology and tumor phenotypic characteristics successfully. Although several imaging modalities (namely optical, positron emission tomography [PET], and MR) can be used for such purposes in the preclinical and clinical settings, this discussion focuses on MR imaging. MR imaging offers two main advantages over modalities that use radiolabeled or optical probes: higher spatial resolution (micrometers) and the ability to obtain anatomic, physiologic, and metabolic information in a single imaging session. Furthermore, the current growth in high-field clinical and micro-MR imaging systems has spurred the development of many technical advances which has driven an ever-increasing number of clinical and research applications that model and phenotype human disease. The application of MR imaging techniques to the diagnosis and treatment of cancer, generally, as well as to site-specific cancers, ultimately will lead to the successful translation of such methods to the practice of a more predictive and preventive medicine; this may culminate in more personalized health care. This translation only can be defined in the context of a systems biology approach. Such an approach embodies the idea that when the genetic make-up of the system (ie, gene and protein regulatory elements) is acted upon by environmental influences, it will generate a variety of gene and protein expression patterns (ie, molecular signatures; see later discussion). The realization of future imaging goals in the clinical setting only can be achieved with continued advances in imaging instrumentation; the synthesis of novel, increasingly specific agents; and the creation of new transgenic animal models of human disease.

Linking cancer biology and imaging

Systems biology and nanotechnology

To understand biology at the systems level, it becomes important to consider the isolated parts of the system (ie, genes, proteins, and metabolites), and to focus on the structure and dynamics of the system as a whole. It is important to identify all of the genes and proteins of a given cell or organism to understand the properties and complexity of the system, and to understand the interconnection of these components and how they interact dynamically [1].

The central components of systems biology are gene and protein regulatory elements (ie, circuits) that comprise cells and cell networks. These circuits, once sufficiently detailed and accurate, dictate cellular organization and function in response to environmental cues. In this context, a given disease may be represented by the gain or loss of specific functions which define the disease process—in essence, the genetic or environmental reprogramming of cells [2].

This assembled network circuitry constitutes a hypothesis of how the system works at the

---

* Corresponding author.

E-mail address: bradburm@mskcc.org
(M. Bradbury).

molecular scale [3]. The hypothesis is tested by a systematic series of perturbations on the system. Several perturbations may be performed in parallel that result in the generation of many molecular signatures of gene and protein expression. With each new set of measurements, the hypothesis can be modified appropriately, in an iterative fashion, to allow the system to be defined more precisely. A large number of such measurements may lead to the construction of a more complete molecular description (model) of the system. In addition to revealing the molecular signatures that define the nature and progression of disease, such a model would elucidate a few critical diagnostic or therapeutic targets (biomarkers) for further testing of the network.

The successful implementation and realization of a systems biology approach for disease diagnosis and drug discovery preferably will be resolved at the single cell or small cell population level to eliminate heterogeneous cell population responses. This effort requires the on-going fabrication of nanodevices for sensitive, real-time detection of genes, mRNAs, and proteins (nanotechnologies), as well as advances in microchip technology (microfluidics) for integration of many pumps, valves, and channels that can perform multiple analyses of small patient sample blood volumes in parallel (ie, cell sorting DNA purification, and single-cell gene expression profiling) [2,4,5]. Such nanotechnology-based labs, or nanolabs, combined with appropriate bioinformatics algorithms and molecular imaging techniques, potentially can identify the molecular signatures of disease and disease progression (ie, critical protein targets) for exposure to candidate pharmaceuticals (Fig. 1). This knowledge—directly translatable to mouse models and patients—may expedite drug development by selecting more appropriate molecular biomarkers as objective end points of treatment efficacy [6,7].

Critical gene and protein targets for molecular imaging

Target selection is critical for developing higher-specificity contrast agents, molecular/genomic imaging, and appropriate therapeutic interventions [8]. As a part of the target selection process, real-time, high-throughput screening techniques are being used to measure many signatures of gene or protein expression simultaneously over the range of disease progression or physiologic responses. Genes or proteins that are expressed at

abnormally high or low levels in a particular disease or developmental process can be selected and subsequently separated and identified using a range of technologies in the fields of functional genomics (eg, DNA microarrays, quantitative polymerase chain reaction) [9–11] and proteomics (eg, two-dimensional gel electrophoresis, mass spectrometry) [12–14]. This process has been performed to separate and identify, for example, certain classes of genes that are responsible for disease initiation or progression. The fabrication of microdevices on a chip-based platform, the so-called "nanolab," is under way in several laboratories to increase the speed of protein identification markedly and the understanding of protein structures and functions. This intensive effort has led to the present investigation of a vast number of potential therapeutic targets in the pharmaceutical industry. Approximately 500 molecular entities can be targeted by currently available drugs; these are mostly proteins, primarily cell-surface receptors and enzymes [8]. Estimates of the number of molecular targets that currently are available for evaluation of potential diagnostic or therapeutic agents are much greater (ie, 5000–10,000 entities); this underscores the unprecedented opportunity which is afforded molecular and genomic imaging in the characterization and validation of such targets for eventual clinic use [15].

To maximize the usefulness and efficiency of molecular and genomic imaging, choosing informative imaging targets of sufficient number and density is paramount to ensure adequate signal. This requires the judicious selection of genes and proteins that represent critical points in the molecular pathway of a disease process. Imaging of proteins or protein function is more feasible, given the much larger number of such targets per cell (eg, protein targets can be as high as 10^6) [15] compared with the number of DNA or mRNA targets per cell. The latter case requires a much more robust signal amplification strategy for target visualization.

Cancer biology and the potential role of molecular imaging

Tumor growth is dependent on the collective manifestation of six essential alterations in cell physiology [16]. This realization has led to the development of novel diagnostic and treatment strategies that are directed at one or more of these properties. These physiologic alterations include self-sufficiency in growth signals, insensitivity to

Step 1. Develop Systems Hypothesis

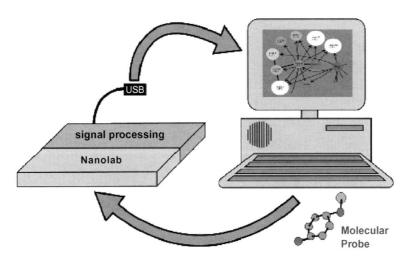

Step 2. Perturb System & Identify Drug Targets

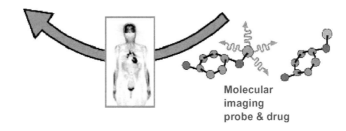

Step 3. Molecular Imaging of Disease & Drug Testing

Fig. 1. Possible methods through which the various tools described might be used to solve a systems biology problem and to apply that solution to a drug discovery process. In Step 1, the nanolab is used to carry out a rapid and informative molecular analysis of a biologic system by way of a global analysis of proteins and mRNA levels in a few cells. The data, coupled with an informatics algorithm, generate a hypothesis of the system. Step 1 also illustrates a means for carrying out an informative molecular-based diagnosis of disease. In Step 2, the hypothesis is tested using molecular probes, and drug targets are identified. In Step 3, the most effective of these molecular probes is turned into an imaging probe (and a drug), and applied toward imaging and treating disease within a living patient. (*Adapted from* Heath JR, Phelps ME, Hood L. NanoSystems biology. Mol Imag Biol 2003;5(5):312–25; with permission.)

growth-inhibitory signals, evasion of programmed cell death (apoptosis), limitless replicative potential, sustained angiogenesis, and tissue invasion and metastasis (Fig. 2). The ability to image molecular events that drive oncology, tumor phenotypic characteristics, and dynamic changes in these processes is essential for optimizing modern cancer care.

There are limitations in the visualization of tumors that are in the very early stages of development, as well as in the ability to monitor tumor phenotype, quantify tumor invasion, or detect real-time in vivo activity of anticancer therapeutics. Conventional diagnostic imaging generally visualizes nonspecific changes that are related to morphology or physiology (ie, blood volume, perfusion), or biochemical changes that usually are caused by alterations in multiple genes and proteins. Conversely, molecular imaging, relies on the ability to target genes and proteins that are known to be linked directly or indirectly to human disease. Cellular-based imaging and phenotypic mouse imaging often are included in this latter definition. Specifically, the location and level at which specific proteins/genes are expressed in the body, as well as temporal variations in these levels and distributions, particularly following an intervention, ultimately are desired.

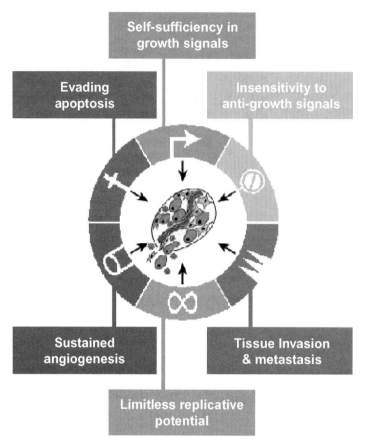

Fig. 2. Acquired capabilities of cancer. Most, if not all cancers, have acquired the same set of functional capabilities during their development, albeit through various mechanistic strategies. (*From* Hanahan D, Weinberg RA. The hallmarks of cancer. Cell 2000;100:57–70; with permission.)

Several factors have led to a major transformation and explosive growth in the imaging sciences [8,15]. A wealth of gene/protein expression data that are associated with molecular mechanisms of disease continues to accrue, in addition to the successful sequencing of the human genome. There has been progress in combinatorial chemistry and mass screening methods for generating a large number of potential candidate molecules for specific target interaction. An ever-increasing number of transgenic animal models have been developed or are under development. Novel approaches for generating protein/gene-specific imaging contrast have been elaborated, and there have been significant improvements in imaging technology. The last two advances are addressed in the context of MR imaging (see later discussion).

All of these factors, along with the expansion of multiple scientific disciplines, have facilitated the transition from in vitro and tissue culture-based systems to in vivo imaging studies within intact, living subjects. With this linkage, the attainment of several important goals in relation to the biomedical and imaging sciences has or will become possible [17]. These goals include the continued development of specific molecular- and cellular-based imaging techniques, cell tracking and targeting methods, molecular assessment of disease progression, and monitoring of therapeutic agents on a molecular/cellular level.

Advances in MR imaging applicable to molecular medicine

Technical issues and developments

The increase in magnetic field strength is just one of the recent advances in MR imaging. The advantages of using higher field strengths include greater signal-to-noise and contrast-to-noise ratios, which permit reductions in overall scan length or improvements in spatial resolution. In addition, enhanced spectral resolution and larger blood oxygenation level–dependent contrast can be achieved. Although moving to higher field strengths introduces several inherent pitfalls, including a potential reduction in image contrast as a result of lengthening the T1 relaxation time, homogeneity of the B0 and B1 magnetic fields, reduced radiofrequency (RF) penetration, higher gradient coil performance and linearity, and increased susceptibility effects, these are outweighed by the ultimate benefits of the technology [18,19].

Although the initially introduced high-field systems were not optimized and required on-site expertise for operation, advances in imaging hardware, software, and physics in the past decade have facilitated the mainstream operation of these magnets. Although 3-T systems are becoming state-of-the-art for clinical applications, several ultrahigh systems have been established for research purposes in humans, including several 7-T magnets and a few 8-T and 9.4-T whole-body systems [18]. Custom-built or whole body coils are being constructed or are now available for many clinical applications.

Although early high-field clinical studies focused on neuroimaging applications, there has been an expansion to other areas of the body. Preliminary abdominal imaging studies, performed on normal volunteers using a 4-T system [20,21], in conjunction with a custom-built transmit/receive six-RF coil set, yielded higher signal-to-noise ratios and improved image contrast in several abdominal viscera, relative to the 1.5-T systems. In addition, several recent structural and functional studies [22,23] of the prostate gland were performed successfully at 3 T using an endorectal or pelvic phased array coil. One additional study [24] revealed the clinical usefulness of high-field prostate MR spectroscopic imaging (MRSI) for accurately delineating and staging prostate cancer.

In parallel with successively increased magnetic field strengths for clinical applications, magnetic field strengths that are used for small animal imaging systems also have been increasing. The highest horizontal bore system for small animal imaging is now at 11.7 T, with 9.4-T systems becoming the standard [25]. These systems have produced near-microscopic resolution (tens of microns range) images for small animal models, and have been used to analyze physiologic and

molecular markers. Given the exploding growth of mouse models, however, the immediate problem of characterizing the effect of specific genetic alterations on morphologic changes (ie, phenotype) has been the primary application of micro-MR imaging or MR microscopy (MRM) [25–27].

MRM dictates the need for much higher field strengths than those that are used conventionally, and depends on the use of special RF coils and improved three-dimensional–encoding strategies. With additional improvements in sensitivity and field-of-view coverage on high-field magnets (9.4 T), a whole mouse is able to be imaged at 100 microns isotropic resolution, albeit over long imaging times (> 12 hours) [25]. More remarkable are the isotropic resolutions of 50 and 25 microns that can be achieved for limited volumes of the intact mouse specimen and excised organs, respectively [25]. The tremendous increase in volumetric resolution that is offered (> 250,000 fold that of a typical image in the human body) results in the visualization of structures that are not seen by conventional means. In this context, MRM also can be expected to have a substantial influence in developmental biology and cell trafficking.

Novel targeted MR contrast agents

Paramagnetic MR contrast agents that have been synthesized to date decrease the T1 and T2 relaxation properties of water protons in the surrounding media. Some agents preferentially reduce T1 without significantly influencing T2 relaxation effects (gadopentetate dimeglumine, GdDTPA), whereas other agents create significant T2* relaxation effects (superparamagnetic iron oxide particles, SPIOs). Typically, multiple iron or gadolinium atoms are attached to the targeting molecules of interest using macromolecules, including albumin [28], polylysine [29], dextran, polyamidoamine dendrimers of different generations [30], or coated liposomes [31]. Generally, gadolinium-based agents exhibit low relativities per unit of metal, particularly upon cellular internalization, in addition to an uncertain toxicity profile following cellular release over time.

SPIOs or ultrasmall SPIOs usually are stabilized with aminated cross-linked dextrans for in vivo administration and are the preferred agents of interest because of several favorable properties [32–39]. These include: (1) the ability to induce large signal changes per unit of metal, particularly on T2*-weighted images; (2) favorable biocompatibility and recycling properties; (3) ease of chemical manipulation/linkage given its typical dextran coating; and (4) the demonstration of variable magnetic properties with size [29]. These iron nanoparticles are used primarily as blood pool or macrophage imaging agents [38,39], although they have been used, more recently, in preclinical stem and T-cell trafficking studies within [40,41] and outside of the central nervous system [42,43]. In addition, they can be conjugated to any number of enzymes, antibodies, or peptides for specific imaging applications.

Many clinical and experimental MR contrast agents are nonspecific and circulate within the vasculature, and often are limited to reporting anatomic information. A new generation of highly-specific, MR-based agents that report on the physiologic status and metabolic activity of cells or organisms recently have been synthesized [8,32,44]. In general, contrast agents or molecular probes, can be categorized as follows [45]: (1) nonspecific or compartmental probes, (2) targeted probes, and (3) activatable or 'smart' probes (Fig. 3). Typically, compartmental, conventional probes are used to measure physiologic processes (eg, perfusion, blood volume), but cannot be targeted to specific cellular or subcellular biologic processes [45] or reveal changes in the early stages of a disease process. Conversely, the use of targeted probes or probes that are bound to antibodies or other substrates offers higher specificity for a particular cellular or subcellular target, such as tumor cell–surface receptors or intracellular enzymes. Large paramagnetic gadolinium complexes, such as paramagnetic polymerized liposomes, have been used successfully to image $\alpha_v\beta_3$ integrin receptors that are expressed on angiogenic endothelium [31]. Activatable or 'smart' probes only can be detected upon interacting with a specific target. This significantly reduces potential background signal relative to that which accompanies simple targeted probes and boosts imaging signal and contrast-to-noise ratios. Examples of this class of agent include activatable paramagnetic chelators, [46,47]; paramagnetic substrates that are polymerized by tyrosinases and peroxidases [48]; and, more recently, magnetic nanosensors [49,50] that interact with DNA or RNA sequences.

MR functional and molecular imaging strategies

Dynamic advances in imaging technology, as well as the production of novel and increasingly specific anticancer therapeutic agents, have fueled the development of molecular and genomic imaging. The need for noninvasive or minimally-invasive methods to obtain quantitative, serial information from tumors and their surrounding environments has increased considerably in clinical and experimental oncology. Furthermore,

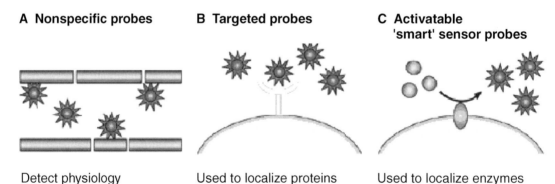

A Nonspecific probes

Detect physiology
(blood volume, angiogenesis)

B Targeted probes

Used to localize proteins
and determine structure

**C Activatable
'smart' sensor probes**

Used to localize enzymes
and determine function

Fig. 3. Probes have been developed to enhance all in vivo imaging techniques, and can be used to highlight internal organs, tumors, or molecular processes selectively. (A) The most commonly used imaging agents simply have compartmental distributions and can be used to image physiologic processes, such as changes in blood volume, perfusion, and blood flow in angiogenesis. With many of these agents, the compartmental distribution changes over time so that fast imaging might be required. (B) Imaging agents can be coupled to molecules, such as antibodies or proteins, and targeted specifically to tumor cells. Depending on the nature of the imaging probe, background noise can be high. (C) 'Smart' sensors reduce signal-to-noise ratios because they only can be detected after they have interacted with their substrate. These agents, primarily developed for MR and optical imaging, are much less detectable in their native injected state. (From Weissleder R. Scaling down imaging: molecular mapping of cancer in mice. Nat Rev Cancer 2002;2:1–8; with permission.)

such imaging methodologies will play an increasingly essential role in studying biology (e.g., developmental biology), as well as in guiding interventions. Clinical imaging techniques, such as perfusion and diffusion imaging, and MR spectroscopy (MRS), are paramount to cancer detection and treatment, from diagnosis and staging to treatment monitoring and delivery.

Of critical importance is the need to use functional or molecular imaging methods that sensitively detect early therapeutic responses, before clinical evidence of such a response. This evaluation traditionally has been performed, using conventional imaging approaches, on the basis of tumor shrinkage. Often, cytotoxic agents that reduce tumor size are administered. An analysis of tumor size, even if using volumetric measurements, may not be applied suitably to the results of targeted, highly-specific therapeutic agents that arrest cancer cell growth (ie, cytostatic agents). In this case, significant changes in tumor size may not occur, particularly early in the process, although a positive treatment response is achieved.

That a variety of targeted agents have yielded disappointing results in clinical trials while proving successful on an experimental basis underscores the potential value of in vivo imaging methods, particularly molecular, for testing novel pharmaceuticals. Furthermore, the ability to identify particular subsets of patients who most likely would benefit from a specific targeted therapy, as well as to monitor the extent to which the agent reaches its target, only can be achieved by some noninvasive means.

To address the above limitations, additional parameters that can monitor the response to new, selective therapies that target one or more levels of tumor biology (i.e., cell proliferation and invasion, angiogenesis, and metastasis) are needed (see Fig. 2). For instance, several new therapeutic strategies [51,52] have targeted angiogenesis and pathologic vascularity; a few are completing phase I trials [53]. Those imaging studies that reveal early evidence of a positive pharmacodynamic response then may be proposed as surrogate end points of drug efficacy. This, in turn, would expedite the selection of more efficacious drug combinations to enter into phase III trials [54].

Because functional clinical imaging techniques and new molecular imaging tools can provide information related to tumor vascularity, microenvironment, and cell metabolism, such functional imaging parameters should be considered and actively investigated as appropriate tumor response variables. This is particularly relevant because such features are interdependent in most solid tumors [55]. Examples of imaging techniques that may act as tumor response variables include ^{1}H MRS and ^{31}P MRS, which permit the assessment of cellular physiology, membrane turnover, or intracellular pH, and dynamic contrast-enhanced (DCE) MR imaging, which reveals information concerning tumor perfusion, capillary permeability, and leakage space [56]. Other MR techniques, such as diffusion imaging, are able to measure water diffusion and cell membrane integrity [57]. Furthermore, molecular imaging techniques will enable processes, such as intracellular signaling, gene delivery and expression, and drug delivery, to be monitored [15].

Perfusion imaging

Perfusion methods ideally are suited as tumor physiologic imaging tools. These techniques offer multiple advantages, including the ability to estimate preoperatively tumor grade, guide stereotactic biopsy, and better delineate tumor margins for surgical and treatment planning purposes [58]. The use of measured perfusion changes as surrogate markers of therapeutic response in clinical trials of newer antiangiogenic agents seems to be promising. Depending on the application, dynamic imaging that uses T2-weighted, "first pass" techniques or T1-based methods is performed. The former, well-established techniques have been used extensively for relative cerebral blood volume measurements of brain neoplasms. Analysis of T1-weighted enhancement, termed DCE MR imaging, mainly reflects lesion permeability, and has been used for lesion characterization; staging; prognosis; and monitoring and predicting the effects of a variety of therapies, particularly antiangiogenic or antivascular treatments [56,59]. This technique has been used frequently for sensitively distinguishing benign from malignant lesions [60]. Generally, malignant tissues enhance early and reveal rapid, large signal intensity increases compared with the slower signal increases in benign lesions. This finding is not demonstrated uniformly, however; an overlap in enhancement rates between benign and malignant breast lesions have been reported, which reduces specificity. Successful staging of gynecologic malignancies and bladder and prostate cancers also has been achieved by using DCE MR imaging [61–63]. For instance, in cases with seminal vesicle invasion or questionable capsular penetration, increased accuracy in prostate cancer staging was shown when DCE MR imaging was used in conjunction with T2-weighted imaging [63].

The use of DCE MR imaging to predict or monitor a wide variety of therapeutic effects has been applied to neoadjuvant chemotherapy in bladder and breast cancers [64,65] and bone sarcomas (Fig. 4) [66]. In addition, several recent studies suggest that the effects of antiangiogenic/antivascular treatments can be assessed [59,67]; a diminished rate of enhancement in successfully treated cases and persistent, abnormal enhancement in poorly-responding cases were noted. That many different types of treatments can result in vascular compromise reflects the relative lack of specificity with regard to tumor response [68]. As such, DCE MR imaging can be considered as an early response indicator.

Diffusion MR imaging

A second interesting application of MR imaging is the quantification of therapy-induced changes in tumor cellularity by evaluating a surrogate marker, such as the diffusivity of water [57,69,70]. The potential clinical usefulness of this

technique for determining the early efficacy of novel, targeted anticancer agents [71], gene therapy [72], and more traditional chemotherapeutic agents [73] is being investigated, particularly in small animal models. Ultimately, this may permit treatments to be tailored on an individual basis and allow alternative therapies to be tested in a more timely fashion. Furthermore, as an early indicator of treatment response, diffusion measurements may provide additional information that is related to the spatial heterogeneity of treatment effects that are beneficial to experimental and clinical trials [71].

The use of diffusion as a potential surrogate marker is based on the dependence of this parameter on several factors, including membrane permeability between the intracellular and extracellular compartments and the directionality of cellular or tissue structures that may promote or retard water motion. Successful treatment of tumors may result in significant tumor cell death, which thereby, alters membrane integrity, increases the effective interstitial space volume fraction, and, subsequently, enhances water

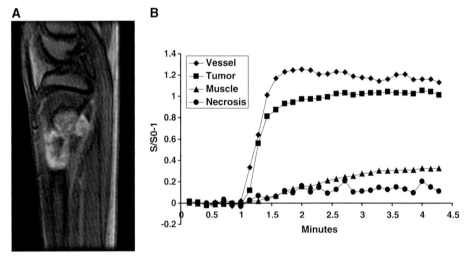

Fig. 4. (*A*) A sagittal MR image is shown 4 minutes after administration of contrast for an osteosarcoma, grade I—30% response. Regions of interest (ROIs) are placed on regions of muscle, vessel, significantly necrotic region, and tumor. (Fast multi-phase spoiled gradient echo sequence, 9 ms/2 ms repetition time/echo time, 256×256 matrix, 24 cm field-of-view, 12-mm thickness). (*B*) Representative time intensity curves from various regions exhibit differences in initial rise time and maximum enhancement. ROI 1 depicts typical muscular uptake and shows a gradual increase in intensity without a noticeable plateau for this scan time. The popliteal artery is shown in ROI 2 having four to five points that characterize the initial arrival of contrast into the vessel over time. ROI 3 depicts a region of significant necrosis, which was characterized by a lesser degree of enhancement than muscle. ROI 4 is indicative of a region of tumor viability showing an enhancement and slope above that of muscle, but less than vessel. Following surgery, this patient was confirmed to be a grade I responder to chemotherapy who exhibited 30% necrosis by single-slice pathology. (Courtesy of D. Panacek, MD, New York, NY.)

mobility throughout the injured tissue region. Typically, diffusion is reported as an apparent diffusion coefficient (ADC), by measuring the degree of signal attenuation that arises from local water mobility in the presence of magnetic field gradients. Several subcutaneous and orthotopic tumor models have demonstrated that diffusion MR imaging may serve as a robust surrogate that can be used to investigate gene therapy or chemotherapeutic regimens [57,74,75]. The ability of the measured ADC values to correlate with, and universally predict antitumoral therapeutic efficacy remains to be established using preclinical models. Several human studies also have been reported [57,70,76,77], with one such case illustrated (Fig. 5).

MR spectroscopy

A wealth of information on tumor physiology and metabolism can be derived from magnetic resonance spectroscopy studies. Depending upon the nucleus that is probed (ie, ^{1}H, ^{19}F, ^{31}P), different metabolic information can be extracted.

The high sensitivity of ^{1}H MRS yields proton spectra of increased spatial and temporal resolution. This has particular relevance in the setting of heterogeneous tumor blood flow, because this heterogeneity is reflected similarly in the tumor oxygenation and pH patterns and the metabolite distribution. By significantly restricting voxel sizes, spatially localized spectra may be obtained; this allows better characterization of the tumor and its response to therapy and permits improved

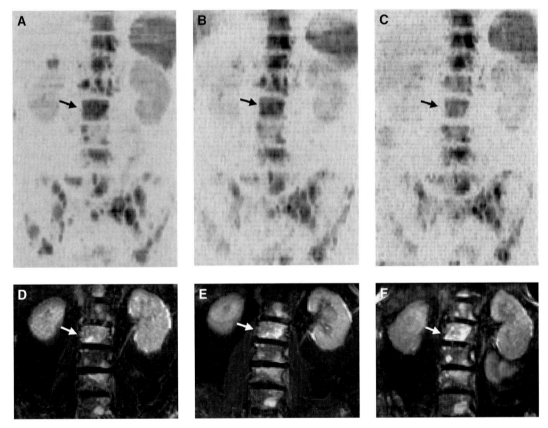

Fig. 5. Data from a 76-year-old man who has prostate cancer metastatic to bone. Coronal maximum intensity projection images are shown at (A) 1 week before the start of chemotherapy, (B) during week 6, and (C) after 12 weeks of therapy. (D–F) Corresponding maximum intensity projection images of the lumbar spine generated from a short TI inversion recovery (STIR) data set at the same time points. Because of overlapping signals in the STIR data set from cerebrospinal fluid, only coronal slices that intersected the lumbar spine anterior to the vertebral foramina were included. The lesion in L2 denoted by dark arrows on the diffusion-weighted series (A–C) and light arrows on the STIR series (D–F) suggests a more positive response to therapy than most other lesions. (From Ballon D, Watts R, Dyke JP, et al. Imaging therapeutic response in human bone marrow using rapid whole-body MRI. Magn Reson Med 2004;52:1234–8; with permission. Courtesy of Eric Lis, MD, and Douglas Ballon, PhD.)

delineation of metabolite distributions. In addition, the contaminating effects of the surrounding tissue is reduced.

Typically, tumor proton spectra contain resonances from taurine, total choline (choline, phosphocholine, and glycerophosphocholine), total creatine (phosphocreatine and creatine), and lactate [78]. Elevated choline and lactate levels generally are exhibited in these tumor spectra [79]. High lactate levels are a reflection of poor tumor blood flow and high glycolytic rates that are associated with tumors. Using high-resolution ^{1}H MRS studies of cell extracts, the high levels of total choline that are detected in breast, prostate, and various brain tumors have been determined to arise primarily from increased phosphocholine levels in tumor cells [80,81]. High levels of phosphocholine and phosphoethanolamine also have been confirmed in several additional in vitro and in vivo ^{1}H and ^{31}P MRS studies of several cancers, including breast, prostate, and brain [82].

The total choline signal usually is measured in ^{1}H MRS tumor experiments (Fig. 6). In conjunction with high-resolution anatomic MR imaging, MRS can improve significantly the analysis of tumor location and aggressiveness. In addition, the application of combined MR imaging and MRSI to pre- and posttreatment studies may reveal directly the presence and spatial extent of cancers, as well as the mechanism and time course of therapeutic response. Detection of elevated choline levels using MR imaging or MRSI has been shown for brain [83], prostate [84], breast [85], and other tumors [79].

Molecular MR imaging of cell-based therapies

Cell-based therapies, in which cells act as therapeutic vehicles for treating disease, is an exciting and rapidly growing field that has broad applicability in biomedicine. Although the field itself is not new and encompasses the use of blood transfusions, bone marrow transplants, and transplantation of embryonic nigral dopaminergic neurons for Parkinson's disease, more recent clinical trials are investigating the feasibility of using purified stem cell populations for treating advanced hematologic diseases and multiple myeloma. In addition, novel cell therapies have been used for the treatment of other types of cancer [86,87], neurodegenerative disease [88], cardiovascular disease [89], diabetes [90], and autoimmune diseases [91], to name but a few of an ever-growing list of potential diseases. This has fueled the demand for noninvasive, quantitative cellular/molecular imaging tools that are able to monitor cellular delivery and therapeutic efficacy sensitively and accurately in patients.

Two evolving areas of particular clinical interest, from the molecular imaging standpoint, are the adoptive transfer of immunocytes and stem

A   **B**

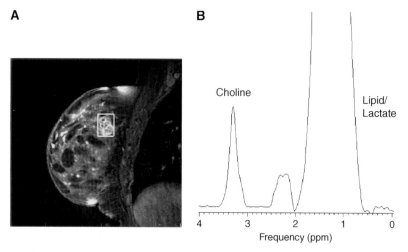

Fig. 6. (*A*) A three-dimensional sagittal fat-suppressed, postcontrast T1-weighted fast spoiled gradient-recalled image reveals a pathologically proven malignant breast tumor along the superior quadrant of the breast. The rectangular box that encompasses the lobulated, enhancing lesion demonstrates the voxel placement for the single-voxel ^{1}H MRS examination. (*B*) ^{1}H MRS obtained from the contrast-enhanced lesion area with a point-resolved spectroscopic sequence (repetition time/echo time = 2000 ms/135 ms, number of excitations = 128) demonstrates an apparent choline peak at 3.23 ppm. (Courtesy of S. Thakur, PhD, W. Huang, PhD, E. Morris, MD, L. Bartella, MD, New York, NY.)

cell therapy. In the first case, adoptively transferred immune effectors with antitumor activity have been infused into the tumor-bearing host (ie, adoptive immunotherapy), mainly using cytotoxic T lymphocytes for the treatment of lymphoma, melanoma, and other malignancies [92–94]. Successful cytotoxic T-lymphocyte tracking and recruitment to an experimental, intact melanoma model recently was reported [95] using high-resolution MR methods (Fig. 7). The second area, therapeutic (stem) cell transplantation, has been referred to—in the broad sense—as regenerative medicine, an area of medicine that encompasses a wide range of disciplines that are devoted to the common goal of repairing or replacing cells, tissues, and organs. The ability to perform high-resolution, three-dimensional MR monitoring of cell populations that are used for therapeutic purposes in space and time would facilitate our understanding of molecular mechanisms that

mediate cellular recruitment, cellular distribution/proliferation, homing, and cell fate, and ultimately, permit the optimization of treatment protocols.

Magnetically labeled cells can be tracked at high temporal and spatial resolution using MR imaging to provide information on the dynamic movements of cells within and among tissues in animal disease models [40–42]. Alternatively, this imaging strategy likely will be translated to the monitoring of (stem) cell therapy or adoptive immunotherapy in patients. Such applications require the in vitro introduction of a suitable biocompatible magnetic label or genetic modification of the cell (see later discussion) [96]. Using the former approach, the cell population of interest is isolated in sufficient quantity and purity for loading of an imaging agent, typically iron oxide particles, because they significantly effect large signal changes per unit mass of metal on

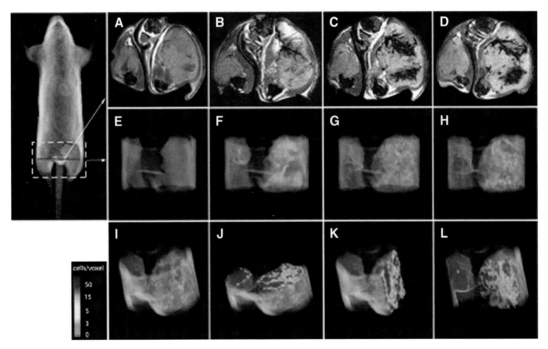

Fig. 7. Time course of CLIO-HD OT-I CD8$^+$ T cell homing to B16-OVA tumor. CLIO-HD is a highly derivatized cross-linked iron oxide nanoparticle. Serial MR imaging was performed after adoptive transfer into a mouse carrying B16F0 (*left*) and B16-OVA (*right*) melanomas. (*A–D*) Axial slices through the mouse thighs before adoptive transfer (*A*) and at 12 hours (*B*), 16 hours (*C*), and 36 hours (*D*), after adoptive transfer of CLIO-HD-labeled OT-I CD8$^+$ T cells. (*E–H*) Three-dimensional color-scaled reconstructions of B16F0 (*left*) and B16-OVA (*right*) melanomas at 0 hours (*E*), 12 hours (*F*), 16 hours (*G*), and 36 hours (*H, I*), after adoptive transfer. Numbers of cells/voxel are color-coded as shown in scale. Axial (*J*), sagittal (*K*), and coronal (*L*) plane slices through the three-dimensional reconstruction shown in *I*. Data are representative of eight individual animals. (*From* Kircher MF, Allport JR, Graves EE, et al. *In vivo* high resolution three-dimensional imaging of antigen-specific cytotoxic T-lymphocyte trafficking to tumors. Cancer Res 2003;63: 6838–46; with permission.)

T2*-weighted imaging. T1-based agents (ie, gadolinium-based) also can be selected, however. While offering the advantage of increased specificity of the label for a given cell population relative to the background tissue (ie, increased signal to noise), several limitations exist, including progressive label dilution with successive cell divisions and "one-time" labeling of the cell population [96]. These limitations restrict the imaging observation period, which, in turn, is dependent on cell type (ie, rapidly or slowly dividing cells).

Molecular MR imaging of gene expression and therapy

The genetic modification of cells requires the introduction of isolated, foreign DNA material that contains the gene of interest (ie, transfection) into a selected cell type in culture. This technique may produce an imagable and stably transfected cell line over the course of the study, but preferably, on a permanent basis. Because visualization by molecular imaging methods is determined genetically, long-term imaging or tracking of these transfected cells can be achieved, assuming that adequate cell numbers are present for detection. The genetic label will be present in the cell progeny; this eliminates the problem of cellular dilution with each cell division. Because the modification is genetic, the possibility of the cell being transformed or immortalized, such that its biologic properties are altered, is a possibility [96]. Furthermore, the long-term consequences of genetic cell modification raise safety concerns and may limit applicability in humans to specific, tumor-directed gene therapies [96]. Such techniques are time-intensive and may result in limited gene expression, particularly on a permanent basis.

MR imaging of genetically altered cells or gene expression relies on creating sufficient image contrast between the cell population of interest and the remainder of the host tissues. One prime difficulty is the small number of MR imaging agents that can be incorporated easily into existing cellular metabolic pathways, compared with PET. Two strategies have been developed to image gene expression [97,98], namely: (1) imaging of introduced enzymes or reporter genes (ie, genes that encode an easily visualized product) into specific cell populations that bind to or metabolize administered paramagnetic substrates (ie, probes); and (2) imaging of unique spectroscopic signals (ie, signatures). As an example of the first approach, tumor cells that express an engineered transferrin receptor (ETR+) or null tumors (ie, ETR⁻) were grown in the flanks of a nude mouse [99]. The mouse was perfused with a (super)paramagnetic transferrin probe (ie, monocrystalline iron oxide nanoparticles bound to transferrin). This amplification strategy generated a large signal intensity difference between the two tumors on in vivo MR imaging 24 hours later. Only the ETR+ tumors demonstrated uptake of the transferrin probe; this confirmed the specificity of the transferrin probe for the engineered receptor. Using the second approach, gene expression has been measured by MRS. In one study, tumor cell lines which express the cDNA that encodes for yeast cytosine deaminase (yCD) were introduced into animal models [100]. Using ^{19}F MRS, the conversion of the nontoxic prodrug, 5-fluorocytosine to the antimetabolite, 5-fluorouracil by yCD could be measured in vivo.

The efficacy of gene therapy also has been evaluated using MR imaging and MRS. For example, improved distal flow was assessed qualitatively using MR angiography in patients who had chronic critical leg ischemia that participated in an intramuscular gene therapy trial that tested the safety and efficacy of vascular endothelial growth factor [101].

Summary

The implementation and integration of systems biology approaches with the emerging nanosciences and microchip technology will revolutionize profoundly molecular imaging and fuel the drive toward a more predictive and individualized health care. In combination with informatics platforms, key gene and protein targets will be identified, and serve as more effective targets for diagnostic and therapeutic interventions. Drug development also will be expedited by the judicious selection of more appropriate molecular biomarkers that will serve as objective end points of treatment efficacy, in addition to facilitating the development of new target-specific therapeutics. Finally, with the more widespread proliferation of high-field magnets and advancements in imaging hardware; acquisition methods; and novel, "smart" MR agents, the ability to achieve higher resolution analyses of tumor biology, cell tracking, and gene expression will be realized more fully.

Although radiologists will continue to serve as diagnostic consultants and assist in management decisions, the contributions from new developments in the biologic and molecular sciences will significantly alter the scope of our profession. Radiologists will be required to participate more actively in the individualized care of the patient and cultivate a deeper understanding of the underlying molecular basis of disease and molecular pharmacology for facilitating selection of the most appropriate combination of imaging studies that address biologically relevant questions. These radical changes in our profession will necessitate the re-education and emergence of a small cadre of professionals that is educated broadly in multiple scientific disciplines, and demonstrate expertise in clinical care and the basic sciences. The optimistic view is that this already is happening.

References

[1] Kitano H. Systems biology: a brief overview. Science 2002;295:1662–4.

[2] Heath JR, Phelps ME, Hood L. NanoSystems biology. Mol Imaging Biol 2003;5(5):312–25.

[3] Ideker T, Thorsson V, Ranish JA, et al. Integrated genomic and proteomic analyses of a systemically perturbed metabolic network. Science 2001;292: 929–34.

[4] Hood L, Heath JR, Phelps ME, et al. Systems biology and new technologies enable predictive and preventative medicine. Science 2004;306:640–3.

[5] Weston AD, Hood L. Systems biology, proteomics, and the future of health care: toward predictive, preventative, and personalized medicine. J Proteome Res 2004;3:179–96.

[6] Hood L, Perlmutter RM. The impact of systems approaches on biological problems in drug discovery. Nat Biotechnol 2004;22(10):1215–7.

[7] Rudin M, Weissleder R. Molecular imaging in drug discovery and development. Nat Rev Drug Discov 2003;2:123–31.

[8] Cherry SR. In vivo molecular and genomic imaging: new challenges for imaging physics. Phys Med Biol 2004;49:R13–48.

[9] Venter JC, Levy S, Stockwell T, et al. Massive parallelism, randomness, and genomic advances. Nat Gen 2003;33:219–27.

[10] Weber BL. Cancer genomics. Cancer Cell 2002;1: 37–47.

[11] Brown PO, Botstein D. Exploring the new world of the genome with DNA microarrays. Nat Genet 1999;21:33–7.

[12] Phizicky E, Bastiaens PIH, Zhu H, et al. Protein analysis on a proteomic scale. Nature 2003;422: 208–15.

[13] Yarmush ML, Jayaraman A. Advances in proteomic technologies. Annu Rev Biomed Eng 2002;4: 349–73.

[14] Martin DB, Nelson PS. From genomics to proteomics: techniques and applications in cancer research. Trends Cell Biol 2001;11:S60–5.

[15] Weissleder R, Mahmood U. Molecular imaging. Radiology 2001;219:316–33.

[16] Hanahan D, Weinberg RA. The hallmarks of cancer. Cell 2000;100:57–70.

[17] Massoud TF, Gambhir SS. Molecular imaging in living subjects: seeing fundamental biological processes in a new light. Genes Dev 2003;17:545–80.

[18] Hu X, Norris DG. Advances in high-field magnetic resonance imaging. Annu Rev Biomed Eng 2004;6: 157–84.

[19] Norris DG. High field human imaging. J Magn Reson Imaging 2003;18:519–29.

[20] Uematsu H, Dougherty L, Takahashi M, et al. Abdominal imaging at 4 T MR system: a preliminary result. Eur J Radiol 2003;47:161–3.

[21] Uematsu H, Takahashi M, Dougherty L, et al. High field body MR imaging: preliminary experiences. J Clin Imag 2004;28:159–62.

[22] Sosna J, Pedrosa I, Dewolf WC, et al. MR imaging of the prostate at 3 Tesla: comparison of an external phased-array coil to imaging with an endorectal coil at 1.5T. Acad Radiol 2004;11(8): 857–62.

[23] Bloch BN, Rofsky NM, Baroni RH, et al. 3T magnetic resonance imaging of the prostate with combined pelvic phased-array and endorectal coils; initial experience (1). Acad Radiol 2004;11(8): 863–7.

[24] Futterer JJ, Scheenen TW, Huisman HJ, et al. Initial experience of 3T endorectal coil magnetic resonance imaging and 1H-spectroscopic imaging of the prostate. Invest Radiol 2004;39(11): 671–80.

[25] Johnson GA, Cofer GP, Gewalt MS, et al. Morphologic phenotyping with MR microscopy: the visible mouse. Radiology 2002;222:789–93.

[26] Benveniste H, Kim K, Zhang L, et al. Magnetic resonance microscopy of the C57BL mouse brain. Neuroimage 2000;11:601–11.

[27] MacKenzie-Graham A, Lee EF, Dinov ID, et al. A multimodal, multidimensional atlas of the C57/6J mouse brain. J Anat 2004;204:93–102.

[28] Schmiedl U, Ogan M, Paajanen H, et al. Albumin labeled with Gd-DTPA as an intravascular blood pool enhancing agent for MR imaging: biodistribution and imaging studies. Radiology 1987;162(1 Pt 1):205–10.

[29] Bogdanov AA, Weissleder R, Frank HW, et al. A new macromolecule as a contrast agent for MR angiography: preparation, properties, and animal studies. Radiology 1993;187:701–6.

[30] Bryant LH, Brechbiel MW, Wu C, et al. Synthesis and relaxometry of high-generation (G = 5, 7, 9,

10) PAMAM dendrimer-DOTA-gadolinium chelates. J Magn Reson Imaging 1999;9:348–52.

[31] Sipkins DA, Cheresh DA, Mahmood R, et al. Detection of tumor angiogenesis *in vivo* by $\alpha_v\beta_3$-targeted magnetic resonance imaging. Nat Med 1998;4(5):623–6.

[32] Pathak AP, Gimi B, Glunde K, et al. Molecular and functional imaging of cancer: advances in MRI and MRS. Methods Enzymol 2004;386: 3–60.

[33] Bjørnerud A, Johansson L. The utility of superparamagnetic contrast agents in MRI: theoretical consideration and applications in the cardiovascular system. NMR Biomed 2004;17:465–77.

[34] Bulte JWM, Kraitchman D. Iron oxide MR contrast agents for molecular and cellular imaging. NMR Biomed 2004;17:484–99.

[35] Berry CC, Curtis ASG. Functionalisation of magnetic nanoparticles for applications in biomedicine. J Phys D Appl Phys 2003;36:R198–206.

[36] Blankenberg FG. Molecular imaging: the latest generation of contrast agents and tissue characterization techniques. J Cell Biochem 2003;90: 443–53.

[37] Shinkai M, Ito A. Functional magnetic particles for medical applications. Adv Biochem Eng Biotechnol 2004;91:191–220.

[38] Artemov D. Molecular magnetic resonance imaging with targeted contrast agents. J Cell Biochem 2003;90:518–24.

[39] Weinmann H-J, Ebert W, Misselwitz B, et al. Tissue-specific MR contrast agents. Eur J Radiol 2003;46:33–44.

[40] Bulte JWM, Douglas T, Witwer B, et al. Magnetodendrimers allow endosomal magnetic labeling and *in vivo* cell tracking of stem cells. Nat Biotechnol 2001;19:1141–7.

[41] Bulte JWM, Zhang S, van Gelderen P, et al. Neurotransplantation of magnetically-labeled oligodendrocyte progenitors: magnetic resonance tracking of cell migration and myelination. Proc Natl Acad Sci USA 1999;96:15256–61.

[42] Hill JM, Dick AJ, Raman VK, et al. Serial cardiac magnetic resonance imaging of injected mesenchymal stem cells. Circulation 2003;108:1009–14.

[43] Dodd CH, Hsu HC, Chu WJ, et al. Normal T-cell response and *in vivo* magnetic resonance imaging of T cells loaded with HIV transactivator-peptide-derived superparamagnetic nanoparticles. J Immunol Meth 2001;256:89–105.

[44] Meade TJ, Taylor AK, Bull SR. New magnetic resonance contrast agents as biochemical reporters. Curr Opin Neurobiol 2003;13:597–602.

[45] Weissleder R. Scaling down imaging: molecular mapping of cancer in mice. Nat Rev Cancer 2002; 2:1–8.

[46] Louie AY, Huber MM, Ahrens ET, et al. *In vivo* visualization of gene expression using magnetic resonance imaging. Nat Biotechnol 2000;18:321–5.

[47] Moats RA, Fraser SE, Meade TJ. A "smart" magnetic resonance imaging agent that reports on specific enzymatic activity. Angew Chem Int Ed Engl 1997;36:726.

[48] Bogdanov A, Matuszewski L, Bremer C, et al. Oligomerization of paramagnetic substrates result in signal amplification and can be used for MR imaging of molecular targets. Mol Imaging 2001;1: 1–9.

[49] Josephson L, Perez M, Weissleder R. Magnetic nanosensors for the detection of oligonucleotide sequences. Angew Chem Int Ed Engl 2001;40: 3204–6.

[50] Perez JM, Simeone FJ, Saeki Y, et al. Viral-induced self-assembly of magnetic nanoparticles allows the detection of viral particles in biological media. J Am Chem Soc 2003;125:10192–3.

[51] Brower V. Tumor angiogenesis—new drugs on the block. Nat Biotechnol 1999;17:963–8.

[52] Pralhad T, Madhusudan S, Rajendrakumar K. Concept, mechanisms, and therapeutics of angiogenesis in cancer and other diseases. J Pharm Pharmacol 2003;55:1045–53.

[53] Dzik-Jurasz ASK. Molecular imaging in oncology. Cancer Imaging 2004;4:162–73.

[54] Padhani AR. Functional MRI for anti-cancer therapy assessment. Eur J Cancer 2002;38:2116–27.

[55] Folkman J. Angiogenesis in cancer, vascular, rheumatoid, and other disease. Nat Med 1995;1: 27–31.

[56] Padhani AR, Husband JE. Dynamic contrast-enhanced MRI studies in oncology with an emphasis on quantification, validation and human studies. Clin Radiol 2001;56:607–20.

[57] Chenevert TL, Stegman LD, Taylor JM, et al. Diffusion magnetic resonance imaging: an early surrogate marker of therapeutic efficacy in brain tumors. J Natl Cancer Inst 2000;92:2029–36.

[58] Covarrubias DJ, Rosen BR, Lev MH. Dynamic magnetic resonance perfusion imaging of brain tumors. Oncologist 2004;9:528–37.

[59] Galbraith SM, Maxwell RJ, Lodge MA, et al. Combretastatin A4 phosphate has tumor antivascular activity in rat and man as demonstrated by dynamic magnetic resonance imaging. J Clin Oncol 2003;21:2831–42.

[60] Knopp MV, Weiss E, Sinn HP, et al. Pathophysiologic basis of contrast enhancement in breast tumors. J Magn Reson Imaging 1999;10:260–6.

[61] Liu PF, Krestin GP, Huch RA, et al. MRI of the uterus, uterine cervix, and vagina: diagnostic performance of dynamic contrast-enhanced fast multiplanar gradient-echo imaging in comparison with fast spin-echo T2- weighted pulse imaging. Eur Radiol 1998;8:1433–40.

[62] Barentsz JO, Jager GJ, van Vierzen PB, et al. Staging urinary bladder cancer after transurethral biopsy: value of fast dynamic contrast-enhanced MR imaging. Radiology 1996;201:185–93.

[63] Jager GJ, Ruijter ET, van de Kaa CA, et al. Dynamic TurboFLASH subtraction technique for contrast-enhanced MR imaging of the prostate: correlation with histopathologic results. Radiology 1997;203:645–52.

[64] Barentsz JO, Berger-Hartog O, Witjes JA, et al. Evaluation of chemotherapy in advanced urinary bladder cancer with fast dynamic contrast-enhanced MR imaging. Radiology 1998;207:791–7.

[65] Knopp MV, Brix G, Junkermann HJ, et al. MR mammography with pharmacokinetic mapping for monitoring of breast cancer treatment during neoadjuvant therapy. Magn Reson Imaging Clin N Am 1994;2:633–58.

[66] Reddick WE, Taylor JS, Fletcher BD. Dynamic MR imaging of microcirculation in bone sarcoma. J Magn Reson Imaging 1999;10:277–85.

[67] Morgan B, Thomas AL, Drevs J, et al. Dynamic contrast-enhanced magnetic resonance imaging as a biomarker for the pharmacological response of PTK787/ZK 222584, an inhibitor of the vascular endothelial growth factor receptor tyrosine kinases, in patients with advanced colorectal cancer and liver metastases: results from two phase I studies. J Clin Oncol 2003;21(21):3955–64.

[68] Padhani AR. Dynamic contrast-enhanced MRI in clinical oncology: current status and future directions. J Magn Reson Imaging 2002;16: 407–22.

[69] Ross BD, Chenevert TL, Rehemtulla A. Magnetic resonance imaging in cancer research. Eur J Cancer 2002;38:2147–56.

[70] Ross BD, Moffat BA, Lawrence TS, et al. Evaluation of cancer therapy using diffusion magnetic resonance imaging. Mol Cancer Ther 2003;2(6): 581–7.

[71] Moffat BA, Hall DE, Stojanovska J, et al. Diffusion imaging for evaluation of tumor therapies in preclinical animal models. MAGMA 2004;17: 249–59.

[72] Hamstra DA, Tychewicz JM, Lee KC, et al. 19F Spectroscopy and diffusion weight MRI predict increased tumor response to cytosine deaminase and uracil phosphoribosyl transferase gene dependent enzyme prodrug therapy. Mol Ther 2004;10(5): 916–28.

[73] Hall DE, Moffat BA, Stojanovska J, et al. Therapeutic efficacy of DTI-015 using diffusion magnetic resonance imaging as an early surrogate marker. Clin Cancer Res 2004;10(23):7852–9.

[74] Jennings D, Hatton BN, Guo J, et al. Early response of prostate carcinoma xenografts to docetaxol chemotherapy monitored with diffusion MRI. Neoplasia 2002;4:255–62.

[75] Poptani H, Puumalainen AM, Grohn OH, et al. Monitoring thymidine kinase and ganciclovir-induced changes in rat malignant gliomas in vivo by nuclear magnetic resonance imaging. Cancer Gene Ther 1998;5:101–9.

[76] Mardor Y, Roth Y, Lidar Z, et al. Monitoring response to convection-enhanced taxol delivery in brain tumor patients using diffusion-weighted magnetic resonance imaging. Cancer Res 2001;61: 4971–3.

[77] Ballon D, Watts R, Dyke JP, et al. Imaging therapeutic response in human bone marrow using rapid whole-body MRI. Magn Reson Med 2004;52: 1234–8.

[78] Howe FA, Maxwell RJ, Saunders DE, et al. Proton spectroscopy in vivo. Magn Reson Q 1993;9:31–59.

[79] Negendank W. Studies of human tumors by MRS: a review. NMR Biomed 1992;5:303–24.

[80] Bhakoo KK, Williams SR, Florian CK, et al. Immortalization and transformation are associated with specific alterations in choline metabolism. Cancer Res 1996;56:4630–5.

[81] Aboagye EO, Bhujwalla ZM. Malignant transformation alters membrane choline phospholipid metabolism of human mammary epithelial cells. Cancer Res 1999;59:80–4.

[82] Ackerstaff E, Glunde K, Bhujwalla ZM. Choline phospholipid metabolism: a target in cancer cells? J Cell Biochem 2003;90:525–33.

[83] Li X, Lu Y, Pirzkall A, et al. Analysis of the spatial characteristics of metabolic abnormalities in newly diagnosed glioma patients. J Magn Reson Imaging 2002;16(3):229–37.

[84] Kurhanewicz J, Vigneron DB, Nelson SJ. Three-dimensional magnetic resonance spectroscopic imaging of brain and prostate cancer. Neoplasia 2000;2: 166–89.

[85] Gribbestad IS, Sitter B, Lundgren S, et al. Metabolite composition in breast tumors examined by proton nuclear magnetic resonance spectroscopy. Anticancer Res 1999;19(3A):1737–46.

[86] Mitchell DA, Fecci PE, Sampson JH. Adoptive immunotherapy for malignant gliomas. Cancer J 2003;9:157–66.

[87] Kipps TJ. Immune and cell therapy of hematologic malignancies. Int J Hematol 2002;76:269–73.

[88] Peaire AE, Takeshima T, Johnston JM, et al. Production of dopaminergic neurons for cell therapy in the treatment of Parkinson's disease. J Neurosci Methods 2003;124:61–74.

[89] Zimmerman WH, Eschenhagen T. Cardiac tissue engineering for replacement therapy. Heart Fail Rev 2003;8:259–69.

[90] Scharfmann R. Alternative sources of beta cells for cell therapy of diabetes. Eur J Clin Invest 2003;33: 595–600.

[91] Shaw T, Quan J, Totoritis MC. B cell therapy for rheumatoid arthritis: the rituximab (anti-CD20) experience. Ann Rheum Dis 2003;62:55–9.

[92] Hanson HL, Donermeyer DL, Ikeda H, et al. Eradication of established tumors by CD8+ T cell adoptive immunotherapy. Immunity 2002;13:265–76.

[93] Chapman AL, Rickinson AB, Thomas WA, et al. Epstein-Barr virus-specific cytotoxic T lymphocyte

responses in the blood and tumor site of Hodgkin's disease patients: implications for a T cell-based therapy. Cancer Res 2001;61:6219–26.

[94] Yee C, Thompson JA, Byrd D, et al. Adoptive T cell therapy using antigen-specific CD8$^+$ T cell clones for the treatment of patients with metastatic melanoma: in vivo persistence, migration, and anti-tumor effect of transferred T cells. Proc Natl Acad Sci USA 2002;99:16168–73.

[95] Kircher MF, Allport JR, Graves EE, et al. *In vivo* high resolution three-dimensional imaging of antigen-specific cytotoxic T-lymphocyte trafficking to tumors. Cancer Res 2003;63: 6838–46.

[96] Schellingerhout D, Josephson L. Molecular imaging of cell-based therapies. Neuroimag Clin N Am 2004;14:331–42.

[97] Allport JR, Weissleder R. *In vivo* imaging of gene and cell therapies. Exp Hematol 2001;29:1237–46.

[98] Shah K, Jacobs A, Breakefield XO, et al. Molecular imaging of gene therapy for cancer. Gene Ther 2004;11:1175–87.

[99] Ichikawa T, Hogemann D, Saeki Y, et al. MRI of transgene expression: correlation to therapeutic gene expression. Neoplasia 2002;4(6):523–30.

[100] Stegman L, Rehemtulla A, Beattie B, et al. Non-invasive quantitation of cytosine deaminase transgene expression in human tumor xenografts with in vivo magnetic resonance spectroscopy. Proc Natl Acad Sci USA 1999;96:9821–6.

[101] Shyu KG, Chang H, Wang BW, et al. Intramuscular vascular endothelial growth factor gene therapy in patients with chronic critical leg ischemia. Am J Med 2003;114(2):85–92.

ELSEVIER
SAUNDERS

Magn Reson Imaging Clin N Am
13 (2005) 241–254

MAGNETIC
RESONANCE
IMAGING CLINICS
of North America

Approach to Abdominal Imaging at 1.5 Tesla and Optimization at 3 Tesla

Diego R. Martin, MD, PhD[a],*, Harry T. Friel, MS[b],
Raman Danrad, MD[a], Jan De Becker, PhD[c],
Shahid M. Hussain, MD[d]

[a]Department of Radiology, Emory University School of Medicine, 1365 Clifton Road NE, Atlanta, GA 30322, USA
[b]Philips Medical Systems, 595 Miner Road, Highland Heights, OH 44143, USA
[c]Philips Medical Systems, P.O. Box 10.000, 5680 DA Best, The Netherlands
[d]Section of Abdominal Imaging, Department of Radiology, Erasmus University Medical Center,
Dr. Molewaterplein 40, 3015 GD Rotterdam, The Netherlands

The magnetic field strength of choice that is used currently for body MR imaging has been based on the 1.5 T systems. At the current state of development, this field strength has provided an optimal combination of signal to noise (SNR) and speed, and allows optimization of rapid acquisition techniques while staying within government institution–determined energy deposition-rate limits. These systems also have provided a good balance between T1 values, that are dependent on field strength, and achievable contrast affects. In addition, field distortion and paramagnetic affects that increase with increasing field strength and can yield undesirable image artifacts remain within tolerable limits at 1.5 T. There are theoretic considerations that have introduced a desire to examine the potential for developing higher field systems for body MR imaging. Current efforts are well underway to transfer techniques that are used at 1.5 T to 3 T; however, several additional considerations have become evident during this process. Approaches that have been successful when migrating techniques from lower to higher fields—up to 1.5 T—have not been successful migrating from 1.5 T to 3 T. Significant

adjustments to these approaches are required. This article reviews fundamental principles and sequence techniques that have been used successfully for imaging diseases of the abdomen and pelvis at 1.5 T, and introduces concepts and specific alteration of sequence parameters for optimization of abdominal–pelvic imaging at 3 T.

Fundamentals of MR imaging techniques applied to the abdomen and pelvis

Image quality, reproducibility of image quality, and good conspicuity of disease require the use of sequences that are robust, reliable, and avoid artifacts [1–5]. Maximizing these principles to achieve high-quality diagnostic MR images usually requires the use of fast scanning techniques, with the overall intention of generating images with consistent image quality that demonstrate consistent display of disease processes. Another advantage of using fast scanning techniques is that, when beneficial to diagnostic yield, a greater number of individual sequences can be used within a reasonably short total examination time. This approach contributes to one of the major strengths of MR imaging, which is comprehensive information on disease processes.

Respiration, bowel peristalsis, and vascular pulsations are related to major artifacts that

---

* Corresponding author.
  E-mail address: diego_martin@emoryhealthcare.org
(D.R. Martin).

have lessened the reproducibility of MRI. Breathing-independent sequences and breath-hold sequences form the foundation of high-quality MR imaging studies of the abdomen. Breathing artifact is less problematic in the pelvis, and high spatial and contrast resolution imaging have been the mainstay for maximizing image quality for pelvic studies.

Disease conspicuity depends on the principle of maximizing the difference in signal intensities between diseased tissues and the background tissue. For disease processes that are situated within or adjacent to fat, this is readily performed by manipulating the signal intensity of fat, which can range from low to high in signal intensity on T1-weighted images (T1WIs) and T2-weighted images (T2WIs). For example, diseases that are low in signal intensity on T1WIs (eg, peritoneal fluid or retroperitoneal fibrosis) are most conspicuous on T1WI sequences in which fat is high in signal intensity (ie, sequences without fat suppression). Conversely, diseases that are high in signal intensity (eg, subacute blood or proteinaceous fluid) are more conspicuous if fat is rendered low in signal intensity with the use of fat suppression techniques. On T2WIs, diseases that are low in signal intensity (eg, fibrous tissue) are most conspicuous on sequences in which background fat is high in signal intensity, such as echo-train spin-echo (SE) sequences. Diseases that are moderate to high in signal intensity (eg, lymphadenopathy or ascites) are most conspicuous on sequences in which fat signal intensity is low, such as fat-suppressed (FS) sequences.

Gadolinium chelate enhancement may be routinely useful because it provides information about diseased tissues that can lead to detection and characterization. After intravenous administration, gadolinium is delivered to the diseased tissues through the blood supply, and within the tissue, may distribute into at least two compartments: (1) into the feeding vessels and capillaries, a rapid process that initially results in an arterial phase bolus of contrast that increases the gadolinium concentration in the vessels to a peak intravascular level, and then diminishes; and (2) into the interstitial space, a slower process that occurs by diffusion of gadolinium chelate through the connections between endothelial cells of the vessel walls and leads to accumulation in the interstitial space. As the gadolinium contrast recirculates in the blood pool, the blood concentration continues to diminish as a result of renal filtration and urinary excretion. Interstitial accumulation of gadolinium diffuses down a concentration gradient back into the blood pool; however, this is a slow process and can be appreciated over a period of minutes after initial gadolinium intravenous administration [6]. Capillary-phase image acquisition is achieved by using a short-duration sequence that is initiated immediately after gadolinium injection. Spoiled gradient-echo (SGE) sequence, performed as multisection two-(2D) or three-dimensional (3D) acquisition, is an ideal sequence to use for capillary phase imaging. Most focal mass lesions are evaluated best in the capillary phase of enhancement, particularly lesions that do not distort the margins of the organs in which they are located (eg, focal liver, spleen, or pancreatic lesions). Images that are acquired 1.5 minutes to 10 minutes after contrast administration are in the interstitial phase of enhancement; the optimal window is 2 minutes to 5 minutes postcontrast. Diseases that are superficial, spreading, or inflammatory in nature generally show well on interstitial phase images. The concomitant use of fat suppression serves to increase the conspicuity of disease processes that are characterized by increased enhancement on interstitial phase images, including peritoneal metastases, cholangiocarcinoma, ascending cholangitis, inflammatory bowel disease, and abscesses [7–11].

Most diseases that affect the chest, abdomen, and pelvis can be characterized by defining their appearance on T1, T2, and early and late postgadolinium images. There are many acronyms used by multiple vendors, and some of these are summarized in Table 1; acronyms are defined in Box 1.

T1-weighted sequences

T1WI sequences are routinely useful for investigating diseases of the abdomen, and they supplement T2WIs for investigating diseases of the pelvis. The primary information that precontrast T1WIs provide includes: (1) information on abnormally increased fluid content or fibrous tissue content that appears low in signal intensity on T1WIs; and (2) information on the presence of subacute blood or concentrated protein, which are high in signal intensity. T1WI sequences that are obtained without fat suppression also demonstrate the presence of fat as high-signal intensity tissue. The routine use of an additional fat attenuating technique facilitates the reliable characterization of fatty lesions.

Table 1
Acronyms for commonly used sequences

| Sequence | Vendor | | |
	Philips	General Electronics	Siemens
Fast spin echo	TSE	FSE	TSE
Single shot fast spin echo	SSh TSE	SSFSE/RARE	HASTE
Snapshot/ultrafast gradient echo	TFE	Rapid SPGR	TurboFlash
		FIRM	MP RAGE
3D turbo field echo with fat suppression	THRIVE	FAME/LAVA	VIBE
Fast field echo	FFE	SPGR	FLASH
		FSPGR	FISP
		GRASSE	GRE
		GRE	
Steady state fast field echo	Balanced FFE (bFFE, bTFE)	FIESTA	True FISP
Saturation bands	REST	SAT	PreSAT
Spectrally selective fat suppression	SPIR	CHEMSAT	FATSAT
	SPAIR		
Water excitation fat suppression	Proset		QuickFatSat

Spoiled gradient-echo sequences

Spoiled gradient-echo sequences are the most important and versatile sequences for studying abdominal disease. These sequences provide T1WIs and, with the use of phased-array multicoil imaging, may be used to replace longer duration sequences, such as the T1WI SE sequence. Image parameters for SGE are: (1) long repetition time (TR; ~150 milliseconds) to maximize signal-to-noise ratio and the number of sections that can be acquired in one multisection acquisition and (2) the shortest in-phase (IP) echo time (TE) (~6.0 milliseconds at 1.0 T and ~4.2–4.5 milliseconds at 1.5 T) to maximize signal-to-noise ratio and the number of sections per acquisition [2]. At 1.5 T, hydrogen protons in a voxel that contains 100% fat will precess approximately 220 Hz to 230 Hz slower than a voxel that is made up of 100% water. That means that every 4.4 milliseconds the fat protons will lag behind by 360°, and regain IP orientation relative to water protons, whereas at 2.2 milliseconds, or at half this time, the fat and water protons will be 180° out-of-phase (OP). Current generation MR control software have incorporated dual-echo breath-hold SGE sequences that can acquire two sets of k-space filled to obtain two sets of images—one set IP and the other set OP—with spatially matched slices. For routine T1WIs, IP TE may be preferable to the shorter OP TEs (4.0 milliseconds at 1.0 T and 2.2–2.4 milliseconds at 1.5 T), to avoid phase-cancellation artifact around the borders of organs and fat-water phase cancellation in tissues that contain fat and water

protons. Flip angle should be approximately 70° to 90° to maximize T1WI signal. With the use of the larger built-in body coil, the signal-to-noise ratio of SGE sequences usually is suboptimal with a section thickness of less than 8 mm, whereas with the phased-array surface coils, a section thickness of approximately 5 mm results in diagnostically adequate images. On new MR imaging machines, more than 22 sections may be acquired in a 20-second breath-hold, or 44 paired sections when using the dual-echo technique.

Application of out-of-phase spoiled gradient-echo sequences

Out-of-phase (opposed-phase) SGE images are useful for demonstrating diseased tissue in which mixtures of fat and water protons are present within the same voxel. A voxel that contains predominantly fat or water will not demonstrate diminished signal on OP images. A TE of 2.2 milliseconds is advisable at 1.5 T, and 4.4 milliseconds is advisable at 1.0 T. A TE of 6.6 milliseconds also is out-of-phase at 1.5 T; however, the shorter TE of 2 milliseconds is preferable because of decreased susceptibility effects (ie, the shorter TE reduces the time for dephasing effects to accumulate, as is caused by metals or gas), more sections can be acquired per sequence acquisition, signal is higher, the sequence is more T1-weighted (T1W), and in combination with a T2-weighted (T2W) sequence, it is easier to distinguish fat and iron in the liver. At 1.5 T, fat and iron cause liver signal decrease on OP images using a TE of 6.6 milliseconds, relative to the IP

Box 1. Acronyms

ceMRA: Contrast-enhanced magnetic resonance angiography
CSE: Conventional spin echo
FID EPI: Echo planar imaging readout of the free induction decay
FIESTA: Fast imaging employing steady state acquisition
FISP: Fast imaging with steady precession
FLASH: Fast low-angle shot
FSE: Fast spin echo
FSPGR: Fast spoiled gradient-recalled acquisition into steady state
GRASE: Gradient and spin echoes
GRASS: Gradient-recalled acquisition in the steady state
GRE: Gradient-echo imaging, gradient-recalled echo
GRE EPI: Echo planar imaging solely using gradient echoes (readout of the free
    induction decay)
HASTE: Half-Fourier acquired single-shot turbo spin echo
HASTIRM: Half-Fourier acquired single-shot turbo spin echo with preceding inversion
    pulse, utilizing only magnitude information
IR: Inversion recovery
MP RAGE (3D): Magnetization prepared rapid acquired gradient echoes
MRCP: Magnetic resonance cholangiopancreatography
RARE: Rapid acquisition with relaxation enhancement
SAR: Specific absorption rate
SE EPI: Echo planar imaging readout module under a spin-echo technique
SPAIR: Spectral attenuated inversion recovery
SPIR: Spectral inversion recovery
SP GRE: Spoiled gradient (recalled) echo
SPGR: Spoiled GRASS
SSFP: Steady-state free precession
TFL: Turbo FLASH
THRIVE: T1-weighted high resolution isotropic volume imaging
TrueFISP: True fast imaging with steady precession
TSE: Turbo spin echo
T1 FFE: T1-weighted fast field echo
T2 FFE: T2-weighted fast field echo

---

images that are acquired with a TE of 4.4 milliseconds, whereas on 2.2-millisecond OP TE images fat is darker and iron is brighter relative to TE 4-millisecond images. Relative sensitivity to magnetic susceptibility effects, which increase with an increase in TE, also can be used to distinguish iron-containing paramagnetic structures (eg, surgical clips, or foci of iron deposition in the spleen or liver) from nonmagnetic signal void structures (eg, calcium). To illustrate this point, the signal void susceptibility artifact from surgical clips increases in size as the TE increases from 2.2 milliseconds to 4.4 milliseconds, whereas the signal void from calcium remains unchanged; however, the most common indications for OP imaging are the detection of abnormal fat accumulation within the liver and the detection of lipid within adrenal masses—a feature that is used to characterize benign adrenal adenomas. Current MR imaging systems can acquire IP and OP images during a single breath-hold SGE acquisition; this feature always should be used on routine imaging of the abdomen.

Intravascular gadolinium-chelate contrast-enhanced spoiled gradient-echo sequences

In addition to its use in precontrast T1WIs, SGE should be used routinely for multi-phase image acquisition after gadolinium administration for investigation of the liver, spleen, pancreas, and kidneys. An important feature of the multisection acquisition of SGE is that the central phase-encoding steps generally are used to fill central k-space, which determines image contrast. This contrast component of the dataset is acquired over a 4-second to 5-second period for the entire data set, and essentially is shared by each individual section. Thus, the data acquisition is sufficiently short for the entire data set to isolate a distinct phase of enhancement (eg, hepatic arterial dominant phase). Furthermore, this ensures that images of organs (eg, liver) are shown in the same phase of contrast enhancement uniformly throughout the volume of the tissue.

Fat-suppressed spoiled gradient-echo sequences

FS SGE sequences are used routinely as precontrast images for evaluating the pancreas and for the detection of subacute blood. Fat suppression generally is achieved on SGE images by selectively stimulating slower precessing hydrogen protons that are associated with fat by using a tuned radiofrequency (RF) pulse—followed by spoiler gradients—before performing the gradient-echo imaging components of the sequence. Image parameters are similar to those for standard SGE. It may be advantageous to use a lower OP TE (2.2–2.5 milliseconds at 1.5 T), which benefits from additional fat-attenuating effects and also increases signal-to-noise ratio and the number of sections per acquisition. On current MR imaging machines, FS SGE may acquire 22 sections in a 20-second breath-hold with reproducible uniform fat suppression. One method that modern systems use to reduce the amount of additional time that fat suppression adds to the SGE sequence—and acquire a greater number of slices per breath-hold—is to perform a fat suppression step only after several phase-encoding steps, instead of after every phase encode. Another approach is to tune the stimulation RF pulse to activate only protons in water, but not in fat; this eliminates the need to add fat saturation pulses.

FS SGE images are used to improve the contrast between intra-abdominal fat and diseased tissues and blood vessels on interstitial-phase gadolinium-enhanced images. Gadolinium enhancement generally increases the signal intensity of blood vessels and diseased tissue, and fat suppression diminishes the competing high signal intensity of background fat.

Three-dimensional gradient-echo sequences

3D SGE imaging has been used extensively for MR angiography, but only recently has it evolved into an accepted useful technique for soft tissue imaging in the abdomen and pelvis. This development has been achieved, in part, simply by reducing the flip angle of 60° to 90° that is used for angiography, down to 10° to 15°. Advantages include the ability to acquire a volumetric data set that can be sectioned into thinner sections than typically are used for 2D images—generally in the 2.5- to 3.0-mm per slice range—with contiguous slices, and with images that can be postprocessed into other imaging planes. Although there are differences between some of the sequence features that are seen with different MR systems, fat suppression tends to be superior with greater uniformity, as compared with 2D SGE. On some MR systems, it also is possible to image a larger volume of tissue during the same breath-hold period, than with 2D SGE. A potential limitation of 3D SGE imaging has been a diminished contrast-to-noise ratio. This has led to concern regarding the use of this technique, other than for gadolinium-enhanced FS interstitial phase imaging, where the gadolinium effectively improves the contrast to noise ratio.

T2-weighted sequences

The predominant information that is provided by T2W sequences include: (1) the presence of increased fluid in diseased tissue, which results in high signal intensity; (2) the presence of chronic fibrotic tissue, which results in low signal intensity; and (3) the presence of iron deposition, which results in very low signal intensity.

Standard spin-echo and fast spin-echo sequences

Standard T2W SE or fast SE are long acquisition methods that require several minutes to acquire slices through the abdomen or pelvis. Advantages include good contrast to noise. With abdominal imaging, breathing-related motion precludes the use of these sequences, unless used in conjunction with a motion correction method (ie, respiratory gating). This will add to the total scan time, and the motion correction is neither reliable nor accurate, and results in at least mild edge blurring which effectively deteriorates resolution. Typical scan times are between 5 minutes and 7 minutes, depending on the respiratory rate and pattern. It is not unusual for the acquisition to fail, which necessitates repetition.

Pelvic imaging can be performed without breath-holding in most patients, with little image deterioration that is due to breathing-related motion relative to the upper abdomen. Motion that is due to contracting bowel can cause image deterioration, and can be reduced by using intravenous or intramuscular glucagon. Latest generation fast SE techniques, including sequences called turbo SE, or fast SE-xl, are based on intermediate-length echo-trains; acquisition time can be reduced to as little as 2.5 minutes for the pelvis.

Echo-train spin-echo sequences

Echo-train SE sequences are termed single shot fast SE, turbo SE, or rapid acquisition with relaxation enhancement (RARE) sequences. The principle of echo-train SE sequences is to summate multiple echoes within the same repetition time interval to decrease examination time, increase spatial resolution, or both. This is a slice-by-slice technique; a single slice-selective excitation pulse is followed by a series of echoes, typically using between 80 and 100 180° pulses, each separated by approximately 3 milliseconds, to fill in k-space for the entire slice. The T2W contrast is achieved by using the echoes that are obtained at approximately 80 milliseconds to 90 milliseconds for filling central k-space, where central k-space is responsible for image contrast. Although the theoretic TR is infinite, each slice requires approximately 1.2 seconds to 1.5 seconds, before continuing to the next slice. The motion-sensitive component represents only a small fraction of the entire acquisition period, which makes this technique insensitive to breathing artifacts. Echo-train SE has achieved widespread use because of these advantages. In contrast, conventional T2 SE sequences are lengthy and suffer from patient motion and increased examination time. The major disadvantage of echo-train sequences is that T2 differences between tissues are decreased. Generally, this is not problematic in the pelvis because of the substantial differences in the T2 values between diseased and normal tissue. In the liver, however, the T2 difference between diseased and background normal liver may be small, and the T2-averaging effects of summated multiple echoes blur this T2 difference. This results in diminished lesion conspicuity for lesions with mildly elevated T2W signal intensity (eg, hepatocellular carcinoma) as compared with

standard SE sequences. Diseases with T2 values that are similar to those of liver generally have longer T1 values than liver, so that lesions that are visualized poorly on echo-train SE generally are well-visualized on SGE or immediate postgadolinium SGE images as low-signal lesions.

Echo-train SE, and T2-weighted sequences, in general, are important for evaluating the abdomen and pelvis. In liver masses, T2WIs predominantly are important for lesion characterization, whereas T1WIs are important for lesion detection sensitivity and characterization. T2WIs also are important for assessment of diffuse liver disease, including iron deposition, edema related to active liver disease, and fibrosis. Echo-train T2W sequences are important for assessment of fluid-filled structures, including bile duct, gall bladder, pancreatic duct, stomach, and bowel; as well as cysts or cystic masses, abscesses, or collections, or free fluid in the abdomen or pelvis. The relative resistance of echo-train images to motion degradation generally yields better resolution of structures internal to cystic masses, such as the septations within a pancreatic serous or mucinous tumor. MR cholangiopancreatography (MRCP) is based on modified echo-train sequences, where the effective TE is made longer, on the order of 250 to 500 milliseconds. Lengthening the TE results in heavily T2W high contrast images that yield most soft tissues dark, and makes fluid in bile ducts, gall bladder, and the pancreatic duct bright. MRCP can be performed in thin sections of 3 mm to 4 mm for higher resolution, or by using a single thick slab of 3 cm to 4 cm, to include most of the pancreatic and bile duct in a single image. Echo-train imaging is well-suited to bowel because of its insensitivity to respiratory motion and bowel peristalsis, and its relative resistance to the distorting paramagnetic effects of intraluminal bowel gas, as a result of repeated refocusing echo pulses.

Fat is high in signal intensity on echo-train SE sequences in comparison with conventional SE sequences, in which fat is intermediate in signal intensity. The MR imaging determination of recurrent malignant disease versus fibrosis for pelvic malignancies illustrates this difference. Recurrent malignant disease in the pelvis (eg, cervical, endometrial, bladder, or rectal cancer) generally appears high in signal intensity on conventional SE sequences because of the higher signal intensity of the diseased tissue relative to the moderately low-signal intensity of fat. In contrast, fat is high in signal intensity on echo-train SE images, and recurrent disease commonly appears lower in signal intensity. The fact that abnormal tissue is not high in signal intensity on echo-train T2WIs relative to fat is not specific for neoplasm; fibrosis can have a similar appearance. This may be particularly problematic in patients who have undergone therapy. Fat also may be problematic in the liver because fatty liver will be high in signal intensity on echo-train SE sequences, and thereby, diminishes contrast with most liver lesions, which generally are high in signal intensity on T2WIs. It may be essential to use fat suppression on T2W echo-train SE sequences for liver imaging. Generally, fat suppression should be applied for at least one set of images of the abdomen or pelvis to ensure optimal contrast between high signal abnormalities, such as fluid collections or cystic masses, and adjacent intra-abdominal or pelvic fat.

General approach to abdominal MR imaging

A comprehensive examination may be based on a combination of rapid acquisition and robust T2W single shot, and T1W SGE combined with IP and OP and fat suppression and 2D or 3D implementations to generate a 15-minute study time [5]. Additionally, forms of balanced echo or steady state precession (balanced field echo or true fast imaging by steady precession) imaging have been developed for cardiac imaging; implementations of these sequences are being evaluated regarding their potential usefulness for abdominal–pelvic applications, including imaging of the bowel and fetal imaging. To evaluate the potential usefulness of abdominal–pelvic imaging at 3 T, these major sequences require optimization of parameters. The remainder of this article evaluates the fundamental principles that face imaging at 3 T, and examines approaches to sequence optimization.

Challenges in body MR imaging at 3 Tesla

Specific absorption ratio (SAR) and RF power deposition: SAR, a measure of RF energy that is deposited in the body, increases four times, and has an undesirable impact on essential image characteristics, including contrast, acquisition time, and resolution at 3 T. The SAR thresholds as per Food and Drug Administration guidelines are 2 W/kg in the normal mode and 4 W/kg in the first level controlled mode [12].

Multiple sources of field distortions: Susceptibility affects, greater at 3 T, in body imaging may arise from air–soft tissue interfaces that arise from the lungs, gastrointestinal tract, irregular skin surfaces, and surgical clips or hardware.

Large field of view: Fields of view in excess of 35 cm to 40 cm are used commonly for body imaging in the Z-direction, which places high demand on static magnetic field homogeneity over a large area. Field homogeneity is significantly more challenging at 3 T.

Motion artifacts: Motion from respiration, heart, and bowel peristalsis may cause marked image deterioration. Certain fast acquisition techniques are limited by SAR, such as single shot SE.

Image contrast: Adjustments are required to adapt to the longer T1 and shorter T2 of soft tissues at 3 T. In addition, sequences have been optimized at 1.5 T to achieve a balance between speed of acquisition and image contrast. At 3 T, image contrast may suffer from a combination of compromises that arise from SAR limitations.

Increased SNR: RF signal that is generated at 3 T is four times stronger than at 1.5 T; however, a simultaneous increase in noise by a factor of 2 results in only a two-fold net increase in SNR. A challenge is to be able to realize this theoretic benefit because the increase in SNR is balanced against losses from adjustments for limitations that are related to SAR.

Magnetohydrodynamic effect (also known as dielectric effect): This phenomenon is seen when the transmitter wavelength approaches the size of the body structure, especially free fluid [13]. For a circular body habitus there is loss of signal at the periphery, whereas for an oval body habitus the signal loss occurs at the periphery of the short axis. To a certain extent this can be corrected by using phantom-derived algorithms like body tuned CLEAR (Philips Medical Systems, Cleveland, Ohio).

RF coils: A smaller variety of RF coils is available for 3 T. The penetration of transmitted RF into the tissue becomes more difficult at higher frequency because of a higher static magnetic field. Surface coils provide greater sensitivity to signal, are critical to image optimization, and can help to reduce sensitivity to the received dielectric effect.

Optimization of sequence parameters at 3 Tesla

The sequences that are used currently for a broad range of tissue disease applications in body imaging include the single shot echo train (SSET), balanced field echo (bFFE), 2D gradient-echo IP and OP (2D GRE IP and OP), and 3D gradient-echo (3D GRE).

Single shot turbo spin-echo sequences

Repetition time

TR is the time between 90° activation RF pulses, with a train of refocusing RF pulses obtained following the 90° activation. The ideal TR for maximizing signal from single shot turbo spin echo (SSh TSE) images is infinite, or at least long enough to allow the longitudinal magnetization to recover fully following the long echo train [14,15]. The down side is that the longer the TR, the longer the entire acquisition. Therefore, on 1.5 T, the compromise that is performed commonly is to obtain the shortest possible TR that allows adequate preservation of T2W signal, typically down to 700 to 1000 milliseconds, or 0.7 to 1.0 seconds per slice. This allows acquisition of a total set of images during a single breath-hold. Another phenomenon is cross-talk, which is the effect of one slice, after receiving an echo train, affecting the tissues on either side, corresponding to the neighboring slices. The neighboring slices suffer from decreased signal as a result of bleeding of the echo train into the adjacent tissue. To reduce this effect, the authors normally stagger the slice acquisition to obtain images from alternate slices starting with even-numbered slices, and the returning to obtain the odd-numbered slices. Staggering of slices in this way is referred to as intercalation or interleaved excitation. On 3 T, unlike 1.5 T, the minimum TR is limited by SAR, and with current optimized parameters is approximately 1500 milliseconds. This is a result of the larger amount of thermal energy that is deposited during the refocusing echo-train at 3 T. The effect is to produce a slice every 1.5 seconds; this requires two breath-holds to acquire the total set of images.

As an alternative to breath-hold imaging, the single shot sequence can be triggered by respiratory gating. A breathing sensor, generally a strap placed around the patient's abdomen which contains a pressure transducer, is used to determine when the patient is at end-expiration. While the patient breathes quietly, one single shot slice is obtained at each end-expiration. With an average respiration rate of 15 breaths per minute, this allows 4 seconds between each slice, and an effective TR of 4000 milliseconds. In this way, 3 T SSh TSE imaging can

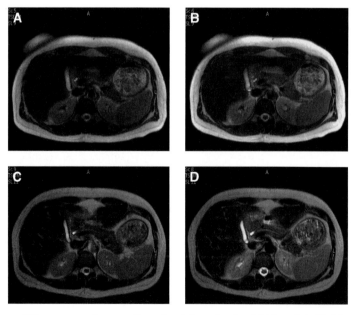

Fig. 1. No significant difference seen between liver signal intensity for 3-T breath-hold (*A*) compared with 3-T respiratory triggered (*B*) single shot turbo spin echo images. Liver intensity is slightly lower for 1.5-T breath hold (*C*) compared with respiratory triggered (*D*).

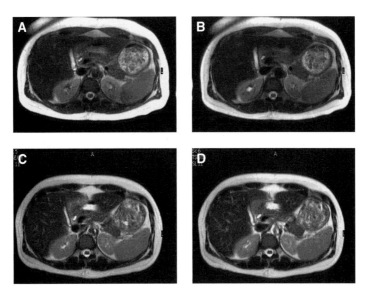

Fig. 2. Liver signal is appreciably diminished on 3-T single shot turbo spin echo if TE is increased from 78 milliseconds (*A*) to 100 milliseconds (*B*). Minimal difference in liver signal is noted on 1.5-T single shot turbo spin echo with TE of 78 milliseconds (*C*) and 100 milliseconds (*D*).

be acquired without hitting SAR limits, and also allows maximization of image signal by allowing sufficient time for reconstitution of the longitudinal magnetization. By using respiratory triggering, cross-talk also becomes a diminished concern. The authors have found that cross-talk is less significant at 3 T (Fig. 1). This seem to be due to the longer TR that is required, a feature which is imposed by SAR limits at 3 T (see Fig. 1).

Echo time

TE is the time delay between the initial 90° slice excitation and the echoes that are used to fill the central part of k-space. The central k-space provides the image contrast and determines the T2W attributes. At 3 T, the rate of T2 decay, or T2-star, occurs more quickly. At 1.5 T, changing TE from 78 milliseconds to 100 milliseconds results in no

appreciable decrease in liver signal, whereas at 3 T, an appreciable signal decrease is seen as darkening of the liver (Fig. 2). This has an impact on routine liver imaging where SSh TSE can be used to detect the presence of elevated liver iron in the setting of hemochromatosis. Liver iron leads to T2-star affects and independently decreases liver signal intensity on SSh TSE images. The authors have found that it is important to keep the TE less than 80 milliseconds at 3 T to avoid the excessive darkening of normal liver, and to maintain sensitivity for elevated liver iron affects.

Single shot turbo spin-echo echo-train length

Because of a higher rate of T2 decay that is seen at 3 T, SSh TSE techniques are more sensitive to blurring as the echo-train length gets longer. Parallel processing, such as SENsitivity ENcoding

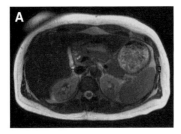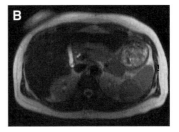

Fig. 3. Improved resolution is seen for 3-T single shot turbo spin echo with SENSE (*A*) compared with the same scan without SENSE that is associated necessarily with longer echo train length (*B*). Also note improved image uniformity on SENSE scan using CLEAR uniformity correction (*A*).

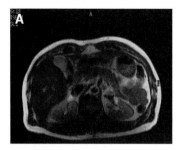 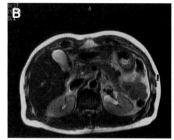

Fig. 4. Noticeable dielectric effect is noted on 3-T single shot turbo spin echo without Body Tuned CLEAR uniformity correction (*A*). Image uniformity is improved with use of Body Tuned CLEAR uniformity correction (*B*).

(SENSE), normally is used for accelerating image acquisition; it essentially is an undersampling method that is based on using the sensitivity profile of a multi-element receiver coil. Through activation of SENSE, another benefit is that echo-train duration is reduced, which results in reduced blurring and sharper image resolution. The authors suggest the use of SENSE for SSh TSE, not for the typical purpose of shortening image acquisition time, but to achieve improved image sharpness (Fig. 3). This finding may be observed on 1.5-T and 3-T images.

Dielectric effect at 3 Tesla

At the higher resonant frequency that is used at 3 T, the wavelength of the transmitted RF is shorter and can result in local changes in RF conduction in the tissue that varies with anatomic geometry [12]. This so-called "dielectric effect" can result in local reduction in signal intensity that can be appreciated readily on SSh TSE scans. Specialized image uniformity correction processing can be performed to adjust localized pixel intensities to improve the uniformity of the image (Fig. 4).

Echo-train refocusing flip angle

At 1.5 T, the SSh TSE echo-train is formed conventionally as a series of 180°-refocusing RF

pulses without the problem of SAR limits being reached; however, this is a problem at 3 T where higher energy RF is required and results in longer TR to keep within allowable SAR limits. To reduce the rate of energy deposition, the refocusing pulses can be reduced (eg, 150° or less). Different iterations of this method have been used by the various 3 T MR imaging vendors and incorporated into the different vendor-recommended imaging protocols.

Balanced-echo sequences

Balanced steady-state precession gradient-echo sequences versus balanced nonsteady-state precession gradient-echo sequences

Balanced steady-state precession gradient-echo techniques (bFFE, FIESTA, true FISP) have proven to be clinically useful techniques for visualization of abdominal anatomy and vasculature. At 1.5 T, the technique typically is run with constant TR to develop and maintain the steady state RF saturation of tissue that is required to generate the balanced gradient-echo contrast and avoid banding-type artifacts [16]. Shorter TR and TE also contribute to reduction in banding and flow artifacts. Higher RF excitation flip angles of 60° or more are used routinely to maximize bright signal of blood relative to static

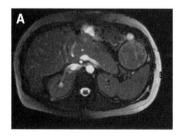 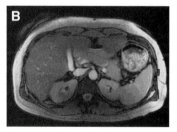

Fig. 5. Brighter blood signal is acquired on 1.5-T bFFE (*A*) compared with 3-T bTFE (*B*).

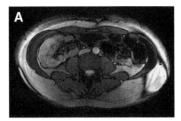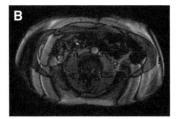

Fig. 6. 3-T bTFE acquired as three stacks of images with table movement to center each stack to magnet isocenter (*A*) significantly reduces banding artifacts compared with same scan acquired with one stack and no table movement (*B*). Slice offset is 4 cm from magnet isocenter (*A*); slice offset is 12 cm (*B*).

tissues. Because of the higher RF power that is used at 3 T, acquiring all slices with uninterrupted constant TR would result in excessively long TR and TE and unacceptable levels of banding and flow artifacts. A nonsteady-state version of the sequence can be run (bTFE) to reduce energy deposition. Instead of running sequence with uninterrupted TR for all slices, each slice is acquired separately, using starter RF pulses to achieve steady-state conditions before the slice is acquired. A short delay follows before the next slice to keep energy deposition per unit time to allowable SAR limits. A consequence of the bTFE sequence is that blood signal is not as bright as the comparable 1.5-T bFFE technique (Fig. 5).

Sensitivity to field homogeneity

Balanced echo steady-state precession gradient-echo imaging is a technique that is highly sensitive to the main B_0 field homogeneity and paramagnetic affects. Resultant image artifacts are characterized by low signal banding, mostly around the outer margins of the field of view but also can be seen around air–tissue interfaces. These artifacts become more evident as the image plane moves further away from the center of B_0 along the Z-axis. Major factors that affect banding artifacts are the TR and TE; the objective is to use the minimum TR and TE achievable to reduce artifact sensitivity to field

homogeneity or paramagnetic affects. Features of an imaging system that determine minimal TR and TE include the gradient performance and bandwidth (BW) of the receiver spectrometer. At higher field strength, these demands increase as a result of increased field inhomogeneity affects. Another approach to reduce this distortion is to split the total number of slices that is required to cover the imaged tissues in the Z-direction into multiple groups of smaller numbers of slices in combination with multiple table movements. The imaging field needs to be recentered in the Z-axis to correspond to the center of the magnet (Fig. 6). The compromise at 3 T that is suggested here is to perform two to three acquisitions to cover the abdomen using multiple table steps in contrast to one acquisition which is achievable at 1.5 T while maintaining banding artifacts to an acceptable degree.

Repetition time, echo time, and flip angle

On balanced field imaging, contrast improves with a decrease in TR and TE and an increase in flip angle. A decrease in flip angle is necessary at 3 T to reduce energy deposition and facilitate imaging below SAR limits. To further overcome SAR limits, a decreased RF pulse amplitude is required at 3 T; this results in an increase in the minimum TR and TE which are achievable and further decreases contrast. To overcome these

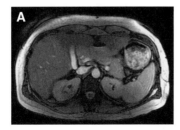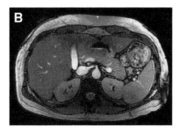

Fig. 7. 3-T bTFE with TE 1.4 milliseconds (*A*) has fewer artifacts compared with TE 1.6 milliseconds (*B*).

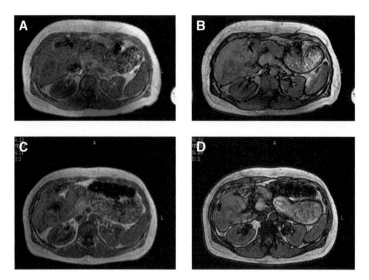

Fig. 8. 3-T IP TE 2.3 milliseconds (*A*) and OP TE 1.15 milliseconds (*B*) compared with 1.5-T IP TE 4.6 milliseconds (*C*) and OP TE 2.3 milliseconds (*D*).

undesirable affects, a lower B1 gradient can be used by increasing slice thickness, and thus, shortening the time that is required for application of the gradient pulses. This, in turn, decreases the combined time that is required to apply the RF and gradient pulses and allows for a shorter TR and TE (Fig. 7).

Two-dimensional gradient-echo sequences

In-phase and out-of-phase echo ordering

Requirements for this sequence are that the OP acquisition is obtained first and the shortest possible TEs are used for both echoes. The first echo needs to be acquired OP to detect fat and discriminate signal decrease from iron

paramagnetic affects. If the OP image is acquired after the IP, iron also may result in relative signal decrease because paramagnetic affects increase as the TE increases. Furthermore, the shortest possible TE reduces the amount of artifacts as the TE increases, and may result from paramagnetic substances that cause artifacts, such as surgical clips. Acquiring the shortest possible TE at 3 T–field strength requires an echo-time of 1.15 milliseconds for OP images and 2.3 milliseconds for IP images. Fig. 8 shows the feasibility of performing these acquisitions at 3 T.

Potential limitation at 3 Tesla

At 3 T, the shortest OP/IP TE is 1.15/2.3 milliseconds, in contrast to twice these TEs at

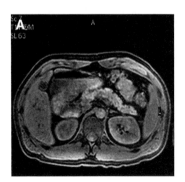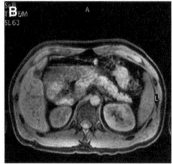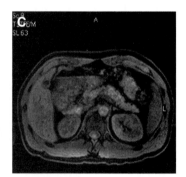

Fig. 9. 3-T THRIVE with TE 1.4 milliseconds and maximum BW (*A*) has better resolution, less susceptibility, and acceptable SNR, compared with TE 2 milliseconds with maximum BW (*B*) and TE 2 milliseconds with minimum BW (*C*). (*A*) is the TE/BW of choice for 3 T.

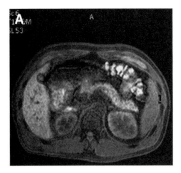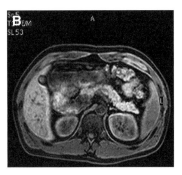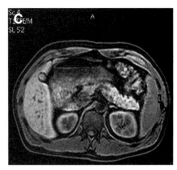

Fig. 10. 1.5-T THRIVE with TE 1.3 milliseconds and maximum BW (*A*) and TE 1.9 milliseconds with maximum BW (*B*) have lower SNR compared with TE 1.9 milliseconds with minimum BW (*C*). (*C*) is the TE/BW of choice for 1.5 T.

1.5 T. This results in a data-stream arriving at twice the rate at 3 T. The authors have found that some systems may not have sufficient data BW to acquire IP/OP echoes as a single scan. If this is not a capability of your specific system, it may be necessary to acquire the IP/OP images as two separate breath-hold acquisitions.

Characteristics of out-of-phase images

Typically, OP images show OP cancellation artifact at soft tissue–fat interfaces; this is seen as a dark thin line circumscribing solid organs, including the liver, spleen, and kidneys. At 3 T, this cancellation artifact appears identical to that seen at 1.5 T (see Fig. 8). Unlike paramagnetic affects that bloom at higher field strength, water–fat cancellation affect depends only on the voxel size and BW.

Three-dimensional gradient-echo T1-weighted high resolution isotropic volume imaging

Echo time, bandwidth, and signal-to-noise ratio

At 3 T, changes in TE have a greater affect on image quality and can be appreciated as image blurring, as shown by decreasing the TE from 2.0 milliseconds to 1.4 milliseconds (Fig. 9) [17]. To achieve the minimum TE at 3 T, the maximum sampling BW should be used. Although increasing BW decreases SNR, the authors have found that the benefits of a decreased TE outweigh this drawback.

Table 2
Summary of approach to 3-T optimization

Sequence	Problems	Optimization
SSFE	Higher TR required because of SAR	Respiratory gating instead of breath hold
	Cross talk	Interleaved slices
	Shorter T2: darkening of liver	Keep TE <80 ms
	Blurring from T2* effect	Parallel SENSE processing to compact the echo-train length and sharpen image
	180° refocusing pulses cause SAR limits	Use <180° refocusing pulses during the echo train
Balanced echo	Steady state flip angle of 60° causes SAR limits	Run noncontinuous TR and lower RF excitation flip angle approximately 35°
	Low signal banding at the periphery	Slices in Z direction are split; table moved to maintain main field isocenter
	Suboptimal contrast because larger flip angle is limited by SAR	Increasing slice thickness lowers minimal TE and TR allowing higher flip angle and improved contrast
2D gradient in-phase and out-of-phase	Dual echo interphase time interval half of 1.5 T with first OP echo = 1.2 ms leading to possible hardware data-stream overload	IP and OP sequences may need to be run separately
3D gradient echo	T2* dephasing	Increase bandwidth to achieve decreased TE with net improvement in contrast and SNR at 3 T; can convert to higher resolution
	Increase susceptibility effects	

This is in contrast to 1.5 T, where a similar increase in BW is more deleterious to image quality (Fig. 10). Furthermore, more marked image deterioration (images may appear noisier with less edge definition) is noted at 3 T for a given TE as compared with 1.5 T (see Figs. 9 and 10), likely because of stronger paramagnetic affects that occur at higher field strength. On precontrast 3-T images, a significantly higher liver-to-spleen contrast ratio is achievable with greater signal. The authors find that this additional signal can be converted to higher in-plane resolution and thinner slice reconstructions to achieve superior image sharpness of the liver as compared with 1.5 T.

Discussion

The relative strengths of higher field imaging at 3 T, in general, are realized more easily when using longer acquisition techniques, such as fast spin-echo T1WIs and T2WIs, or multi-excitation gradient-echo with oversampling. This explains the relative ease with which implementation of 3-T imaging has occurred for brain, spine, and musculoskeletal applications where longer acquisition imaging is used predominantly (minutes) and the relative difficulty in implementing abdominal imaging where faster acquisition sequences are used (seconds). Fundamental approaches that may be used for optimization of the sequences that are required for abdominal imaging are summarized in Table 2.

References

[1] Brown MA, Semelka RC. Clinical applications. In: Brown MA, Semelka RC, editors. MRI: basic principles and applications. 3rd edition. New York: Wiley-Liss; 1999. p. 223–46.

[2] Semelka RC, Willms AB, Brown MA, et al. Comparison of breath-hold T1-weighted MR sequences for imaging of the liver. J Magn Reson Imaging 1994;4:759–65.

[3] Semelka RC, Kelekis NL, Thomasson D, et al. HASTE MR imaging. Description of technique and preliminary results in the abdomen. J Magn Reson Imaging 1996;6:698–9.

[4] Gaa J, Hutabu H, Jenkins RL, et al. Liver masses: replacement of conventional T2-weighted spin echo MR imaging with breath-hold MR imaging. Radiology 1996;200:459–64.

[5] Semelka RC, Balci NC, Op de Beeck B, et al. Evaluation of a 10-minute comprehensive MR imaging examination of the upper abdomen. Radiology 1996; 211:189–95.

[6] Semelka RC, Helmberger T. Contrast agents for MR imaging of the liver: state-of-the-art. Radiology 2001;218:27–38.

[7] Low RN, Semelka RC, Worawattanakul S, et al. Extrahepatic abdominal imaging in patients with malignancy: comparison of MR imaging and helical CT in 164 patients. J Magn Reson Imaging 2001; 12:269–77.

[8] Low RN, Semelka RC, Worawwattanakul S, et al. Extrahepatic abdominal imaging in patients with malignancy: comparison of MR imaging and helical CT, with subsequent surgical correlation. Radiology 1999;210:625–32.

[9] Rofsky NM, Lee VS, Laub G, et al. Abdominal MR imaging with a volumetric interpolated breath-hold examination. Radiology 1999;212:876–84.

[10] Lee VS, Lavelle MT, Rofsky NM, et al. Hepatic MR imaging with a dynamic contrast-enhanced isotropic volumetric interpolated breath-hold examination: feasibility, reproducibility, and technical quality. Radiology 2001;215:365–72.

[11] Semelka RC, Balci NC, Wilber KP, et al. Breath-hold 3D gradient-echo MR imaging of the lung parenchyma: evaluation of reproducibility of image quality in normals and preliminary observations in patients with disease. J Magn Reson Imaging 2000; 11:195–200.

[12] Brix B, Seebass M, Hellwig G, et al. Estimation of heat transfer and temperature rise in partial-body regions during MR procedures: an analytical approach with respect to safety considerations. Magn Reson Imaging 2002;20:65–76.

[13] Tropp J. Image brightening in samples of high dielectric constant. J Magn Reson 2004;167:12–24.

[14] Li T, Mirowitz SA. Fast T2-weighted MR imaging: impact of variation in pulse sequence parameters on image quality and artifacts. Magn Reson Imaging 2003;21:745–53.

[15] Thomas DL, De Vita E, Roberts S, et al. High-resolution fast spin echo imaging of the human brain at 4.7 T: implementation and sequence characteristics. Magn Reson Med 2004;51:1254–64.

[16] Reeder SB, Herzka DA, McVeigh ER. Signal-to-noise ratio behavior of steady-state free precession. Magn Reson Med 2004;52:123–30.

[17] Li T, Mirowitz SA. Fast multi-planar gradient echo MR imaging: impact of variation in pulse sequence parameters on image quality and artifacts. Magn Reson Imaging 2004;22:807–14.

ELSEVIER
SAUNDERS

Magn Reson Imaging Clin N Am
13 (2005) 255–275

MAGNETIC
RESONANCE
IMAGING CLINICS
of North America

Liver Masses

Shahid M. Hussain, MD[a],*, Richard C. Semelka, MD[b]

[a]Section of Abdominal Imaging, Department of Radiology, Erasmus University Medical Center,
Dr. Molewaterplein 40, 3015 GD Rotterdam, The Netherlands
[b]Department of Radiology, University of North Carolina,
2006 Old Clinic Building, CB #7510, Chapel Hill, NC 27599-7510, USA

Annually, thousands of patients undergo imaging for the work-up of suspected or known liver masses. At imaging, several types of liver masses can be observed. The main goals of imaging are to assess: (1) the number and size of the liver abnormalities; (2) the location of abnormalities relative to the liver vessels; (3) the nature of the lesions (benign versus malignant); and (4) the origin (primary versus secondary) of abnormalities.

The exact prevalence of benign liver masses is unknown, but some studies suggest that they may be found in more than 20% of the general population [1]. Recent studies suggest that small (<15 mm) liver lesions that are seen at CT are benign in more than 80% of patients who have known malignancy [2]. With the application of multi-row detector CT and thinner collimation, it is likely that more liver lesions will be detected that will need additional imaging for characterization, most likely with MR imaging [3–5].

It is particularly important to distinguish benign lesions from metastatic and primary malignant lesions. Several malignancies, such as breast, pancreas, and colorectal tumors, tend to metastasize to the liver. The colorectal liver metastases occur most frequently. In the United States, more than 50% of patients (in 1998, 56,000 of 131,600 patients) who died of colorectal cancer had liver metastases at autopsy [6,7]. Of those who have colorectal liver metastases, 10% to 25% are candidates for surgical resection; the 5-year survival rate following resection of isolated colorectal liver metastases can be as high as 38% [7]. Without any treatment, the survival rate is less than 1% [7]. For the remaining 75% to 90% of patients who have liver metastases who are not candidates for surgery, several new therapies have been developed [7–9]. Generally, 1% to 2% of patients who have cirrhosis develop hepatocellular carcinoma (HCC). With treatment, the 5-year survival rate of patients who have HCC can be as high as 75%, whereas without treatment, it is less than 5% [9].

There is no consensus concerning the optimal strategy for imaging the liver. Imaging modalities often are applied based upon the availability and the experience of the radiologists. MR imaging can provide comprehensive and highly accurate diagnostic information concerning liver lesions, which makes the use of other imaging modalities unnecessary. Until recently, MR imaging had been used as a problem-solving modality because it is considered to be an expensive technique. In the near future, MR imaging may be applied as first-line imaging modality with similar or greater accuracy, may enable a faster diagnosis and decision-making, and may be more cost-effective.

In this article, MR imaging features of liver masses are described on current state-of-the-art MR imaging sequences. Liver masses are divided into solid and nonsolid lesions. Description of nonsolid masses includes cysts, biliary hamartomas, and hemangiomas. Description of solid lesions includes liver metastases; and primary liver lesions, such as focal nodular hyperplasia, hepatocellular adenomas, and hepatocellular carcinomas. Finally, MR imaging is compared with other modalities.

* Corresponding author.
E-mail address: s.hussain@erasmusmc.nl
(S.M. Hussain).

Nonsolid liver masses

Liver cysts

Hepatic cysts are common lesions and usually are divided into unilocular (95%) or multilocular varieties. Although the pathogenesis of these cysts is not clear, developmental and acquired causes are postulated [1]. Pathologically, the lining of the cyst shows a single layer of cuboidal to columnar epithelial cells. Lining epithelium rests on an underlying fibrous stroma.

At MR imaging, cysts are low in signal intensity on T1-weighted images, high in signal intensity on T2-weighted images, and retain signal intensity on longer echo time (eg, > 120 millisecond) T2-weighted images. Because cysts do not

enhance with gadolinium on MR images (Fig. 1), delayed postgadolinium images (up to 5 min) may be useful to ensure that lesions are cysts and not poorly vascularized metastases that show gradual enhancement [10]. An advantage of MR imaging over CT imaging in the characterization of cysts is that on gadolinium-enhanced MR images, cysts are nearly signal void, whereas cysts on contrast-enhanced CT images are a light gray in attenuation (see Fig. 1). Single-shot breathing-independent T2-weighted sequences (eg, single-shot turbo spin-echo) are especially effective at showing small (5 mm) cysts. MR imaging is particularly valuable when lesions are small and the patient has a known primary malignancy. Hemorrhagic or protein-containing cysts may

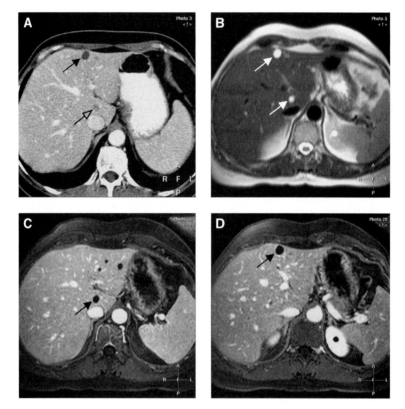

Fig. 1. Typical cyst. (*A*) Axial CT in portal phase shows the subcapsular cyst as an unenhanced hypodense lesion with sharp margins (*arrow*). The second lesion (*open arrow*) that is closer to the inferior vena cava is difficult to recognize as a cyst because of its partial volume and other effects. (*B*) Axial single-shot T2-weighted image shows both cysts with very high signal intensity and sharp margins (*arrows*), which leave no doubt that these are nonsolid lesions. In addition, several smaller cysts also are recognizable that were characterized at CT as "too small to characterize." (*C, D*) Two axial three-dimensional T1-weighted thin-section (4 mm) images from the delayed phase show the larger and smaller cysts as unenhanced lesions with sharp margins (*arrows*). Because of the combination of heavily T2-weighted sequences and contrast-enhanced T1-weighted images, the ability of MR imaging is unparalleled for the characterization of particularly small liver lesions.

have a high signal on T1-weighted images and lower signal on T2-weighted images, but the enhancement should be similar to that of a simple cyst. Otherwise, the cyst should be considered as a complex cyst or a cystic malignancy.

Biliary hamartomas (Von Meyenburg complexes)

Biliary hamartomas are benign biliary malformations that are considered to be part of the spectrum of fibropolycystic diseases of the liver that are caused by ductal plate malformation [11]. This entity is common and is estimated to be present in approximately 3% of patients. At pathology, biliary hamartomas consist of a collection of small—sometimes dilated—irregular and branching bile ducts that are embedded in a fibrous stroma. A few of the ducts may contain inspissated bile. In general, biliary hamartomas contain few vascular channels. Tumors may be solitary or multiple; multiple tumors can be extensive.

At MR imaging, tumors are small (usually <1 cm) and well-defined. The high fluid content renders these lesions low signal on T1, high signal on T2, and negligible enhancement on early and late postgadolinium images. Although this appearance resembles simple cysts, biliary hamartomas demonstrate a thin rim of enhancement on early and late postcontrast images (Fig. 2). The major potential diagnostic error is to misclassify these lesions as metastases because of the presence of faint ring enhancement. The thin enhancing rim of biliary hamartomas that is visualized on

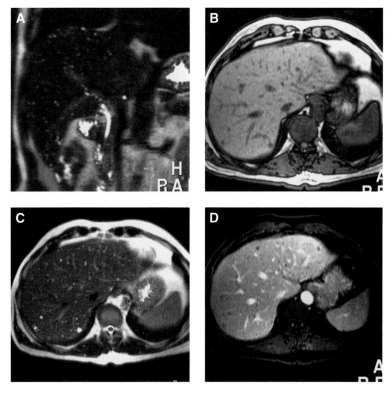

Fig. 2. Biliary hamartomas. (A) Coronal T2-weighted single-shot fast spin-echo (SSFSE) image with a long echo time (TE) of 180 milliseconds shows multiple small hyperintense cystic lesions scattered throughout the liver. Note that many lesions are in the subcapsular location. (B) Axial T1-weighted opposed-phase gradient echo image shows the biliary hamartomas as low signal intensity lesions. (C) Axial T2-weighted SSFSE image (TE = 80 milliseconds) shows that the bright fluid-like lesions vary from millimeters to less than a centimeter in diameter. (D) Axial three-dimensional T1-weighted thin-section (4 mm) image from the delayed phase shows the larger and smaller cysts as unenhanced lesions with a faint rim of enhancement around the hamartomas. This persistent faint rim of enhancement in hamartomas, which is caused by compressed liver parenchyma or inflammation, also usually is present in the arterial phase (not shown).

imaging may be correlated histopathologically with the presence of compressed hepatic parenchyma which border the lesion [11]. In contrast, the pattern of ring enhancement that is displayed by metastases relates histopathologically with the outermost vascularized portion of the tumor. Peritumoral enhancement also is observed in some metastases (see later discussion) [12].

Hemangiomas

Hemangiomas are the most common benign hepatic neoplasm, with an autopsy incidence between 0.4% and 20% [1]. Hemangiomas are more frequent in women. They coexist, not uncommonly, with focal nodular hyperplasia (FNH), particularly in the setting of multiple FNH syndrome [13]. Most of these benign vascular lesions are cavernous hemangiomas. Pathologically, hemangiomas are characterized grossly as well-circumscribed, sponge-like, blood-filled mesenchymal tumors. Microscopically, hemangiomas reveal numerous large vascular channels that are lined by a single layer of flat endothelial cells which are separated by slender fibrous septa. Foci of thrombosis, extensive fibrosis, and calcification may be present.

At MR imaging, hemangiomas have long T1 and T2 values, so they are low in signal intensity on T1-weighted images, high in signal intensity on T2-weighted images, and maintain signal intensity on longer echo times (eg, >120 milliseconds) [14,15]. Hemangiomas have well-defined round or lobular borders. Typically, small lesions appear round, whereas larger lesions have a lobular margin. T2 measurements are less than those of cysts. Typically, hemangiomas enhance in a peripheral nodular fashion on dynamic serial gadolinium-enhanced MR images (Fig. 3). The enhancement usually is slow, progressive, complete or nearly complete fill-in of the entire lesion by 10 min [15–17]. This enhancement pattern is characterized by enlargement and coalescence of enhancing nodules. Serial gadolinium-enhanced spoiled gradient-echo images are effective in distinguishing benign from malignant hepatic masses [15,17–19].

The MR imaging appearances of small (<1.5 cm), medium (1.5–5.0 cm), and large (>5.0 cm) hemangiomas were reported in a multi-institutional study [17]. All lesions were high in signal intensity on T2-weighted images. Three types of enhancement patterns were observed: (1) uniform high signal intensity immediately following contrast (type 1), (2) peripheral nodular enhancement with centripetal progression to uniform high signal intensity (type 2), and (3) peripheral nodular enhancement with centripetal progression and a persistent central scar (type 3). Type 1 enhancement was observed only in small tumors. Types 2 and 3 enhancements were observed in all size categories. In many centers, the gadolinium-enhanced gradient-echo sequence in the delayed phase is performed 2 to 3 min after contrast injection; therefore, types 2 and 3 enhancement patterns often may not be seen. If a typical peripheral nodular enhancement is present in the arterial or portal phases, a complete fill-in of the entire hemangioma is not necessary for diagnosis.

Fast-enhancing hemangiomas show enhancement patterns that can resemble other tumors; metastases are the most difficult to distinguish. Fast-enhancing hemangiomas also can demonstrate perilesional high signal on T2 and perilesional increased enhancement that likely reflects high flow in efferent veins. These findings are rare in hemangiomas and are observed more commonly in metastases, especially colon cancer metastases. A recent study showed that 19% of hemangiomas had temporal peritumoral enhancement; this was more common in hemangiomas with rapid enhancement (41%). The mean diameter of hemangiomas with peritumoral enhancement was not significantly different from hemangiomas without peritumoral enhancement [20]. Small hemangiomas most commonly demonstrate type 2 enhancement. The peripheral nodules of enhancement typically are small.

Giant hemangiomas most frequently have a central scar [17,21]. Virtually all giant hemangiomas have type 3 enhancement (peripheral nodular enhancement with persistent central scar). Absence of a central scar should raise the concern that the mass may represent another lesion (Fig. 4). Very large hemangiomas frequently have mildly complex signal intensity on T2-weighted images with the frequent presence of low signal strands; this reflects the internal network of fibrous stroma that is observed histologically. In rare instances, large hemangiomas may compress adjacent portal veins and result in transient segmental increased enhancement on immediate postgadolinium images secondary to autoregulatory-increased hepatic arterial supply. The most distinctive imaging feature of hemangiomas is the demonstration of a discontinuous ring of nodules immediately after gadolinium administration [15,17,19].

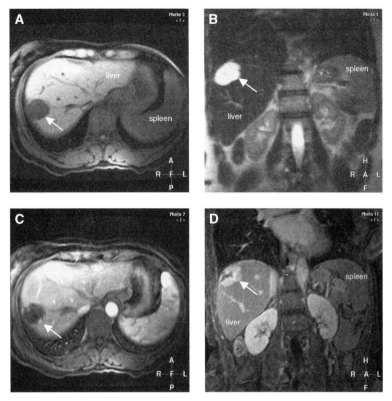

Fig. 3. Medium-sized hemangioma. (*A*) Axial fat-suppressed T1-weighted gradient-echo image shows the hemangioma (*arrow*) as a low signal intensity (SI) lesion with slightly lobulated and sharp margins to the liver. Note that the SI of the hemangioma is lower than that of the spleen. (*B*) Coronal heavily T2-weighted single-shot fast spin-echo image shows the hemangioma (*arrow*) as a bright (fluid-like) structure with lobulated and sharp margins to the liver. The SI is much higher than the spleen which indicates the high fluid content, and hence, nonsolid nature of the lesion. (*C*) Axial T1-weighted three-dimensional gradient-echo image in the arterial phase (no enhancement of the liver veins, heterogeneous enhancement of the spleen) shows a small nodule (*arrow*) in the periphery of the lesion. This peripheral nodular enhancement pattern is typical for most hemangiomas. (*D*) Coronal three-dimensional T1-weighted thin-section (4 mm) gradient-echo image from the delayed phase shows almost complete enhancement of the hemangioma (*arrow*). This indicates that the lesion retains its contrast within the large vascular channels for several minutes after contrast injection. For the diagnosis of hemangioma, a combination of high signal on T2-weighted images and the peripheral nodular enhancement is sufficient; there is no need for complete filling-in of the lesion.

Reports have shown that hemangiomas may be distinguished reliably from metastases on T2-weighted images based on the smooth lobular margins and the higher calculated T2 values of hemangiomas (mean of 140 milliseconds) [14]. Although this may be true in most patients, cumulative experience from many centers has shown that T2-weighted images alone may not allow characterization of small tumors nor allow reliable distinction between hemangiomas and hypervascular malignant tumors (eg, leiomyosarcoma and islet-cell tumors). It should be kept in mind that hypervascular and mucinous metastases also may show long T2 values.

Solid liver masses

Liver metastases

Metastases are the most common malignant tumors of the liver in western countries. Liver metastases usually appear as solitary or multiple nodules; rare appearances include confluent masses or small, infiltrative lesions which mimic cirrhosis. Tumors may be complicated by central necrosis or cystic change. Several malignancies, such as breast, pancreas, and colorectal tumors, tend to metastasize to the liver.

Optimal hepatic imaging involves detection and characterization of focal lesions [2,16,18,

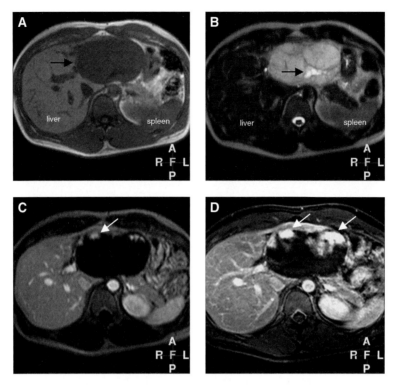

Fig. 4. Giant hemangioma. (*A*) Axial in-phase T1-weighted gradient-echo image shows the hemangioma (*arrow*) as a low signal intensity (SI) lesion with lobulated and sharp margins to the liver. Note that the SI of the hemangioma is lower than that of the spleen. (*B*) Axial T2-weighted single-shot fast spin-echo image shows a bright lesion that contains a brighter central scar (*arrow*). The large size, high SI, and a brighter central scar are typical for giant hemangiomas. (*C*) Axial T1-weighted three-dimensional gradient-echo image in the portal phase shows typical peripheral nodular enhancement of the hemangioma (*arrow*). (*D*) Axial three-dimensional T1-weighted gradient-echo image from the delayed phase shows progressive peripheral nodular enhancement of the hemangioma (*arrows*) which indicates that the lesion retains its contrast within the large vascular channels for several minutes after contrast injection. For the diagnosis of giant hemangiomas, there is no need for complete filling-in of the lesion. Often, the central scar of the giant hemangiomas will not show enhancement on delayed contrast-enhanced images.

22–26]. Detection involves identification of the presence of lesions and the segmental extent of liver involvement [25]. Demonstration that malignant disease has limited hepatic involvement may have a substantial impact on patient management [7].

Metastases show variable signal intensity on T1- and T2-weighted images, and variable patterns and extent of contrast enhancement, unlike most benign lesions. Transient tumor blush in the arterial phase of a dynamic contrast-enhanced examination, however, is observed commonly in small (<2 cm) hypervascular metastases [15,16,26–28].

Colorectal metastases

Unlike many other cancers, the presence of distant metastases from colorectal cancer does not preclude curative treatment [7]. Approximately 25% of patients who have colorectal liver metastases have no other distant metastases. Of these, 10% to 25% are candidates for surgical resection. For the 75% to 90% of patients who have liver metastases that are not amenable to surgery, several new therapies have been developed (eg, minimal invasive treatments, such as radiofrequency ablation, stereotactic radiation therapy, and systemic chemotherapy) [7].

Optimal hepatic imaging evaluation involves detection and characterization of focal lesions [7,29,30]. Demonstration that malignant disease has limited hepatic involvement may have a substantial impact on patient management. Survival of patients who have colorectal metastases may be improved by surgical or other forms of treatment. In most comparative studies, MR imaging is superior to CT in the evaluation of the liver

[16,17,22,25–27,31–35]. The current challenge is whether the superior performance of MR imaging translates into a beneficial effect on patient management, disease outcome, and health care costs. New MR sequences, phased-array surface coils, and tissue-specific MR contrast agents suggest that MR imaging may exceed further the diagnostic ability of CT.

At MR imaging, most colorectal carcinoma metastases show several typical findings (Fig. 5). The lesions appear as low signal intensity on T1-weighted images without revealing the internal tumor anatomy, and moderately high signal intensity (usually comparable to spleen) on T2-weighted images with fat suppression [28]. On T2-weighted images, the internal tumor anatomy of medium- to large-sized colorectal metastases has a target-like configuration: (1) highest (fluid-like) signal intensity is in the center of the lesion as a result of coagulative necrosis; (2) lower signal intensity is in a broad zone outside the center because of the presence of a desmoplastic reaction that facilitates the formation of the tumor matrix in which strands of tumor cells can grow; and (3) a slightly higher signal intensity is in the outermost zone as a result of more compact tumor cells with more vessels and less desmoplasia [28]. The outermost zone is only a few millimeters thick and consists of the growing edge of the colorectal metastases. In addition, colorectal metastases also

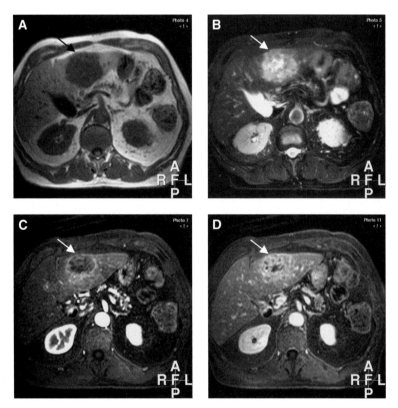

Fig. 5. Colorectal metastasis. (*A*) Axial in-phase T1-weighted gradient-echo image shows the metastasis as a low signal intensity (SI) lesion (*arrow*) with sharp margins to the liver. (*B*) Axial T2-weighted single-shot fast spin-echo image shows the target-like configuration of the lesion (*arrow*) with moderately high SI in the periphery and a fluid-like SI centrally. This configuration represents the more compact and solid tissue in the periphery of the lesion and coagulative necrosis centrally. (*C*) Axial T1-weighted three-dimensional gradient-echo image in the arterial phase shows typical continuous irregular ring-shaped peripheral enhancement of the metastasis (*arrow*). This enhancement pattern indicates that the metastasis is more vascularized in the most peripheral part of the lesion (ie, the growing edge of the lesion). (*D*) Axial three-dimensional T1-weighted gradient-echo image in the delayed phase shows progressive filling-in of the lesion (*arrow*). This indicates that the lesion has less vessels centrally, and therefore, it takes more time to enhance these parts. This finding also illustrates that the filling-in of lesions can be seen in malignant (metastases) and benign (hemangiomas) liver tumors and should not be used as a distinctive feature.

may be surrounded by perifocal edema within the compressed liver tissue immediately around the lesions [28]. After administration of gadolinium, most colorectal metastases show an irregular, continuous, ring-shaped (as opposed to the broken ring or peripheral nodular enhancement of hemangioma) enhancement in the arterial phase [15,26,32]. This ring-shaped enhancement reveals the growing edge of the lesion. In the portal and delayed phase, the metastases often show washout in the outer parts and a progressive enhancement toward the center of the lesions. Larger lesions may show cauliflower-like enhancement. The smaller lesions often lack the coagulative

necrosis, and hence, the fluid-like signal in the center of metastases.

Based on the intrinsic soft tissue contrast of T2-weighted images and a higher sensitivity of MR imaging to gadolinium than the sensitivity of CT for iodine-contrast media, MR imaging is more accurate in detection and characterization than CT, particularly for small liver metastases. Especially, the ability of MR imaging to distinguish small cysts from small metastases by (heavily) T2-weighted sequences is unparalleled (Fig. 6).

Ill-defined increased perilesional and subsegmental enhancement are common with colorectal cancer and pancreatic ductal adenocarcinoma

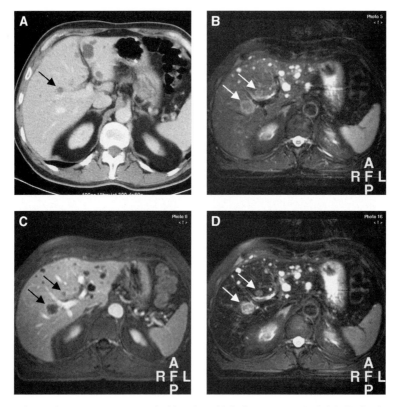

Fig. 6. Multiple colorectal metastases versus coincidental multiple liver cysts. (*A*) Axial CT in the portal phase in a patient who has known colon carcinoma showed a possible slight increase in the size of one of the lesions (*arrow*). Patient was known to have multiple liver cysts and had several follow-up CT examinations. Note that there is little difference in density between the cysts and the questionable lesion. (*B*) Axial T2-weighted fast spin-echo (FSE) image shows two metastases (*arrows*) that have moderately high signal intensity (comparable to the spleen) compared with the liver and much lower signal intensity than the bright fluid-like signal intensity of the cysts. (*C*) Axial T1-weighted three-dimensional gradient-echo image in the delayed phase shows a typical continuous irregular ring-shaped peripheral enhancement of the metastases (*arrows*). This enhancement pattern indicates that the metastases are more vascularized in the most peripheral part of the lesions (ie, the growing edge of the lesions). (*D*) Axial T2-weighted FSE image after uptake of a superparamagnetic iron oxide (SPIO) contrast medium by Kupffer cells within the liver and spleen shows the two metastases (*arrows*) with improved conspicuity that is due to the decreased signal intensity of the liver (and spleen) by the T*-effect of the SPIO contrast medium.

metastases, but are uncommon with other metastases. Typically, perilesional enhancement with colon cancer is ill-defined and circumferential, whereas with pancreatic ductal adenocarcinoma, it often is a wedge-shaped enhancement that is demarcated more sharply. A recent publication reported that microscopic examination of liver tissue that surrounds metastases showed variable degrees of hepatic parenchyma compression, desmoplastic reaction, and inflammatory infiltrates [36].

Other types of metastases

At MR imaging, other metastases vary substantially in appearance on T1- and T2-weighted images. Borders usually are ill-defined, but may be sharp. Frequently, lesion shape is irregular but may be regular, round, or oval. Generally, metastases are moderately low in signal intensity on T1-weighted images and modestly high in signal intensity on T2-weighted images. Some metastases, particularly hypervascular metastases from islet-cell tumors, leiomyosarcoma, pheochromocytoma, renal-cell carcinoma, necrotic metastases, or cystic metastases from ovarian cancer, may be high in signal intensity on T2-weighted images; this renders the distinction from hemangiomas difficult [27].

Homogeneous enhancement may be observed in large metastases; however, in noncirrhotic livers, this enhancement pattern is characteristic of hepatocellular adenomas and FNH. The most common enhancement feature of such metastases is a peripheral ring of enhancement on immediate postgadolinium spoiled gradient-echo images with central progression or wash-out in the later phases after contrast injection (Fig. 7).

Melanoma metastases may represent a mixture of high- and low-signal intensity lesions on T1- and T2-weighted images as a result of the

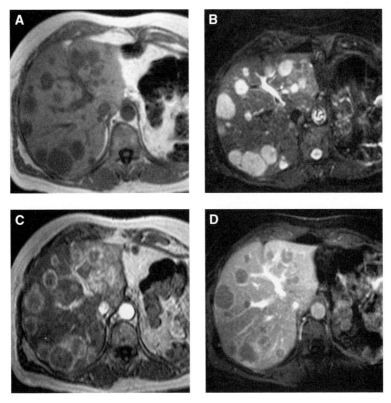

Fig. 7. Multiple neuroendocrine metastases. (*A*) Axial T1-weighted gradient-echo shows multiple hypointense metastases. (*B*) Axial T2-weighted fast spin-echo image shows the metastases that are variable in size; have sharp margins to the liver; and high, almost fluid-like, signal intensity. (*C*) Axial T1-weighted two-dimensional gradient-echo image in the arterial phase shows typical continuous, irregular, ring-shaped enhancement of the metastases. (*D*) Axial T1-weighted three-dimensional gradient-echo image in the delayed phase shows wash-out of contrast from the metastases.

paramagnetic property of melanin [28]. Melanoma metastases usually are hypervascular and show intense enhancement in the arterial phase (Fig. 8). Melanoma metastases must be highly pigmented, well-differentiated lesions to produce this paramagnetic effect. Amelanocytic malignant melanomas or poorly differentiated tumors do not produce the paramagnetic effect and appear mildly hypointense on T1, and mildly hyperintense on T2.

Metastases from mucin-producing tumors, such as ovarian cancer or mucinous cystadenocarcinoma of the pancreas, may result in liver metastases that are high in signal intensity on T1-weighted images as a result of the protein content. Metastases that are active in protein synthesis, such as in the production of enzymes or hormones (eg, carcinoid tumors), also may be high in signal intensity on T1-weighted images because of the presence of a high concentration of protein (Fig. 9).

Hepatic nodules

Various parenchymal liver diseases may lead to hepatitis, fibrosis, and eventually, to cirrhosis. Cirrhotic liver contains regenerative nodules and also may contain dysplastic nodules and HCCs [9,37].

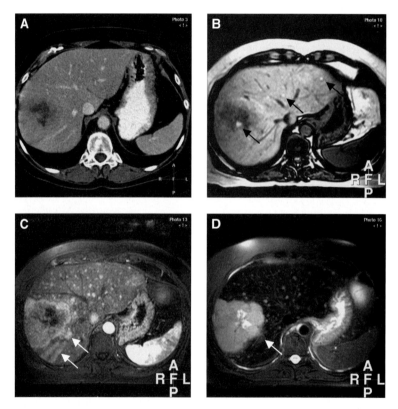

Fig. 8. Melanoma metastases. (*A*) CT in the portal phase shows a large lesion with central necrosis and solid enhancing tissue in the periphery. These findings are nonspecific and can be seen in almost all large metastatic liver lesions. (*B*) Axial T1-weighted opposed-phase gradient-echo image shows in addition to the larger lesion, numerous smaller bright lesions (*arrows*). The larger lesion also contains areas with bright signal. These findings were compatible with melanin-containing liver metastases in this patient who was operated on for a melanoma in the past. (*C*) Axial T1-weighted MR gradient-echo image in the arterial phase shows numerous hypervascular small lesions throughout the liver. The larger lesion shows enhancement in the periphery. A mid-sized lesion in the vicinity of the larger lesion shows concomitant wedge-shaped enhancement due to liver vascular compression (*arrows*). (*D*) Axial T2-weighted fast spin-echo image after uptake of a superparamagnetic iron oxide contrast medium that decreases the signal of the normal liver (and spleen) and improves the conspicuity of the liver metastases. Note the medium-sized lesion in the vicinity of the larger lesion (*arrow*). MR imaging was performed only 3 weeks after the CT examination.

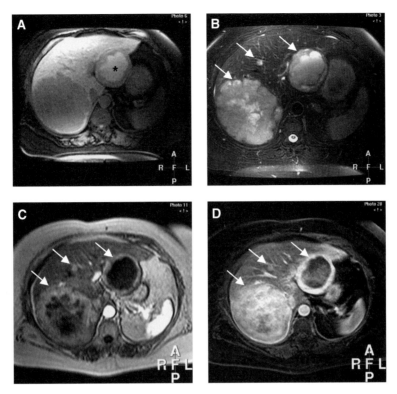

Fig. 9. Carcinoid metastases. (*A*) Axial fat-suppressed T1-weighted gradient-echo image before injection of gadolinium shows two large liver lesions. The larger lesion has a low SI (comparable to the spleen) and the smaller lesion has a higher signal in the central part (*) that most likely is due to protein-containing fluid. (*B*) Axial T2-weighted fast spin-echo image shows a third smaller lesion in addition to the larger lesions (*arrows*). The solid areas of the lesions have intermediate signal intensity, between that of the liver and the spinal fluid. (*C*) Axial two-dimensional T1-weighted gradient-echo image in the arterial phase shows enhancement of the solid parts of the lesions (*arrows*). (*D*) Axial MR T1-weighted gradient-echo image in the delayed phase shows persistent enhancement of the solid areas of the lesions (*arrows*). The lesions were proven pathologically to be carcinoid metastases.

Except for FNH, hepatic nodules usually develop in previously damaged livers. Damage to the liver can be caused by several factors: (1) endemic: aflatoxin, a product of the fungus *Aspergillus flavus* is an important cause of HCC in Africa and Asia; (2) metabolic and genetic disorders, including hemochromatosis, Wilson's disease, and α_1-antitrypsin deficiency; (3) dietary: obesity, diabetes (type II), and alcoholism can lead to fatty infiltration of the liver (steatosis), steatohepatitis, and cirrhosis; and (4) viral: viral hepatitis, mainly caused by hepatitis B and C viruses.

Since 1995, a modified nomenclature categorizes hepatic nodules into two groups—the regenerative and the dysplastic or neoplastic lesions [37]. Regenerative nodules result from a localized proliferation of hepatocytes and their supporting stroma. Regenerative lesions include regenerative nodules, cirrhotic nodules, lobar or segmental hyperplasia, and FNH. Dysplastic or neoplastic lesions are composed of hepatocytes that show histologic characteristics of abnormal growth (caused by presumed or proved genetic alteration). Such lesions include hepatocellular adenoma, dysplastic focus, dysplastic nodule, and HCC [9,37,38].

A step-wise carcinogenesis of HCC has been proposed based on gradually increasing size and cellular density among the following lesions: regenerative nodule, dysplastic nodule, small HCCs, and large HCCs (Fig. 10). Several investigators have proposed a de novo pathway for HCC, mainly in noncirrhotic livers [9]. According to this pathway, hepatocytes give rise to a focus of a small HCC that will grow into a large HCC. Neoangiogenesis is important for sustained growth of HCCs and facilitates early detection.

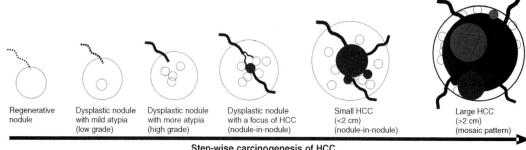

Step-wise carcinogenesis of HCC
With increasing size, cellularity, and angiogenic activity within the nodules

Fig. 10. Step-wise carcinogenesis of HCC. In a liver with an underlying parenchymal liver disease (eg, hepatitis, fibrosis, cirrhosis), HCC develops according to a step-wise carcinogenesis from regenerative nodules through dysplastic nodules to HCC. During this process, neoangiogenesis (formation of tumor vessels) plays an important role.

Focal nodular hyperplasia

FNH is a benign liver tumor that occurs predominantly in women during their reproductive years, but cases have been reported in men and children [13]. FNH often is an incidental finding on imaging studies and needs to be differentiated from other focal liver lesions, such as HCC, hepatocellular adenomas, and hypervascular metastases. Most FNHs do not require treatment.

FNH is lobulated and well-circumscribed, although unencapsulated. The pathognomonic macroscopic feature is the presence of a central stellate scar with radiating septa; this divides the lesion into numerous nodules of normal hepatocytes that are arranged abnormally. The central scar contains thick-walled vessels with its sources from the hepatic artery that provides excellent arterial blood supply to the lesion. At histology, the classic FNH is characterized by the presence of abnormal nodular architecture, malformed appearing vessels, and cholangiolar proliferation. Nonclassic FNHs lack one of the following classic features—nodular abnormal architecture or malformed vessels—but always show bile ductular proliferation [13].

At MR imaging, FNH is slightly hypointense on T1-weighted images and slightly hyperintense on T2-weighted images [9,13,37]. FNHs also may be nearly isointense on T1- and T2-weighted sequences. Unlike liver cell adenomas, FNHs rarely have higher signal intensity than liver on T1-weighted images. FNH is said to contain fat in up to 20% of cases at histopathology; however, in the authors' experience, the amount of fatty infiltration in FNH—as opposed to adenoma—probably is too small to detect with confidence on the current chemical shift imaging sequences. The central scar usually is high on T2-weighted images. FNHs show intense homogeneous enhancement during the arterial phase of the dynamic contrast-enhanced sequence. The central scar and radiating septa in FNHs show enhancement on delayed images (Fig. 11). The specific contrast media, such as the superparamagnetic iron oxide (SPIO)-based and manganese-based, are targeted at the Kupffer cells and hepatocytes, respectively. These contrast media can be used to demonstrate the hepatocellular origin of the lesions. The Kupffer cells show uptake of SPIO and lower signal intensity of the lesions and the surrounding liver on T2- and T2*-weighted images. MR imaging has a higher sensitivity (70%) and specificity (98%) for FNH than ultrasound and CT. The central scar was detected more often by using MR imaging than CT (78% and 60%, respectively) [13].

Hepatocellular adenomas

Hepatic adenomas are benign neoplasms that occur most often in young women who have a history of oral contraceptive use; the annual incidence is 3 or 4 per 100,000. Occasionally, hepatic adenomas are found in men who use anabolic steroids or in patients with glycogen storage disease or liver adenomatosis. Most patients who have hepatic adenomas are clinically asymptomatic and have normal liver function. Large adenomas may cause symptoms of pain and may present with hemorrhage. Typically, liver adenomas occur in young women who use oral contraceptives. Association with other conditions (eg, familial diabetes mellitus, galactosemia, glycogen storage disease type 1) or hepatocellular-

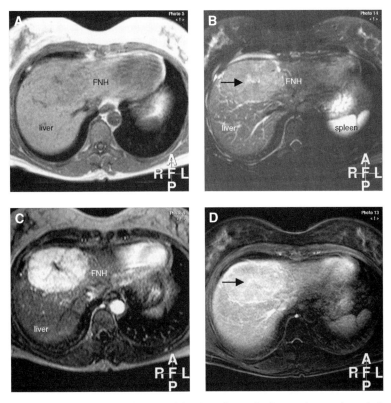

Fig. 11. Focal nodular hyperplasia. (*A*) Axial T1-weighted gradient-echo image shows a large lesion (FNH) that is almost isointense to the liver with a darker central scar and septae. (*B*) Axial T2-weighted fast spin-echo image shows FNH that is slightly hyperintense to the liver with a brighter central scar and septae (*arrow*). Note that FNH is surrounded by a thin pseudocapsule that is composed of compressed liver parenchyma and vessels. (*C*) Axial two-dimensional T1-weighted gradient-echo image in the arterial phase shows intense homogeneous enhancement of the entire FNH, except for the central scar and septae. (*D*) Axial MR T1-weighted gradient-echo image shows FNH that has become almost isointense to the liver with enhancement of the central scar (*arrow*), the septae, and the pseudocapsule.

stimulating agents (eg, anabolic steroids) has been reported. Liver cell adenomas are composed of sheets of cells that may resemble normal hepatocytes [38]. Unlike FNHs, liver cell adenomas lack the central scar and radiating septa. Necrosis and hemorrhage are frequent causes of pain. In addition, according to the currently used terminology, hepatocellular adenomas are classified as premalignant nodules [37]. Because of their potential for malignant degeneration, it is preferred to treat larger (> 5 cm) adenomas surgically.

Hepatic adenomas are solitary in 70% to 80% of cases. Multiple lesions are observed frequently in patients who have type 1 glycogen storage disease and liver adenomatosis. Histologically, hepatic adenomas are composed of sheets of cells that closely resemble normal hepatocytes that are arranged in plates which are separated by sinusoids. Kupffer's cells are present, but usually in lower numbers than in normal liver parenchyma. Bile ducts and portal tracts are absent in adenomas.

On T1- and T2-weighted images, liver cell adenomas typically do not differ much in their signal intensity from the surrounding liver parenchyma. The lesions are mildly hypointense to moderately hyperintense on T1-weighted images, and mildly hyperintense on T2-weighted images [38]. They show a blush of homogeneous enhancement on arterial phase and fade to near isointensity on later phases of dynamic gadolinium-enhanced images. Adenomas may be hyperintense to the liver on fat-suppressed T1-weighted and T2-weighted images. Hyperintensity on T1-weighted images may be due, in part, to the fatty contents of the adenomas. In the case of abundant steatosis of the liver, the liver is more suppressed than the lesion; this gives adenomas a higher signal intensity than the liver on T2-weighted images with fat suppression.

Fatty infiltration of the liver and the lesion can be demonstrated on in- and opposed phase T1-weighted gradient-echo imaging (chemical shift imaging). A complete or partial pseudocapsule that presents as a rim of low signal intensity on T1 may be seen in some adenomas. This pseudocapsule usually is much thinner and has a high signal on T2-weighted images than the true fibrotic tumor capsule of HCC.

On dynamic gadolinium-enhanced gradient-echo MR images, adenomas show early arterial enhancement and become nearly isointense relative to liver on delayed images. The intensity of the arterial enhancement often is lower than in the classic types of FNH. In the delayed phase, the central scar and septae are absent (Fig. 12).

Regenerative nodules

Typically, regenerative nodules in cirrhotic liver have low signal intensity on T2-weighted images, variable signal intensity on T1-weighted images, and do not enhance in the arterial phase of dynamic gadolinium-enhanced images (Fig. 13).

Dysplastic nodules

The signal intensity and enhancement characteristics of dysplastic nodules are not well-established. Because of the gradual step-wise transition from a regenerative nodule into HCC, the hepatocytes within hepatic nodules undergo numerous changes that might not be reflected in their signal intensity or vascularity. Therefore, current MR imaging sequences might not be able to distinguish regenerative nodules from dysplastic

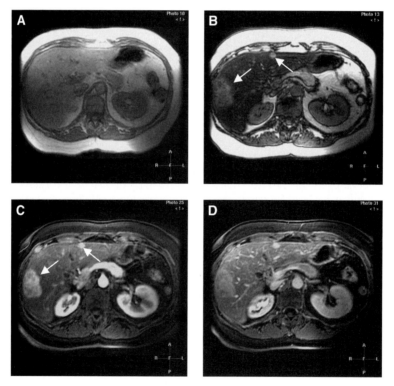

Fig. 12. Hepatocellular adenomas. (*A*) Axial in-phase T1-weighted gradient-echo image does not show any distinct lesions. This indicates that the lesions are almost completely isointense to the liver, and hence, most likely are composed of liver tissue. (*B*) Axial opposed-phase T1-weighted gradient-echo image shows marked decrease of the signal of the liver due to diffuse severe fatty infiltration. Two focal lesions that also show evidence of fatty infiltration remain high in signal intensity (*arrows*). (*C*) Axial MR T1-weighted gradient-echo image shows moderately intense homogeneous enhancement (blush) of both lesions (*arrows*). (*D*) Axial MR T1-weighted gradient-echo image in the delayed phase shows that both lesions become almost isointense to the liver. These findings are compatible with multiple adenomas. Because of suspicions of malignancy and the size, the larger lesion was resected and the diagnosis of liver cell adenoma was confirmed.

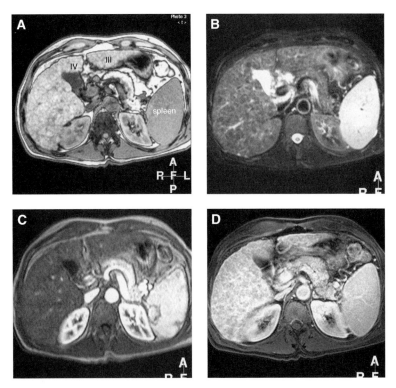

Fig. 13. Regenerative nodules. (*A*) Axial opposed-phase T1-weighted gradient-echo image shows multiple bright nodules within a cirrhotic liver with irregular contours, atrophy of segments III and IV with expanded gallbladder fossa. Note also that the spleen is enlarged which indicates portal hypertension. (*B*) Axial T2-weighted fast spin-echo image shows multiple cirrhotic nodules that are low in signal intensity with brighter septae surrounding most of the nodules. (*C*) Axial two-dimensional T1-weighted gradient-echo image in the arterial phase shows no enhancing nodules or other lesions within the liver. Regenerative nodules usually show negligible arterial enhancement. (*D*) Axial MR T1-weighted gradient-echo image in the delayed phase shows septal enhancement that is typical of cirrhosis.

nodules with certainty. Some MR imaging features of high-grade dysplastic nodules and small HCCs were described [9,37]. Most high-grade dysplastic lesions (formerly adenomatous hyperplasia) and well-differentiated small HCCs may have high signal intensity on T1-weighted MR images.

Hepatocellular carcinoma

HCC is a malignant neoplasm that is composed of cells with hepatocellular differentiation. A small HCC is defined as measuring up to 2 cm in diameter. At pathology, the criteria that are used to distinguish HCCs from high-grade dysplastic nodules are not defined clearly. Criteria that favor malignancy include: (1) prominent nuclear atypia, (2) high nuclear-cytoplasmic ratio with nuclear density twice that of normal, (3) plates three or more cells thick, with numerous unaccompanied arteries, (4) mitoses in moderate

numbers, and (5) invasion of stroma or portal tracts. Most small HCCs cannot be distinguished histologically from dysplastic nodules with certainty [39].

At MR imaging, HCC is a focal liver lesion with high signal intensity on T2-weighted images and variable signal intensity on T1-weighted MR images. It shows intense enhancement during the arterial phase and wash-out in the portal and later phases of dynamic gadolinium-enhanced MR imaging (Fig. 14).

Small HCCs (≤ 2 cm) may have a nodule within a nodule appearance on MR images, especially if a focus of HCC originates within a siderotic regenerative nodule [9]. On T2-weighted images, small HCCs also may appear as small areas of slightly higher signal intensity than the surrounding liver. On T1-weighted images, such areas may be isointense, hypointense, or hyperintense to the liver. On arterial phase dynamic

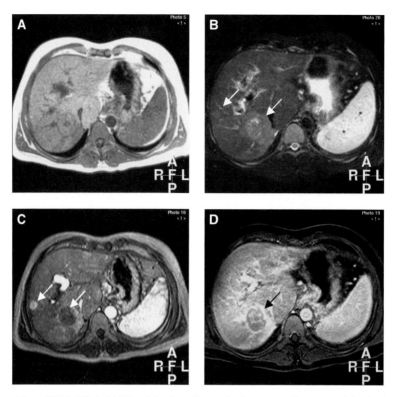

Fig. 14. Small and large HCC. (*A*) Axial T1-weighted gradient-echo image reveals some nodules in the right liver that clearly show signs of cirrhosis with enlarged segment I and splenomegaly. (*B*) Axial T2-weighted fast spin-echo image shows at least two areas with slightly increased signal intensity (*arrows*) within the liver. (*C*) Axial two-dimensional T1-weighted gradient-echo image in the arterial phase shows almost homogeneous enhancement of a small nodule and heterogenous enhancement of a large nodule (*arrows*). (*D*) Axial MR T1-weighted gradient-echo image in the delayed phase shows wash-out in both lesions with septal enhancement in the liver which indicates cirrhosis. The larger HCC has an enhancing tumor capsule (*arrow*). The smaller HCC is difficult to distinguish from the surrounding nodules.

gadolinium-enhanced MR images, most small HCCs show heterogeneous, or sometimes, homogeneous, enhancement.

Large HCCs (>2 cm) may have several additional characteristic features, such as mosaic pattern; tumor capsule; extracapsular extension with the formation of satellite nodules; vascular invasion; and extrahepatic dissemination, including lymph node and distant metastases [9].

The mosaic pattern is a configuration of confluent small nodules that are separated by thin septa and necrotic areas within the tumor. This appearance most likely reflects the histopathology and the characteristic growth pattern of HCC. In one study, 88% of the lesions with a mosaic pattern were larger than 2 cm. On T1- and T2-weighted MR images, the mosaic pattern appears as areas of variable signal intensities, whereas on gadolinium-enhanced images, the

lesions enhance in a heterogeneous fashion during the arterial and later phases (Fig. 15).

Tumor capsule, a characteristic sign of (large) HCCs, is present in 60% to 82% of cases. In one study, 56 of 72 HCCs showed a capsule at histology, and 75% of the lesions with a capsule were larger than 2 cm. The tumor capsule becomes thicker with increasing tumor size. The tumor capsule is hypointense on T1- and T2-weighted images in most cases. Extracapsular extension of tumor, with partial projections or formation of satellite nodules in the immediate vicinity, is present in 43% to 77% of HCCs.

Vascular invasion occurs frequently in HCCs and can affect the portal and hepatic veins. In a recent study of 322 patients who underwent curative resection of HCC, 15.5% showed macroscopic venous invasion and 59.0% showed microscopic venous invasion that was proved at

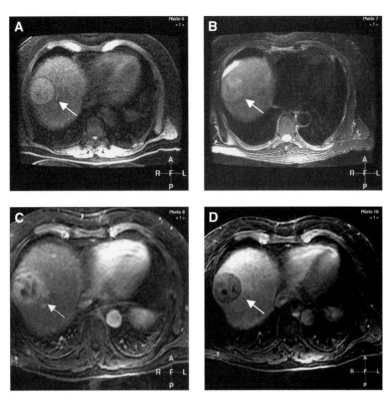

Fig. 15. Large HCC. (*A*) Axial T1-weighted gradient-echo image shows a large round lesion that is predominantly brighter than the liver and is surrounded by a low signal intensity tumor capsule (*arrow*). (*B*) Axial T2-weighted fast spin-echo image shows the lesion that is predominantly bright with some darker areas (mosaic pattern), that is surrounded by a low signal intensity tumor capsule (*arrow*). This T2 low signal intensity indicates that the capsule is composed of fibrous tissue, a typical sign of tumor capsule, as opposed to a pseudocapsule of benign lesions. (*C*) Axial MR T1-weighted gradient-echo image in the arterial phase shows intense heterogeneous enhancement of the entire lesion with a tongue-like extension of enhancement (*arrow*) outside of the contours of the lesion; this most likely represents vascular invasion. (*D*) Axial MR T1-weighted gradient-echo image in the delayed phase shows wash-out in lesions with capsular enhancement (*arrow*).

histopathology. In a meta-analysis of seven reports with 1497 patients, portal vein invasion was found in 24% of the patients who had HCC [9]. At MR imaging, vascular invasion can be seen as a lack of signal void on multislice T1-weighted gradient echo images and flow-compensated T2-weighted fast spin-echo images (1). On gadolinium-enhanced MR images, the tumor thrombus typically shows enhancement in the arterial phase and a filling defect on images that are acquired during later phases. Larger and diffuse HCCs often are associated with vascular invasion (Fig. 16).

Hepatocellular carcinoma in a noncirrhotic liver

In western countries, up to 40% of cases of HCC occur in a noncirrhotic liver. In contrast, in South-East Asia (with endemic viral hepatitis)

only 10% of patients with HCC have a noncirrhotic liver [9]. In patients who do not have cirrhosis or other underlying liver disease, HCC usually is diagnosed at a late stage [9]. In one study of HCC in noncirrhotic liver, the medium tumor diameter was 8.8 cm. The lesions in noncirrhotic livers were significantly larger, more often solitary, and contained a central scar more frequently (Fig. 17). HCC in a noncirrhotic liver is more amenable to surgical resection with a much better prognosis than HCC in a cirrhotic liver [9].

Differential diagnosis of hepatocellular carcinoma

In a noncirrhotic liver, HCC should be distinguished from hepatocellular adenomas, FNH, intrahepatic cholangiocarcinomas, fibrolamellar carcinomas, and hypervascular metastases. Intrahepatic cholangiocarcinomas (<10% of all

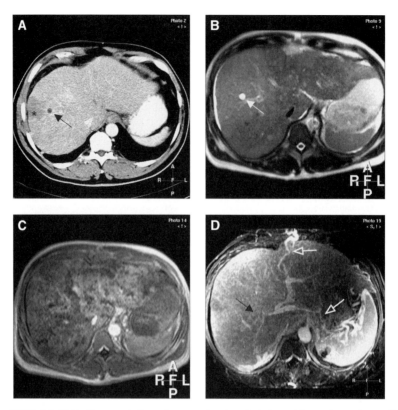

Fig. 16. Diffuse HCC. (*A*) CT in the portal phase from another hospital showed less enhanced area (*) within a liver with known cirrhosis that was interpreted as part of vascular changes. A cyst (*arrow*) was seen as an incidental finding. HCC was not recognized. (*B*) Axial T2-weighted SSFSE image shows increased abnormal signal intensity throughout the liver. The increased signal intensity is partly diffuse (right side of the liver) and partly multifocal (left liver). The liver clearly is cirrhotic with irregular contours and is surrounded by ascites. MR imaging confirms the presence of a small cyst (*arrow*). (*C*) Axial two-dimensional T1-weighted gradient-echo image in the arterial phase shows intense heterogeneous enhancement throughout the liver, but slightly more in the left, than in the right, liver. The combination of heterogeneous high signal intensity on T2 with heterogeneous enhancement in a cirrhotic liver with increased levels of alfa-fetoprotein is compatible with diffuse HCC. (*D*) Axial maximum-intensity projection based on the subtraction images from the portal phase shows invasion by the tumor in the right portal vein (*solid arrow*), multiple collaterals (*open arrows*), and splenomegaly. This patient died from uncontrollable variceal bleeding a few days after the MR imaging examination.

cholangiocarcinomas) may present with a large mass that is associated with some intrahepatic biliary obstruction, umbilication (due to tumor capsular retraction), and enhancement pattern that overlaps with large colorectal metastases and HCC [40]. Mixed HCC-cholangiocarcinoma may occur; the imaging appearance generally is indistinguishable from HCC. Fibrolamellar carcinoma is a malignant hepatocellular tumor with distinct clinical and pathologic differences from conventional HCC [9]. Therefore, fibrolamellar carcinomas should be considered as a separate entity. Cirrhosis, hepatitis, α-fetoprotein or other typical risk factors for HCC usually are absent. At

histology, the lesions consist of large eosinophilic, polygonal neoplastic cells that are arranged in sheets, cords, or trabeculae and are separated by parallel sheets of fibrous tissue (ie, lamellae). Vascular invasion occurs in less than 5% of cases. Regional adenopathy may be present in 50% to 70% of patients, and distant metastases are uncommon (20%). At MR imaging, fibrolamellar carcinomas are hypointense on T1-weighted images, hyperintense on T2-weighted images, and show heterogeneous enhancement.

In cirrhotic livers, HCC should be distinguished from the so-called "early enhancing hepatic lesions" (EHLs). In a recent study, 75

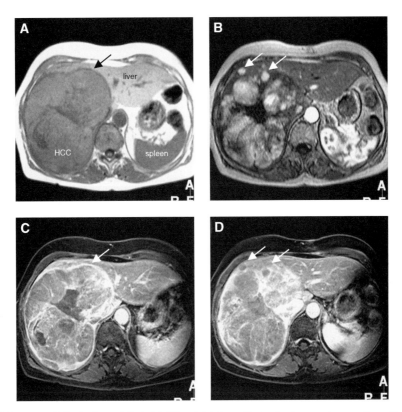

Fig. 17. HCC in a noncirrhotic liver. (*A*) Axial T1-weighted gradient-echo image shows a large liver lesion with predominantly low signal intensity that is surrounded by a thick tumor capsule (*arrow*). (*B*) Axial two-dimensional T1-weighted gradient-echo image in the arterial phase shows intense heterogeneous enhancement of the HCC with enhancement of at least two satellite nodules (*arrows*). (*C*) Axial MR T1-weighted gradient-echo image in the delayed phase shows wash-out of contrast with enhancement of the thick tumor capsule (*arrow*). (*D*) At a slightly lower anatomic level, the ruptured tumor capsule with the satellite nodules (*arrows*) with wash-out of contrast is visible. Note that the liver has a smooth contour and parenchyma with normal homogenous enhancement. The spleen also is a normal size. The lesion was resected and proven to be HCC at pathology. A biopsy from the liver showed no evidence of cirrhosis.

(36%) of 208 patients showed 158 EHLs [41]. Most EHLs were round or oval, whereas others were wedge-shaped, geographic, or triangular. Such lesions should be followed with imaging to exclude high-grade dysplastic nodules and small HCC. Small EHLs that show no interval growth or disappear most likely are vascular shunts or pseudolesions. Budd Chiari nodules often are multiple, may show intense homogeneous enhancement in the arterial phase, and become almost isointense with the surrounding parenchyma in the later phases.

MR imaging versus other modalities

A systematic review of the current literature shows that the sensitivity of MR imaging is between 80% and 100% [22,25,32,42,43] for focal liver lesions, that of CT is 53% to 87% [22–24,30,35,42,44], and that of CT arterio-portography (CTAP) is 87% to 100% [23,30,32]. The specificity of MR imaging and CT was comparable (up to 96%), whereas CTAP had a much lower specificity (~80%), mainly because of the false positive findings that are caused by pseudolesions and the presence of benign lesions. At the authors' hospitals, the state-of-the-art MR imaging protocol for evaluation of the liver is based on T1-weighted, T2-weighted, and dynamic gadolinium-enhanced two-dimensional or three-dimensional spoiled gradient-echo sequences. Imaging with specific contrast media is performed in selected cases. Recent studies show that SPIO-enhanced MR imaging has a better diagnostic performance (higher areas-under-the-curve) than CT [30,35], whereas gadolinium-enhanced MR imaging has a better diagnostic performance than SPIO-enhanced MR imaging for focal liver lesions, including small HCC (<2 cm) [24,45]. A recent comparative study concluded that the sensitivity and specificity of positron emission tomography (PET) for the detection of primary and secondary liver lesions are superior to ultrasound and CT, but not MR imaging. PET has a limited spatial resolution compared with CT and MR imaging, and therefore, most likely will play a role in the exclusion of extrahepatic disease.

Summary

In summary, MR imaging is superior to other imaging modalities, including CT, for the work-up of liver masses. The current challenge is whether the superior performance of MR imaging translates into a beneficial effect on patient management, disease outcome, and health care costs. New MR sequences, phased-array surface coils, and tissue-specific MR contrast agents suggest that MR imaging may exceed further the diagnostic ability of CT.

References

[1] Karhunen PJ. Benign hepatic tumours and tumour-like conditions in men. J Clin Pathol 1986;39:183–8.

[2] Schwartz LH, Gandras EJ, Colangelo SM, et al. Prevalence and importance of small hepatic lesions found at CT in patients with cancer. Radiology 1999;210:71–4.

[3] Francis IR, Cohen RH, McNulty NJ, et al. Multidetector CT of the liver and hepatic neoplasms: effect of multiphasic imaging on tumor conspicuity and vascular enhancement. AJR Am J Roentgenol 2003;180:1217–24.

[4] Haider MA, Amital MM, Rappaport DC, et al. Multi-detector row helical CT in preoperative assessment of small (≤1.5 cm) liver metastases: is thinner collimation better? Radiology 2002;225:137–42.

[5] Valls C, Andia E, Sanchez A, et al. Hepatic metastases from colorectal cancer: preoperative detection and assessment of resectability with helical CT. Radiology 2001;218:55–60.

[6] La Vecchia C, Lucchini F, Franceschi S, et al. Trends in mortality from primary liver cancer in Europe. Eur J Cancer 2000;36:909–15.

[7] Yoon SS, Tanabe TK. Surgical treatment and other regional treatments for colorectal cancer liver metastases. Oncologist 1999;4:197–208.

[8] Kim YK, Kim CS, Lee YH, et al. Comparison of superparamagnetic iron oxide-enhanced and gadobenade dimeglumine-enhanced dynamic MRI for detection of small hepatocellular carcinomas. AJR Am J Roentgenol 2004;182:1217–23.

[9] Hussain SM, Semelka RC, Mitchell DG. MR imaging of hepatocellular carcinoma. Magn Reson Imaging Clin N Am 2002;10:31–5.

[10] Semelka RC, Shoenut JP, Greenberg HM, et al. The liver. In: Semelka RC, Shoenut JP, editors. MRI of the Abdomen with CT correlation. New York: Raven Press; 1993. p. 13–41.

[11] Semelka RC, Hussain SM, Marcos HB, et al. Biliary hamartomas: solitary and multiple lesions shown on current MR techniques including gadolinium enhancement. J Magn Reson Imaging 1999;10:196–201.

[12] Semelka RC. Letter of response. Radiology 2001;219:299–300.

[13] Hussain SM, Terkivatan T, Zondervan PE, et al. Focal nodular hyperplasia: a spectrum of findings at the state-of-the-art MR imaging, ultrasound, CT and pathology. Radiographics 2004;24:3–19.

[14] McFarland EG, Mayo-Smith WW, Saini S, et al. Hepatic hemangiomas and malignant tumors: improved differentiation with heavily T2-weighted conventional spin-echo MR imaging. Radiology 1994;193:43–7.

[15] Mitchell DG, Saini S, Weinreb J, et al. Hepatic metastases and cavernous hemangiomas: distinction with standard- and triple-dose gadoteridol-enhanced MR imaging. Radiology 1994;193:49–57.

[16] Semelka RC, Shoenut JP, Kroeker MA, et al. Focal liver disease: comparison of dynamic contrast-enhanced CT and T2-weighted fat-suppressed, FLASH, and dynamic gadolinium-enhanced MR imaging at 1.5 T. Radiology 1992;184:687–94.

[17] Semelka RC, Brown ED, Ascher SM, et al. Hepatic hemangiomas: a multi-institutional study of appearance on T2-weighted and serial gadolinium-enhanced gradient-echo MR images. Radiology 1994;192:401–6.

[18] Hamm B, Thoeni RF, Gould RG, et al. Focal liver lesions: characterization with nonenhanced and dynamic contrast material-enhanced MR imaging. Radiology 1994;190:417–23.

[19] Whitney WS, Herfkens RJ, Jeffrey RB, et al. Dynamic breath-hold multiplanar spoiled gradient-recalled MR imaging with gadolinium enhancement for differentiating hepatic hemangiomas from malignancies at 1.5 T. Radiology 1993;189:863–70.

[20] Jeong MG, Yu JS, Kim KW. Hepatic cavernous hemangioma: temporal peritumoral enhancement during multiphase dynamic MR imaging. Radiology 2000;216:692–7.

[21] Choi BI, Han MC, Park JH, et al. Giant cavernous hemangioma of the liver: CT and MR imaging in 10 cases. AJR Am J Roentgenol 1989;152:1221–1226.

[22] Bluemke DA, Paulson EK, Choti MA, et al. Detection of hepatic lesions in candidates for surgery: comparison of ferumoxides-enhanced MR

imaging and dual-phase helical CT. AJR 2000; 175:1653–8.

[23] Jang H-J, Lim JH, Lee SJ, et al. Hepatocellular carcinoma: are combined CT during arterial portography and CT hepatic arteriography in addition to triple-phase helical CT all necessary for preoperative evaluation? Radiology 2000;215:373–80.

[24] Kim T, Federle MP, Baron RL, et al. Discrimination of small hepatic hemangiomas from hypervascular malignant tumors smaller than 3 cm with three-phase helical CT. Radiology 2001;219:699–706.

[25] Reimer P, Jahnke N, Fiebich M, et al. Hepatic lesion detection and characterization: value of nonenhanced MR imaging. Superparamagnetic iron oxide-enhanced MR imaging, and spiral CT—ROC analysis. Radiology 2000;217:152–8.

[26] Semelka RC, Shoenut JP, Ascher SM, et al. Solitary hepatic metastasis: comparison of dynamic contrast-enhanced CT and MR imaging with fat-suppressed T2-weighted, breath-hold T1-weighted FLASH, and dynamic gadolinium-enhanced FLASH sequences. J Magn Reson Imaging 1994;4:319–23.

[27] Larson RE, Semelka RC, Bagley AS, et al. Hypervascular malignant liver lesions: comparison of various MR imaging pulse sequences and dynamic CT. Radiology 1994;192:393–9.

[28] Outwater E, Tomaszewski JE, Daly JM, et al. Hepatic colorectal metastases: correlation of MR imaging and pathologic appearance. Radiology 1991;180: 327–32.

[29] Penna C, Nordlinger B. Surgery of liver metastases from colorectal cancer: new promises. Br Med Bull 2002;64:127–40.

[30] Schmidt J, Strotzer M, Fraunhofer S, et al. Intraoperative ultrasonography versus helical computed tomography and computed tomography with arterioportography in diagnosing colorectal liver metastases: lesion-by-lesion analysis. World J Surg 2000; 24:43–8.

[31] Semelka RC, Schlund JF, Molina PL, et al. Malignant liver lesions: comparison of spiral CT arterial portography and MR imaging for diagnostic accuracy, cost, and effect on patient management. J Magn Reson Imaging 1996;1:39–43.

[32] Semelka RC, Cance WG, Marcos HB, et al. Liver metastases: comparison of current MR techniques and spiral CT during arterial portography for detection in 20 surgically staged cases. Radiology 1999; 213:86–91.

[33] Seneterre E, Taorel P, Bouvier Y, et al. Detection of hepatic metastases: ferumoxides-enhanced MR imaging versus unenhanced MR imaging and CT during arterio-portography. Radiology 1996;200:785–92.

[34] Soyer P, de Givry SC, Gueye C, et al. Detection of focal hepatic lesions with MR imaging: prospective comparison of T2-weighted fast spin-echo with and without fat suppression, T2-weighted breath-hold fast spin-echo, and gadolinium chelate-enhanced 3D gradient-recalled imaging. AJR Am J Roentgenol 1996;166:1115–21.

[35] Ward J, Naik KS, Guthrie IA, et al. Comparison of MR imaging after the administration of superparamagnetic iron oxide with dual-phase CT by using alternative-free response operating characteristic analysis. Radiology 1999;210:459–66.

[36] Semelka RC, Hussain SM, Marcos HB, et al. Perilesional enhancement of hepatic metastases: correlation between MR imaging and histopathologic findings—initial observations. Radiology 2000;215: 89–94.

[37] Hussain SM, Zondervan PE, IJzermans JN, et al. Benign versus malignant hepatic nodules: MR imaging findings with pathologic correlation. RadioGraphics 2002;22:1023–36.

[38] Grazioli L, Federle MP, Brancatelli G, et al. Hepatic adenomas: imaging and pathologic findings. Radiographics 2001;21:877–92.

[39] International Working Party. Terminology of nodular hepatocellular lesions. Hepatology 1995;22: 983–93.

[40] Choi BI, Lee JK, Han JK. Imaging of intraductal and hilar cholangiocarcinoma. Abdom Imaging 2004;29:548–57.

[41] Shimizu A, Ito K, Koike S, et al. Cirrhosis or chronic hepatitis: evaluation of small ($\leq$2-cm) early-enhancing hepatic lesions with serial contrast-enhanced dynamic MR imaging. Radiology 2003; 226:550–5.

[42] Bohm B, Voth M, Geoghegan J, et al. Impact of PET on strategy in liver resection for primary and secondary liver tumors. J Cancer Res Clin Oncol 2004;130: 266–72.

[43] Coulam CH, Chan FP, Li KC. Can a multiphasic contrast-enhanced three-dimensional fast spoiled gradient-recalled echo sequence be sufficient for liver MR imaging? AJR Am J Roentgenol 2002;178: 335–41.

[44] Laghi A, Iannaccone R, Rossi P, et al. Hepatocellular carcinoma: detection with triple-phase multidetector row helical CT in patients with chronic hepatitis. Radiology 2003;226:543–9.

[45] Kim M-J, Kim JH, Chung J-J, et al. Focal hepatic lesions: detection and characterization with combination gadolinium- and superparamagnetic iron oxide-enhanced MR imaging. Radiology 2003;228: 719–26.

ELSEVIER
SAUNDERS

Magn Reson Imaging Clin N Am
13 (2005) 277–293

MAGNETIC
RESONANCE
IMAGING CLINICS
of North America

MR Imaging of Diffuse Liver Diseases

Raman Danrad, MD, Diego R. Martin, MD, PhD*

*Department of Radiology, Emory University School of Medicine,
1365 Clifton Road NE, Atlanta, GA 30322, USA*

It is the objective of all cross-sectional imaging techniques to have the ability to evaluate the anatomic configuration of normal and abnormal tissues. In addition, it has become increasingly evident that MR imaging can demonstrate normal and pathologic processes that represent tissue cellular and intracellular architecture, and intracellular processes. Using intravenously injected contrast agent can provide further information regarding the vessels that perfuse normal and abnormal tissues, in regards to the origin of the vessels, the number and size of vessels, and the integrity of the vessel walls. Although CT and ultrasound have some of the abilities that are found in MR imaging, the examples that are discussed in this article show applications of MR imaging of the liver that are uniquely suited to MR; the combination of different sequences that make up a routine MR examination are capable of elucidating important and common disease processes and MR is an evolving anatomic and molecular imaging tool with the capacity to allow realization of the aim to have techniques that represent noninvasive pathology assessment.

The routine MR imaging examination of the liver should use a combination of single shot T2-weighted (T2W) and breath-hold T1-weighted (T1W) images, and include gadolinium enhancement with acquisition of multiple phases. MR provides superior characterization of liver masses than CT, and multiphase gadolinium enhancement, including a properly timed arterial phase, is

critical. The T1W precontrast images must include in-phase and out-of-phase acquisitions to assess hepatic lipid or iron content, and dynamically enhanced postgadolinium images. Timing of the arterial phase images also is critical for demonstration of acute hepatitis. The timing of the venous and equilibrium phase images are less critical, and are important for grading more severe acute hepatitis, demonstration of fibrosis, and for delineating vascular abnormalities. In cirrhosis, dynamic postgadolinium images are critical for detection and characterization of regenerative or dysplastic nodules and hepatocellular carcinoma (HCC). The same sequences that are useful for liver evaluation provide a comprehensive evaluation of all of the soft tissues of the abdomen, and allow depiction of most of the important diseases, and thus, facilitate use of a universal protocol for abdominal imaging.

The following sections discuss MR imaging sequences that are used for the evaluation of diffuse liver diseases, including processes that lead to abnormal lipid metabolization, iron deposition disease, and perfusion abnormalities that are related to inflammation, fibrosis, vascular occlusion or infarction, and hemorrhage.

Fatty liver

Lipid accumulation in hepatocytes can occur as a result of impaired liver function secondary to a variety of etiologies [1]. In the United States, fatty liver can be detected in more than 20% of the population; the most common association with fatty liver is obesity. There has been further association of fatty liver with development of hepatitis that results from nonalcoholic acute

---
* Corresponding author.
E-mail address: diego_martin@emoryhealthcare.org
(D.R. Martin).

steatohepatitis (NASH), and potential progression to cirrhosis. In the setting of liver transplantation, a living related donor liver assessment must include evaluation for the presence of fatty infiltration; this is considered a contraindication to transplantation when severe and can lead to failure of the transplant.

Abnormal lipid accumulation in liver can be detected on MR imaging [2–6], and can be evaluated on the basis of comparing liver signal on spoiled gradient echo (SGE) images that are acquired in-phase and out-of-phase. Hydrogen protons in a voxel that contains 100% fat will precess 220 Hz to 230 Hz slower than a voxel that is made up of 100% water, at 1.5 T. That means that every 4.4 milliseconds the fat protons will migrate 360° and regain in-phase orientation relative to water protons, whereas at 2.2 milliseconds, or at half this time, the fat and water protons will be 180° out-of-phase. Current generation MR systems have incorporated dual-echo

breath-hold SGE sequences that can acquire two sets of k-space filled to obtain two sets of images —one set in-phase, the other out-of-phase—with spatially matched slices. Liver containing lipid results in image voxels with a physical mixture of water and lipid, which when imaged out-of-phase, results in phase cancellation and diminished signal (Fig. 1). Spleen does not accumulate fat, and therefore, can be used as a control against which liver signal can be assessed as a ratio to test for relative diminishment in liver signal on out-of-phase images. Spleen signal can change as a result of iron deposition, however, and use of kidney or skeletal muscle within the image may be more reliable for assessment of relative liver signal changes between in- and out-of-phase images. Fat accumulation in liver can be diffuse (see Fig. 1), diffuse with focal sparing (Fig. 2), or focal. Typical regions that are affected by focal fatty accumulation occur around the falciform ligament, gallbladder fossa (see Fig. 2), and

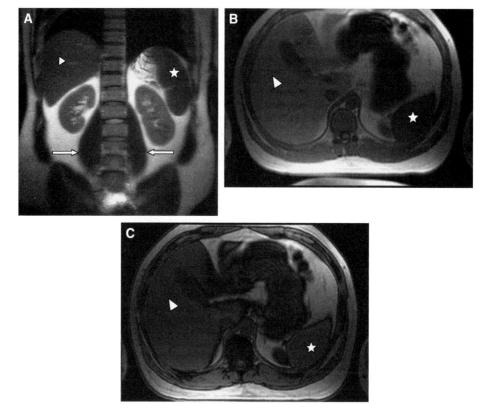

Fig. 1. Fatty infiltration of the liver. Normal liver has signal midway between muscle and spleen. In this patient, coronal T2-weighted single shot fast spin echo image (*A*) shows liver signal (*arrowhead*) that is greater than psoas muscle (*arrows*), and abnormally greater than spleen (*star*). Liver signal diffusely diminishes in signal intensity comparing in-phase (*B*) with out-of-phase (*C*) images of liver, in relation to spleen and muscle.

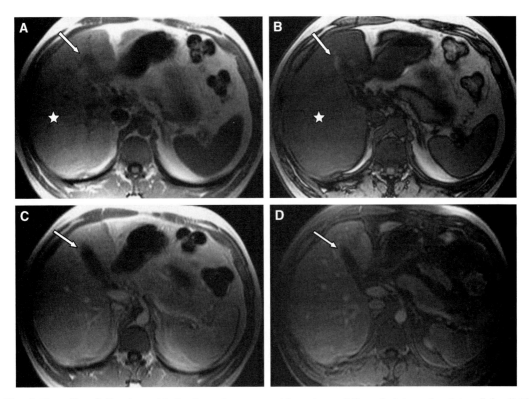

Fig. 2. Fatty liver infiltration with focal sparing: geographic regions of liver that have less intracellular lipid accumulation. Two patients are shown with different etiologies for focal fatty sparing. In a patient who has fatty liver and physiologic sparing around the gallbladder fossa (*A–D*), axial breath-hold in-phase SGE image (*A*) shows normal liver (*star*) and gall bladder fossa (*arrow*). On out-of-phase SGE imaging (*B*), there is marked reduction of liver signal which indicates fatty infiltration. The region surrounding the gallbladder fossa shows no signal drop (*arrow*) and appears higher in signal than adjacent fatty liver, which represents focal fatty sparing. (*C*) Postgadolinium in-phase SGE (repetition time [TR], 180 milliseconds; echo time [TE] 4.2 milliseconds) shows normal signal enhancement around the gallbladder fossa (*arrow*). (*D*) On three-dimensional volumetric interpolated breath-hold examination SGE postgadolinium imaging (TR, 3.7 milliseconds; TE, 1.7 milliseconds) shows apparent increased enhancement surrounding the gall bladder fossa (*arrow*). This perception results from postgadolinium imaging using a sequence with out-of-phase TE, and shows the possible confounding effect in the setting of variable fatty accumulation in the liver. In another patient (*E–G*), diffuse fatty infiltration is demonstrated throughout the liver parenchyma (*E–G, star*) on comparison of in-phase (*E*) and out-of-phase (*F*) axial SGE images. A mass (*E–G, arrow*) shows preservation of signal on out-of-phase imaging (*F*), and appears high in signal compared with fatty liver, which indicates focal fatty sparing within the mass. The mass has low T1-weighted signal relative to normal liver on in-phase imaging (*E*), and demonstrates peripheral interrupted nodular enhancement on postgadolinium in-phase imaging (*G, arrow*) which is typical of a benign hemangioma.

around the inferior vena cava. One possible explanation is that these areas of liver are prone to irritation or stimulation which results in local changes in carbohydrate–lipid metabolism. Contrast-enhanced CT and standard ultrasound are nonspecific and less sensitive for assessment of fatty liver, and can confuse irregularly accumulated lipid with a mass [5–14]. Fatty liver can lead to reduced CT density, and diminish contrast between a low density mass and adjacent liver which makes the mass less conspicuous [15–17].

Iron deposition disease

Iron can accumulate within the liver through two basic mechanisms: accumulation within hepatocytes through normal metabolic chelation mechanisms, or through uptake within the phagocytic Kupffer cells which represents part of the reticuloendothelial system (RES) [18,19]. Serum iron and transferrin saturation are correlated poorly with the degree of iron overload. Although serum ferritin can be used to estimate body iron stores, a variety of etiologies can lead

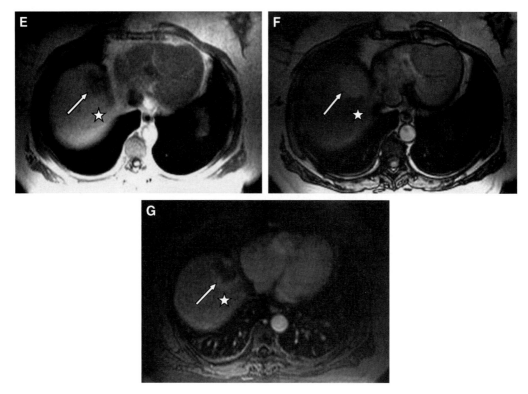

Fig. 2 (*continued*)

to elevation of serum levels, independent of total body iron.

In primary hemochromatosis, the defect seems to be due to inappropriately regulated small bowel increased uptake of dietary iron which results in excess total body iron accumulation [18,19]. Hepatocytes chelate the iron that accumulates within the cytosol. Pancreas also has chelation mechanisms within acinar cells, and can accumulate excess intracellular iron [20]; however, to some degree, iron accumulation can occur in most tissues, typically as a late feature that occurs after hepatic stores have reached high levels [21]. Important examples include the pituitary and heart, where this can result in impaired pituitary function, fatal cardiac arrhythmias, or congestive heart failure. Patients who present with a first-time diagnosis of primary hemochromatosis with the combined findings of elevated liver and cardiac iron deposition and congestive heart failure, have a poor prognosis with a 6-month life expectancy [22,23]. There has been rapid recent development of understanding of the genetic basis of this disease, and that there is a defective genetic hemochromatosis (GH) gene.

The defective GH gene seems to represent the most common inherited genetically communicated disease among people of European descent, and has approximately a 1 in 40 occurrence among Americans, with a 1 in 400 incidence of homozygosity [22,23]. The phenotypic expression of this disease is more complicated, however, and seems to follow a polygenetic penetrance pattern. An inexpensive genetic test is clinically available that could be used for screening purposes.

In secondary hemochromatosis, iron overload can occur secondary to excess red cell turnover from exogenously derived red cells as a result of blood transfusion therapy; this is seen in patients who have underlying red cell or bone marrow abnormalities, such as thalassemia, mastocytosis, or myelofibrosis. Alternatively, endogenously derived excess iron from red cell turnover can result from polycythemia rubra vera, from myoglobin in rhabdomyolysis, or from siderosis that is related to alcoholic liver disease. In secondary hemochromatosis, the mechanism of iron accumulation is different than in primary hemochromatosis. It results from increased uptake of iron that is derived from hemoglobin that arises from dying or abnormal red cells that is taken up by the RES; this leads to iron accumulation in Kupffer cells within liver sinusoids. Similarly, the splenic RES phagocytoses abnormal red cells and actively accumulates iron from hemoglobin. In contrast to primary hemochromatosis, the pancreas typically does not accumulate iron. Clinical significance of hemochromatosis includes the observation that many patients develop cirrhosis and approximately 25% of patients develop HCC. These processes also may be evaluated by MR imaging of the liver.

Liver biopsies have been used for biochemical determination of liver iron overload and have been used as the basis for therapy management in patients who are treated by periodic phlebotomy and iron chelation therapy; however, this method has bleeding risks that are associated with the invasive procedure, and is susceptible to sampling error in patients who have heterogeneous iron deposition in the liver. The sensitivity of CT is insufficient, with a minimum threshold for liver iron detection that is more than five times greater than the normal liver iron load, particularly in cases with fatty liver.

MR imaging is sensitive to iron concentration in the liver because of the paramagnetic properties of iron. This results in T2 or T2-star affects that diminish the signal intensity on single shot breath-hold T2 images (Fig. 3), and on breath-hold T1W multiecho SGE images (Fig. 4) [24–30]. Quantitative assessment of liver iron concentration was demonstrated using SGE and spin echo sequences, and relied on measurements of T2-star and T2 decay. Coronal breath-hold T2W single shot fast spin echo images—which should be obtained as part of a routine abdominal MR examination—are useful for rapid visual evaluation because they provide slices that include liver, psoas muscle, and spleen within the same image (see Fig. 3). Normally, liver signal intensity is near the midpoint in between the lower signal intensity of muscle, and the higher signal intensity of spleen. In iron overload disease, the liver signal intensity becomes as low or lower than skeletal muscle. In secondary iron overload, spleen similarly becomes dark. In cases in which there is bone marrow abnormality, such as in myelofibrosis (see Fig. 3), normal high signal marrow fat becomes replaced with low signal cellular marrow hypertrophy and sclerosis. Chronic iron overload can lead to cirrhosis, and increase risk for HCC; these complications can be assessed on MR imaging [31]. For more sensitive and potentially quantitative

noninvasive measurement of liver iron, T2-star and T2 decay rate measurements can be performed [32]. T2-star decay is a measure of how quickly protons lose phase coherence without the use of refocusing pulses. T2 decay is a measure of proton dephasing rates after application of refocusing pulses, and measures only dephasing affects that are not correctable. Generally, the T2-star decay rate is more sensitive to lower levels of intracellular iron accumulation. Intracellular iron accumulation can cause localized magnetic field distortion that leads to susceptibility affects that result in more rapid loss of phase-dependent signal. One method that is used to detect this affect is based on multiecho gradient echo imaging to measure T2-star decay, whereas a spin echo single shot or echo-planar technique with increasing echo times (TEs) may be used for T2 decay measurements. When performing imaging that is dedicated to iron measurement, a series of gradient echo images are acquired with increasing increments of TE. As the TE lengthens, the proton dephasing leads to progressive increased loss of signal intensity; this process was shown to be proportionately increased in relation to intracellular liver iron concentration. When performing a dedicated T2-star analysis of liver iron, the TEs may be selected to correspond to in-phase echoes to avoid potential out-of-phase affects from fat; this is a potential spurious affect in the setting of fatty liver infiltration. At a minimum, however, routine imaging of the abdomen and liver should include a dual-echo SGE acquisition (see Fig. 3) that can be used in conjunction with the coronal single shot T2. The longer second echo image (TE = 4.4 milliseconds) should show darkening of the liver compared with the shorter echo image (TE = 2.2 milliseconds) in the setting of elevated liver iron concentration (Fig. 5). The sensitivity to liver iron may be increased on SGE imaging by increasing the TE to include, for example, echoes at 8.8 milliseconds and 13.2 milliseconds. If only routine shortest possible dual echo out-of-phase (TE = 2.2 milliseconds) and in-phase (TE = 4.4 milliseconds) imaging is used, the relative sensitivity of the single shot spin echo technique is more sensitive. With this approach, demonstration of low liver signal on single shot spin echo alone would indicate a lower liver iron concentration; demonstration of low liver signal on single shot spin echo and on the longer echo dual echo SGE indicate higher liver iron burden. Other investigators showed that liver iron concentration may be calculated and that noninvasive

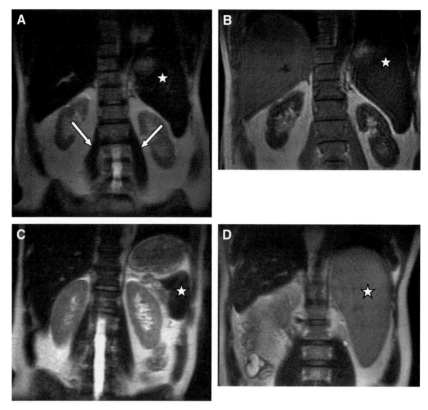

Fig. 3. Iron deposition disease. Different patterns of iron deposition are shown in three different patients. (*A, B*) A patient who underwent a bone marrow transplant and has received multiple blood transfusions shows abnormally low signal intensity of the liver and spleen (*star*) on T2-weighted single shot spin echo image (*A*) as referenced to psoas muscle (*arrows*). This finding is less apparent on short echo gradient echo (repetition time, 180 milliseconds; TE, 4.2 milliseconds) image (*B*). This demonstrates that using these imaging parameters, single shot echo train imaging is more sensitive to the T2* effects of paramagnetic intracellular iron than the gradient echo sequence. (*C*) A second patient shows diminished liver and spleen signal intensity on coronal T2-weighted single shot echo train image which is consistent with hemosiderosis from repeated blood transfusions related to myelofibrosis. In this case, the normally high-signal fatty bone marrow has been replaced by myelofibrosis and red marrow expansion that resulted in diffusely low bone marrow signal. (*D*) Another patient who has hemochromatosis demonstrates diminished signal that only affects the liver, and not the spleen (*star*), with splenomegaly secondary to cirrhosis and portal venous hypertension, a complication of hemochromatosis.

tissue iron concentration may be feasible. This represents the only noninvasive technique that is available for liver iron quantitation, and could be used, for example, for following patients who have hemochromatosis who are on therapy and minimize the need for liver biopsy. Although it is tempting to suggest the use of MR for GH screening, it was noted that the recent development of a genetic marker test is accurate and inexpensive. Regardless, the ability to determine tissue iron concentration quantitatively by MR is a clinically valuable test, and there are attempts to develop useful methodology for routine clinical imaging. In one study, T2W imaging was

performed and ratios between liver and skeletal muscle were used to develop a calculation that corresponded to the quantitative measurement of liver iron [32]. It showed a sensitivity of 89% and specificity of 80% for detection of liver iron in excess of 60 μmol/g using a prescribed liver:-muscle ratio. Normal liver iron concentration is less than 36 μmol/g. In another landmark study, a series of four GRE and one spin echo sequence was developed to provide a series of images—each sensitive over a different range of iron concentration—to develop an algorithm for iron quantitation. This method could detect iron levels that were greater than 85 μmol/g with a positive

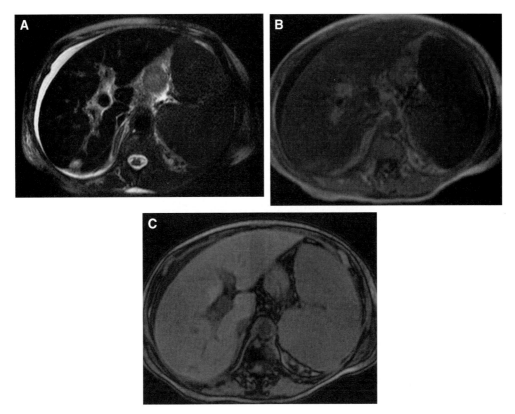

Fig. 4. Iron deposition disease in liver and spleen on gradient echo imaging in a patient who has chronic liver disease, splenomegaly, and hemosiderosis. (*A*) Axial T2-weighted single shot spin echo fat-suppressed image shows that the liver and spleen signal is diminished markedly compared with paraspinal muscles. Ascites is noted around the liver margins. T1-weighted dual echo TE 2.2 milliseconds (*B*) and TE 4.4 milliseconds (*C*) single breath-hold acquisition demonstrates a conspicuous diminishment of liver and spleen signal intensity on the longer echo image.

predictive value of 100%, or levels that were less than 40 μmol/g with a negative predictive value of 100% [33].

Acute hepatitis

Inflammatory liver disease can result from several etiologies, including idiopathic, drug-induced, viral, alcoholic, and gallstone bile duct obstruction [31,34,35]. It was noted that MR imaging may be sensitive to acute hepatitis [36]. On MR imaging, the most sensitive images are the postgadolinium breath-hold SGE images that are acquired during arterial phase (Fig. 6) [31,36]. In a recent report, this abnormal enhancement becomes more marked and can persist into the venous and delayed phases as the severity of disease increases, and can resolve in cases when the hepatitis resolves [36]. Furthermore, the

arterial phase timing critically determines sensitivity to mild acute hepatitis. By performing SGE imaging every 5 seconds after administration of gadolinium in a patient who has mild acute hepatitis, the authors found that irregular liver enhancement was detectable only during the time when the portal veins were filling with contrast, and the hepatic veins were unenhanced. In cases of mild hepatitis, images that are acquired before portal venous filling were too early, and images that were acquired when the hepatic veins were filled were too late. For most patients, the optimal timing falls between 18 seconds and 22 seconds after initiation of the gadolinium injection into an antecubital vein, administered at 2 mL per second, followed by a 20-mL saline wash-in bolus. The parameters for the breath-hold SGE acquisition also must be taken into account, with the above timing based upon a gradient echo sequence that uses linear ordering of k-space—which fills central

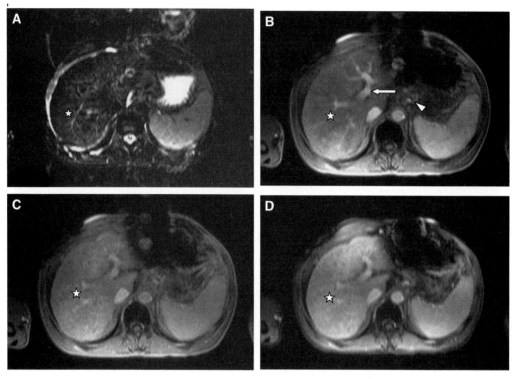

Fig. 5. Cirrhosis. Axial breath-hold T2-weighted single shot fast spin echo (*A*), and breath-hold T1-weighted SGE arterial (*B*), venous (*C*), and fat-suppressed delayed phase (*D*) images through the liver. T2-weighted image (*A, star*) shows irregular increased signal with areas of linear and reticular pattern toward the periphery (*B, star*); these indicate areas of edema that correspond to coarse linear and fine reticular patterns of enhancement that progressively increase in venous (*C*) and delayed phase (*D*) images. These are consistent with areas of late enhancing fibrosis. Numerous tiny parenchymal liver nodules that measure 3 mm to 4 mm enhance mildly in the venous phase (*B, star*) and persist into the delayed phase (*D, star*); these are consistent with small regenerative nodules. Portal hypertension manifests in portal vein dilation and formation of paraesophageal varices (*B, arrowhead*).

k-space in the middle of the acquisition time—with a total acquisition time of 18 seconds. If, for example, the acquisition scan time is decreased by 4 seconds to 14 seconds, then the delay time between the start of the injection and the start of the acquisition should be increased by 2 seconds (eg, from 20 seconds to 22 seconds). This will ensure that the center lines of k-space are filled at the peak of the hepatic arterial tissue perfusion phase. Conversely, if the acquisition time is increased by 4 seconds to 22 seconds scan time, the delay should be decreased by 2 seconds to 18 seconds. The authors have found that there is an approximately 3- to 4-second window before and after the optimal peak, beyond which an abnormality that is seen only during the arterial phase of enhancement may become inconspicuous.

It should be emphasized that no other imaging technique has been shown sensitive for detection of acute hepatitis, and that previously, we relied on serum liver enzyme levels, in combination with percutaneous liver biopsy. MR imaging could be used as a diagnostic aid in patients who have equivocal liver enzyme elevation and nonspecific symptoms, and in patients who present with fatty infiltration. Findings that are suggestive of acute hepatitis (seen as irregular arterial phase gadolinium enhancement) in the setting of fatty liver (seen as signal drop on out-of-phase gradient echo images) are consistent with steatohepatitis and raise the possible diagnosis of NASH. NASH is a recently recognized disease entity that is believed to represent a hepatitis that is related directly to excess intracellular fat accumulation within hepatocytes. This disease has a strong association with obesity and has a risk of progression to chronic hepatitis and cirrhosis. Given that obesity is an epidemic in the United States, the health

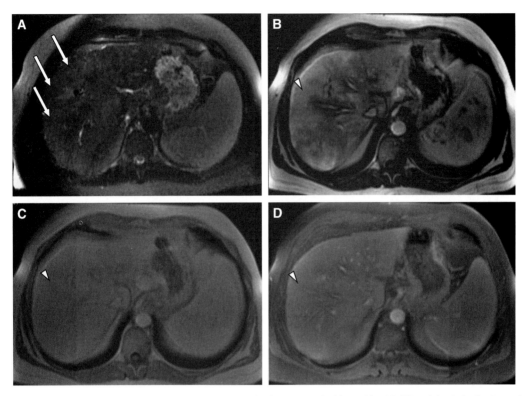

Fig. 6. Findings related to acute hepatitis in a patient who has acute viral hepatitis. (*A*) T2-weighted single shot spin echo image shows patchy hyperintensity (*arrows*) in the peripheral right lobe. (*B*) Postcontrast gradient echo technique shows patchy peripheral irregular enhancement (*arrowhead*) on 20-second arterial phase image that is due to regions with increased perfusion from hepatic artery. (*C*) 60-second and (*D*) 180-second postcontrast images show patchy enhancement (*arrowhead*) has blended with the adjacent, more normally enhancing liver parenchyma.

concern regarding NASH is significant. MR has greater sensitivity and specificity for detection of fatty liver, and is the only imaging test that is sensitive for milder cases of hepatitis.

Multiple causes of transient hepatic perfusion abnormalities have been described [37–39]; however, in cases that present clinically with right upper quadrant pain and abnormal liver arterial phase perfusion, acute hepatitis should be the major diagnostic consideration. It may be argued that patients who have right upper quadrant abdominal symptoms are examined preferentially by MR imaging over CT. MR imaging has potential relative strengths, in regard to contrast sensitivity, and can provide excellent temporal resolution because of the small contrast volume used, in combination with the acquisition of contrast data for the entire liver over approximately a 4- to 5-second period, usually in the center of a two-dimensional T1W gradient echo sequence using interleaved phase acquisition [40]. The safety

profile of gadolinium agents and nonionizing radiation imaging for a multi-phase examination also are attractive characteristics of MR imaging. A three-dimensional (3D) gradient echo T1W sequence may used here for the arterial or venous phase of the examination, with the same potential advantages of temporal resolution. It is possible that the relative contrast sensitivity may not be as high as for the 3D gradient echo technique, particularly if only thinner slicing reconstructions are used for the 3D technique.

The reasons for heterogeneous liver enhancement in acute hepatitis have not been determined fully. Hypothetically, it may be that the areas of relative arterial phase hyperenhancement represent regions of abnormality. In this case, periportal inflammation may compress differentially the lower pressure portal vein intrahepatic branches and lead to preferential segmental hepatic arterial perfusion. Alternatively, the inflammation may lead to altered vascular regulatory affects, with vasodilation and increased hepatic arterial flow to the involved regions. Pathologic correlation is challenging given that histopathologic correlation lacks the ability to determine pathophysiologic in vivo processes that are involved in hemodynamics, an advantage that is inherent to contrast enhanced imaging.

Chronic hepatitis and cirrhosis

A major complication of chronic hepatitis is cirrhosis [31]. In Western nations, the most common etiology has been alcohol-induced hepatitis; however, viral hepatitis has become the most common cause, and globally, viral hepatitis is the most common association with chronic hepatitis, cirrhosis, and hepatocellular carcinoma.

MR imaging feature of fibrosis that is associated with cirrhosis is progressive enhancement on delayed images (see Fig. 4; Fig. 7) [31]; this results from leakage of gadolinium contrast agent from the intravascular into the interstitial space within the fibrotic regions. The typical patterns of cirrhosis include fine reticular and coarse linear, with the fibrotic bands outlining foci of regenerative nodules (see Figs. 4 and 7). If active hepatitis is present, the fibrotic tissue bands may have edema, and appear high in signal on T2W (see Fig. 4) [31]; the liver tissue may develop irregular patchy areas of enhancement that is seen mostly on the arterial phase images.

Regenerative nodules occur in the setting of cirrhosis [41,42] and represent relatively more normal hepatic parenchyma that derives the major blood supply from the portal venous system. Thus, these nodules maximally enhance during portal venous phase postgadolinium SGE images, and usually are less than 1 cm in diameter [27]. These nodules can accumulate iron, and appear low in signal on SGE T1W and single shot fast spin echo T2W images, with little

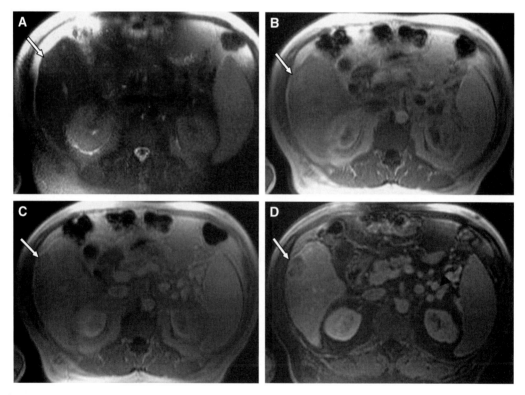

Fig. 7. Hepatocellular carcinoma in a cirrhotic liver. Axial T2-weighted breath-hold fast spin echo (*A*), and gadolinium-enhanced SGE T1-weighted arterial (*B*), venous (*C*), and fat-suppressed delayed phase (*D*) images though the liver. A mass (*arrow*) has a high T2 signal (*A*) and central irregular enhancement on arterial phase imaging (*B*), with rapid wash-out and peripheral capsular enhancement developing in the venous (*C*) and delayed phase (*D*) images. Fine reticular late enhancement pattern in liver represents fibrosis (*D*). Portal hypertension manifests in splenic hilar varices, mild splenic enlargement, and peri-hepatic ascites (*A*).

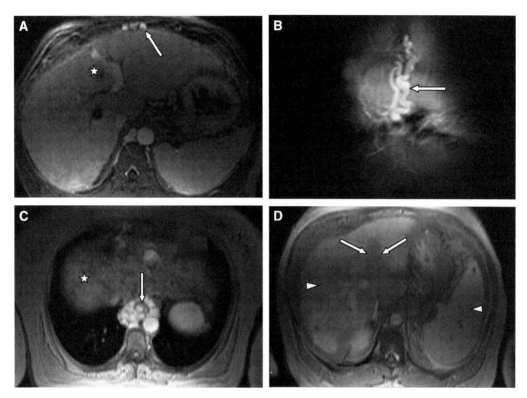

Fig. 8. Venous abnormalities related to complications of chronic liver disease and cirrhosis. Axial (*A*) and coronal (*B*) T1-weighted breath-hold SGE fat-suppressed postgadolinium delayed phase images show recanalized periumbilical vein arising from the left portal vein (*arrow*) and extending to the anterior midline peritoneum. A mass that represents HCC is present (*A, star*). (*C*) Another example of varices demonstrates coarse late enhancing linear and reticular hepatic fibrosis (*star*) which are findings of advanced cirrhosis. This patient presented with esophageal bleeding and prominent varices that encased and lifted the distal esophagus (*arrow*). (*D*) Another patient who has cirrhosis and HCC has marked distension of the left portal vein (*arrows*) and filling with enhancing soft tissue in keeping with vascularized tumor thrombus. Siderotic nodules in the liver and spleen are indicated (*arrowheads*).

enhancement appreciated on postgadolinium SGE images [31].

Dysplastic nodules are premalignant, and are believed to have the potential to transform into progressively higher grades of dysplasia, and finally, into HCC. Dysplastic nodules typically are larger than regenerative nodules, and can be seen to grow over a period of weeks or months. These lesions can show overlap with HCC, and may show mildly elevated T1W signal and low T2W signal. Features that help to distinguish HCC include elevated T2W signal, transient marked arterial phase postgadolinium enhancement, capsular peripheral rim enhancement on venous and equilibrium phase images, and size greater than 2 cm to 3 cm (see Fig. 7). It may be that higher-grade dysplastic nodules overlap more with the HCC features; however, this distinction may be of small clinical significance because the

higher-grade dysplasia has the potential to transform to HCC rapidly.

Portal hypertension may result from obstruction at presinusoidal, sinusoidal, postsinusoidal, or a combination of these sites, and correspond to abnormalities of portal venous, hepatic fibrosis, hepatic venous, or mixed diseases [43]. MR images that are optimal for visualizing changes that are related to portal hypertension are obtained on equilibrium phase SGE images with fat suppression (Fig. 8). In early or mild portal hypertension, MR images show dilation of the portal vein, and possibly splenic vein (see Fig. 8). In more severe and chronic cases, the portal vein can occlude and become thin or inapparent, with the development of multiple, smaller-caliber collaterals seen within the porta hepatis (so-called "cavernous transformation"). Furthermore, porto-systemic collaterals can form and be seen

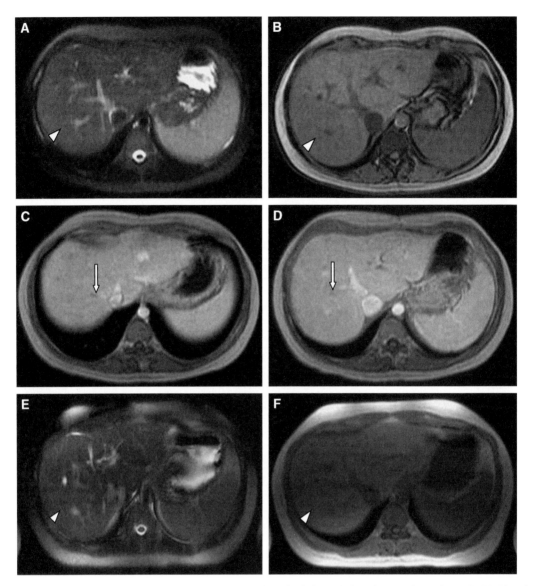

Fig. 9. Budd-Chiari syndrome hepatic segmental venous thrombosis in evolution that was imaged acutely (*A–D*) and after 6 months (*E, F*). (*A*) Axial T2-weignted breath-hold single shot fast spin echo image demonstrates abnormally elevated signal in the right lobe (*arrowhead*). (B) T1-weighted unenhanced breath-hold SGE demonstrates diminished signal in the same distribution (*arrowhead*). (*C, D*) Venous phase gadolinium-enhanced images at two axial levels demonstrate a thrombosed segmental branch of the right hepatic vein (*arrow*). Follow-up imaging in the subacute-chronic stages show diminishment in the elevated signal on T2-weighted imaging (*E* versus *A, arrowhead*), and restoration of T1-weighted signal (*F* versus *B, arrowhead*) that correspond to decreased edema in the hepatic segments that are drained by the involved intrahepatic venous branch. There is development of abnormal patchy increased peripheral enhancement on the arterial phase image (*G, arrowhead*) that becomes more uniform on venous phase (*H*). The thrombosed vessel (*C, D; arrow*) has become inapparent (*H* versus *C, arrow*); this is consistent with collateralization and with altered perfusion to the involved liver segment that likely is related to chronic delayed venous drainage.

as increased number and size of retroperitoneal vessels in the region of the splenic hilum, gastro-hepatic ligament, paraesophageal region (see Fig. 8), and with demonstration of spleno–renal venous connections. Canalization of the perium-bilical vein can be seen as a vessel—sometimes massive—that extends from the left portal vein anteriorly along the falciform ligament toward

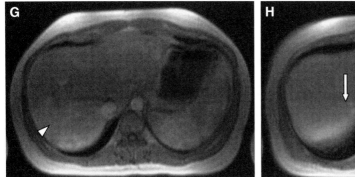
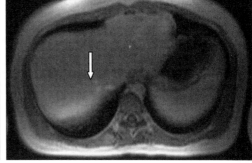

Fig. 9 (*continued*)

the anterior abdominal wall umbilical region (see Fig. 8). Ascites is seen commonly in combination with more advanced portal hypertension as simple uniform high-signal T2W fluid in the free intraperitoneal space.

Budd-Chiari syndrome (hepatic vein thrombosis)

The original description of Budd-Chiari syndrome related to a severe, often fatal, acute form of hepatic vein thrombosis [44]. Currently, Budd-Chiari syndrome is used to describe any form of pathology that is related to hepatic venous thrombosis [44]. Thrombosis within hepatic veins occurs most commonly as a result of hypercoagulable states; occurs more commonly in women; and can be associated with underlying conditions, including pregnancy or post partum state, lupus, sepsis, polycythemia, and neoplasm, particularly HCC.

In Budd-Chiari syndrome, hepatic venous outflow obstruction results in congestion and ischemia that can lead, over time, to atrophy and fibrosis [44]. Depending on degree of involvement, spared segments of liver will undergo compensatory hypertrophy. The caudate lobe characteristically has separate drainage to the inferior vena cava and usually is spared, and commonly can be seen to hypertrophy over time [44]. Hepatic venous drainage is variable, and other segments of liver commonly are spared as well which leads to variable regions of hypertrophy.

The characteristic liver MR imaging pattern (Fig. 9) of Budd-Chiari syndrome in the acute, subacute, and chronic states has been described [44]. In the acute state, central liver shows low T1W, and mildly elevated T2W signal secondary to edema, with irregular increased enhancement in the arterial postgadolinium phase images [44]. In the subacute phase, this pattern of T1W and T2W signal intensity and postgadolinium enhancement is seen to migrate toward the periphery of the liver [44]. In acute and subacute states, hepatic vein thrombosis is visualized best on postgadolinium venous or delayed phase breath-hold SGE images (see Fig. 9). In the chronic phase, visualization of the hepatic vein thrombus may become less apparent; however, there is a characteristic hypertrophy of the caudate lobe that often is massive, as well as hypertrophy of other spared segments [44]. The liver segments that are affected by chronic hepatic venous obstruction show atrophy and fibrosis. Fibrotic regions may show progressively increasing enhancement on delayed postgadolinium images, with regenerative nodules showing higher T1W signal, and intermediate to low T2W signal, with marked enhancement on arterial-venous phase postgadolinium SGE images.

When hepatic venous thrombosis results from direct invasion by tumor, this is related most commonly to HCC. In the case of tumor thrombosis, demonstration of soft tissue enhancement on postgadolinium breath-hold T1W SGE images is diagnostic.

Hepatic congestion due to heart failure

Persistent elevation in central venous pressure secondary to right-side cardiac failure can lead to hepatic congestion with pathologic changes that are seen as nutmeg liver. In chronic cases, some patients go on to develop cirrhosis. On MR imaging, hepatic congestion can be diagnosed on demonstration of the constellation of findings, including cardiac enlargement, dilated hepatic

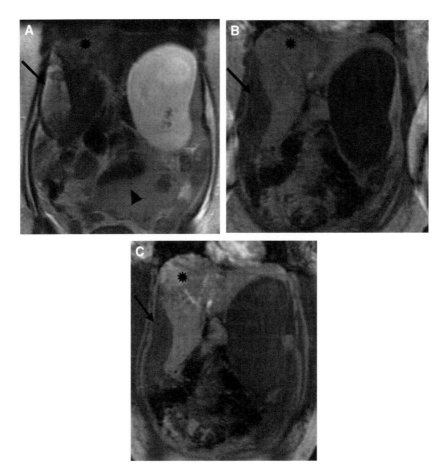

Fig. 10. Post partum woman with toxemia of pregnancy and hepatic infarction and hemorrhage. Coronal breath-hold T2-weighted single shot fast spin echo (*A*) and T1-weighted SGE pre- (*B*) and post-gadolinium (*C*) images show a subcapsular fluid collection (*arrow*) that is consistent with a subcapsular hemorrhage. Extrahepatic hemorrhage is pooling in the left lower quadrant, which is shown as low-signal fluid that surrounds bowel loops (*A, triangle*). Within hepatic parenchyma, a patchy increased focal T2-weighted signal (*A, star*) that is associated with elevated T1-weighted signal on pregadolinium images (*B, star*) is consistent with intrahepatic hemorrhage and edema. This region was noted to enhance progressively on delayed postgadolinium images (*C, star*) and likely represents a vascular leak.

veins, hepatic edema, and irregular postgadolinium hepatic enhancement. In addition, findings of enhancement with a fine and course reticular and linear pattern that develops progressively in more delayed images is consistent with the development of cirrhosis.

Toxemia of pregnancy

Uncontrolled hypertension in late third-trimester pregnancy can be associated with a syndrome that includes hemolytic anemia, elevated liver serum enzymes, and low platelets (HELLP) [45,46]. Liver injury is common in HELLP, as

a result of platelet abnormality and microvascular occlusions in the liver that can lead to ischemic injury and hemorrhage. Pathologically, fibrin deposits are found in the sinusoids, with hemorrhage extending into the subendothelial space. Hemorrhage can extend along the portal triads and form small pools of blood. In more severe cases, the hemorrhage can be more extensive and dissect through the hepatic parenchyma into the subcapsular space, and rupture through the capsule into the free intraperitoneal space (Fig. 10) [45,46]. In severe cases, hemorrhage can be life threatening. Precontrast MR images can show areas of irregular high and low T1W and T2W signal that correspond to areas of edema and blood products

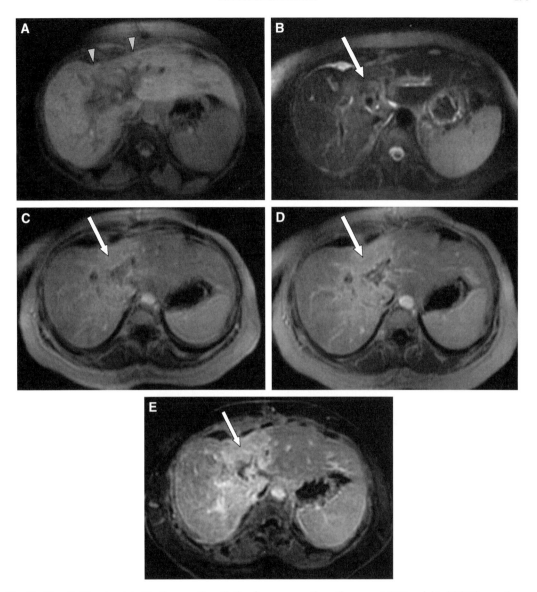

Fig. 11. Hepatic fibrosis related to therapeutic radiation for a pancreatic malignancy. (*A*) T1-weighted SGE image shows a well-demarcated band of liver with decreased signal that involves parts of hepatic segments 4 and 5 corresponding to a radiation portal (*arrowheads*). (B) T2-weighted single shot spin echo image shows mild elevated signal in the same distribution (*arrow*) in keeping with edema. Arterial 20-second (*C*), venous 60-second (*D*), and delayed 3-minute (*E*) postgadolinium enhanced images demonstrate progressive enhancement of the involved region, with evidence of retraction of the overlying capsule, in keeping with fibrosis. The well-delineated margins of involved liver, corresponding to the radiation portal, supports the diagnosis.

(see Fig. 10). MR imaging can provide superb characterization of perfusion abnormalities on dynamically enhanced postgadolinium SGE images, with evidence of active microhemorrhage that is seen as areas of slowly pooled accumulation of gadolinium (see Fig. 10), and characterization of blood products in fluid-filled spaces that is seen as fluid with irregular elevated T1W and variable decreased T2W signal intensity. Ultrasound has been used as a screening tool, but sensitivity and specificity are unknown. CT imaging of liver changes in HELLP have been reported [45,46], but a nonionizing imaging test clearly is preferred in this patient population.

Postradiation fibrosis

When a therapeutic radiation portal includes liver within the exposure field there is a risk of developing postradiation fibrosis. The acute phase is associated with inflammation and edema, and chronic changes include fibrosis and tissue retraction (Fig. 11). The imaging features can be characterized based on abnormal liver signal with distribution following well-delineated linear margins and the margins of the external radiation beam, but not following anatomic liver segments. Acute phase changes show elevated signal on T2W images and low signal on T1W images. Chronic changes are characteristic, and show slightly elevated signal on T2W images, with increased enhancement on arterial phase postgadolinium images that persist and may become more intense on delayed phase. This may be due to the greater susceptibility of the portal venous branches to radiation fibrosis, retraction, and occlusion, with subsequent preferential hepatic arterial supply to the involved hepatic tissue. Hepatic veins also may be affected preferentially and result in impaired and delayed gadolinium outflow. In addition, gadolinium chelate may have increased interstitial distribution in fibrotic tissues as a result of the increased leakiness of blood vessels in the setting of fibrosis. Both factors would contribute to elevated contrast concentration on delayed phase images.

References

[1] Brenner DJ, Elliston CD. Estimated radiation risks potentially associated with full body CT screening. Radiology 2004;232:735–8.

[2] Coates GG, Borrello JA, McFarland EG, et al. Hepatic T2-weighted MRI: a prospective comparison of sequences, including breath-hold, half-Fourier turbo spin echo (HASTE). J Magn Reson Imaging 1998;8:642–9.

[3] Helmberger TK, Schroder J, Holzknecht N, et al. T2-weighted breathold imaging of the liver: a quantitative and qualitative comparison of fast spin echo and half Fourier single shot fast spin echo imaging. MAGMA 1999;9:42–51.

[4] Semelka RC, Martin DR, Balci C, et al. Focal liver lesions: comparison of dual- phase CT and multisequence multiplanar MR imaging including dynamic gadolinium enhancement. J Magn Reson Imaging 2001;13:397–401.

[5] Martin DR, Semelka RC, Chung JJ, et al. Sequential use of gadolinium chelate and mangafodipir trisodium for the assessment of focal liver lesions: initial observations. Magn Reson Imaging 2000;18:955–63.

[6] Naganawa S, Jenner G, Cooper TG, et al. Rapid MR imaging of the liver: comparison of twelve techniques for single breath-hold whole volume acquisition. Radiat Med 1994;12:255–61.

[7] Bradley WG. Optimizing lesion contrast without using contrast agents. J Magn Reson Imaging 1999;10:442–9.

[8] Siewert B, Muller MF, Foley M, et al. Fast MR imaging of the liver: quantitative comparison of techniques. Radiology 1994;193:37–42.

[9] Chien D, Edelman RR. Ultrafast imaging using gradient echoes. Magn Reson Q 1991;7:31–56.

[10] Rofsky NM, Lee VS, Laub G, et al. Abdominal MR imaging with a volumetric interpolated breath-hold examination. Radiology 1999;212:876–84.

[11] Semelka RC, Brown ED, Ascher SM, et al. Hepatic hemangiomas: a multi-institutional study of appearance on T2- weighted and serial gadolinium-enhanced gradient-echo MR images. Radiology 1994;192:401–6.

[12] Kelekis NL, Semelka RC, Worawattanakul S, et al. Hepatocellular carcinoma in North America: a multiinstitutional study of appearance on T1-weighted, T2-weighted, and serial gadolinium- enhanced gradient-echo images. AJR Am J Roentgenol 1998;170:1005–13.

[13] Low RN. Current uses of gadolinium chelates for clinical magnetic resonance imaging examination of the liver. Top Magn Reson Imaging 1998;9:141–66.

[14] Reimer P, Rummeny EJ, Daldrup HE, et al. Enhancement characteristics of liver metastases, hepatocellular carcinomas, and hemangiomas with Gd-EOB-DTPA: preliminary results with dynamic MR imaging. Eur Radiol 1997;7:275–80.

[15] Thu HD, Mathieu D, Thu NT, et al. Value of MR imaging in evaluating focal fatty infiltration of the liver: preliminary study. Radiographics 1991;11:1003–12.

[16] Rofsky NM, Weinreb JC, Ambrosino MM, et al. Comparison between in-phase and opposed-phase T1-weighted breath-hold FLASH sequences for hepatic imaging. J Comput Assist Tomogr 1996;20:230–5.

[17] Kier R, Mason BJ. Water-suppressed MR imaging of focal fatty infiltration of the liver. Radiology 1997;203:575–7.

[18] Mitchell DG. Chemical shift magnetic resonance imaging: applications in the abdomen and pelvis. Top Magn Reson Imaging 1992;4:46–63.

[19] Siegelman ES, Mitchell DG, Semelka RC. Abdominal iron deposition: metabolism, MR findings, and clinical importance. Radiology 1996;199:13–22.

[20] Torres CG, Lundby B, Sterud AT, et al. MnDPDP for MR imaging of the liver. Results from the European phase III studies. Acta Radiol 1997;38:631–7.

[21] Semelka RC, Lee JK, Worawattanakul S, et al. Sequential use of ferumoxide particles and gadolinium

chelate for the evaluation of focal liver lesions on MRI. J Magn Reson Imaging 1998;8:670–4.

[22] Bulte JW, Miller GF, Vymazal J, et al. Hepatic hemosiderosis in non-human primates: quantification of liver iron using different field strengths. Magn Reson Med 1997;37:530–6.

[23] Ernst O, Sergent G, Bonvarlet P, et al. Hepatic iron overload: diagnosis and quantification with MR imaging. AJR Am J Roentgenol 1997;168:1205–8.

[24] Thomsen C, Wiggers P, Ring-Larsen H, et al. Identification of patients with hereditary haemochromatosis by magnetic resonance imaging and spectroscopic relaxation time measurements. Magn Reson Imaging 1992;10:867–79.

[25] Mitchell DG. Hepatic imaging: techniques and unique applications of magnetic resonance imaging. Magn Reson Imaging 1993;9:84–112.

[26] Engelhardt R, Langkowski JH, Fischer R, et al. Liver iron quantification: studies in aqueous iron solutions, iron overloaded rats, and patients with hereditary hemochromatosis. Magn Reson Imaging 1994;12:999–1007.

[27] Gandon Y, Guyader D, Heautot JF, et al. Hemochromatosis: diagnosis and quantification of liver iron with gradient-echo MR imaging. Radiology 1994;193:533–8.

[28] Keevil SF, Alstead EM, Dolke G, et al. Noninvasive assessment of diffuse liver disease by in vivo measurement of proton nuclear magnetic resonance relaxation times at 0.08 T. Br J Radiol 1994; 67:1083–7.

[29] Bonetti MG, Castriota-Scanderbeg A, Criconia GM, et al. Hepatic iron overload in thalassemic patients: proposal and validation of an MRI method of assessment. Pediatr Radiol 1996;26:650–6.

[30] Ernst O, Sergent G, Bonvarlet P, et al. Hepatic iron overload: diagnosis and quantification with MR imaging. AJR Am J Roentgenol 1997;168:1205–8.

[31] Semelka RC, Chung JJ, Hussain SM, et al. Chronic hepatitis: correlation of early patchy and late linear enhancement patterns on gadolinium-enhanced MR images with histopathology initial experience. J Magn Reson Imaging 2001;13:385–91.

[32] Gandon Y, Olivie D, Guyader D. Non-invasive assessment of hepatic iron stores by MRI. Lancet 2004;363:357–62.

[33] Alustiza JM, Artetxe J, Castiella A. MR quantification of hepatic iron concentration. Radiology 2004; 230:479–84.

[34] Matsui O, Kadoya M, Takashima T, et al. Intrahepatic periportal abnormal intensity on MR images: an indication of various hepatobiliary diseases. Radiology 1989;171:335–8.

[35] Marzola P, Maggioni F, Vicinanza E, et al. Evaluation of the hepatocyte-specific contrast agent gadobenate dimeglumine for MR imaging of acute hepatitis in a rat model. J Magn Reson Imaging 1997;7:147–52.

[36] Martin DR, Seibert D, Yang M, et al. Reversible heterogeneous arterial phase liver perfusion associated with transient acute hepatitis: findings on gadolinium-enhanced MRI. J Magn Reson Imaging 2004;20:838–42.

[37] Semelka RC, Worawattanakul S, Kelekis NL, et al. Liver lesion detection, characterization, and effect on patient management: comparison of single-phase spiral CT and current MR techniques. J Magn Reson Imaging 1997;7:1040–7.

[38] Kreft BP, Tanimoto A, Baba Y, et al. Diagnosis of fatty liver with MR imaging. J Magn Reson Imaging 1992;2:463–71.

[39] Kier R, Mason BJ. Water-suppressed MR imaging of focal fatty infiltration of the liver. Radiology 1997;203:575–7.

[40] Rofsky NM, Weinreb JC, Ambrosino MM, et al. Comparison between in-phase and opposed-phase T1-weighted breath-hold FLASH sequences for hepatic imaging. J Comput Assist Tomogr 1996;20: 230–5.

[41] Kreft B, Dombrowski F, Block W, et al. Evaluation of different models of experimentally induced liver-cirrhosis for MRI research with correlation to histopathologic findings. Invest Radiol 1999;34:360–6.

[42] King LJ, Scurr ED, Murugan N, et al. Hepatobiliary and pancreatic manifestations of cystic fibrosis: MR imaging appearances. Radiographics 2000;20: 767–77.

[43] Koolpe HA, Koolpe L. Portal hypertension. angiographic and hemodynamic evaluation. Radiol Clin N Am 1986;24:369–81.

[44] Noone TC, Semelka RC, Siegelman ES, et al. Budd-Chiari syndrome: spectrum of appearances of acute, subacute, and chronic disease with magnetic resonance imaging. J Magn Reson Imaging 2000;11: 44–50.

[45] Rooholamini SA, Au AH, Hansen GC, et al. Imaging of pregnancy-related complications. Radiographics 1993;13:753–70.

[46] Zissin R, Yaffe D, Fejgin M, et al. Hepatic infarction in preeclampsia as part of the HELLP syndrome: CT appearance. Abdom Imaging 1999;24: 594–6.

ELSEVIER
SAUNDERS

Magn Reson Imaging Clin N Am
13 (2005) 295–311

MAGNETIC
RESONANCE
IMAGING CLINICS
of North America

MR Imaging of the Gallbladder and Biliary System

Samantha L. Heller, MD, PhD, Vivian S. Lee, MD, PhD*

Department of Radiology, New York University Medical Center, 530 First Avenue, New York, NY 10016, USA

Imaging of the gallbladder and biliary system traditionally relies upon a combination of modalities. Sonography offers rapid assessment of clinical symptoms, but does not offer functional information and may be limited in visualization of certain regions, such as the distal common bile duct (CBD). Cholescintigraphy is the traditional means of evaluating gallbladder physiologic function, but does not give anatomic information and cannot elucidate pathology outside of the biliary system. Endoscopic retrograde cholangiopancreatography/cholangiography (ERCP/ERC), initially the gold standard for imaging the biliary tree, is an invasive procedure with well-described risks, including radiation exposure and postoperative complications, such as pancreatitis (3%–5%), sepsis, and hemorrhage. For these reasons, ERCP now exists mainly as a therapeutic, rather than diagnostic, modality [1–5]. Conventional CT, has re-emerged as a technique for visualizing biliary pathology with the reintroduction of intravenous (IV) hepatobiliary contrast material, such as iodipamide meglumine (Cholografin, Bracco Diagnostics, Princeton, New Jersey), albeit with the attendant risks of contrast-based allergic reactions and radiation exposure [3].

Magnetic resonance cholangiopancreatography/cholangiography (MRCP/MRC), in use since the 1990s [3], is an accepted noninvasive and low-risk means of imaging the biliary system. In contrast to other modalities, increasingly sophisticated adaptations of MRC offer the possibility of safely acquiring anatomic, cross-sectional, and functional information through one imaging examination.

MR techniques for imaging gallbladder and biliary disease

Conventional MRC technique uses T2-weighting, which acts to increase contrast between fluid and other structures. Bile, which has high water content, appears bright with its long T2 relaxation times, whereas parenchymal tissues are lower in signal intensity [6]. Although early MRC was a slow process that was susceptible to respiratory, bowel, and vascular motion-artifact [3,7], current conventional MR techniques, such as thick-slab heavily T2-weighted turbo spin echo (TSE) and half-Fourier acquisition single-shot TSE (HASTE), also referred to as half-Fourier rapid acquisition relaxation enhancement (RARE), have increased the speed of imaging dramatically, and allow imaging of the biliary system to occur within a single breath-hold [1,8,9].

Thick-slab (30–80 mm thickness) heavily T2-weighted TSE imaging offers high-signal, ERCP-like views of the biliary system and pancreatic ducts that can be performed quickly without requiring postprocessing [3,7,10]. Images are acquired in the coronal and coronal-oblique planes to mitigate the capture of overlapping fluid structures [7]. For images with tomographic detail, thin slice (3–4 mm) HASTE offers rapid acquisition—each slice is acquired in less than 1 second—and has become the standard technique for MRCP/MRC [11,12].

Conventional MRC methods are highly accurate and allow the diagnosis of stones and strictures as well as other pathologies, often in conjunction with conventional unenhanced T1- and T2-weighted MR images and gadolinium-enhanced images [7,13]. These imaging techniques are not without disadvantages; HASTE, for example, demonstrates low signal-to-noise ratios and offers speed at the expense of resolution

---

* Corresponding author.

E-mail address: vivian.lee@med.nyu.edu (V.S. Lee).

1064-9689/05/$ - see front matter © 2005 Elsevier Inc. All rights reserved.
doi:10.1016/j.mric.2005.03.003

mri.theclinics.com

which can impair, for example, the preoperative examination of intrahepatic biliary anatomy in living liver donors [14]. Thick-slab technique may obscure small intraductal filling defects because of volume averaging of signal intensities [15]. The limited number of projection views of thick-slab technique mean that certain anatomic details may be defined poorly.

Additional pitfalls in MR imaging of the biliary system and gallbladder have been reported. Gas, blood, or other material in the ducts may decrease bile signal intensity and cause the appearance of disease [10]. High signal from fluid collections, ascites, and soft tissue edema, not uncommon in postoperative situations, may interfere with desired biliary signal [16]. Conventional MRC also may result in pseudo-lesions, including a through-plane flow artifact that may mimic choledocholithiasis (Fig. 1). Using fat-suppressed coronal single-shot TSE with maximum intensity projection (MIP) reconstruction of fat-suppressed coronals, Watanabe et al [17] noted pseudo-obstruction of the extrahepatic bile duct that was due to arterial pulsatile compression in 14% of their study population, most commonly at the common hepatic duct (75%) and most frequently due to the right hepatic artery (67%). Sugita et al [18], in a phantom study that examined the influence of shape and velocity of flow on MRCP with multisection half-Fourier RARE with phased array coil, described a flow artifact that appeared as decreased signal which may mimic a true filling defect. The artifact was most pronounced when speed of flow exceeded 5 mm/s. They cautioned that in certain cases,

a dilated bile duct itself may cause such an artifact and emphasized the need to review coronal source MR images and transverse T2-weighted images (see Fig. 1).

Conventional T1- and T2-weighted MR imaging should be performed as part of a routine MRC examination. These images can be helpful for diagnosing causes of biliary obstruction and pathology other than stones. Conventional gadolinium-enhanced T1-weighted imaging can be useful in the setting of suspected neoplasm or inflammatory disease, such as cholangitis, cholecystitis, and pancreatitis.

Newer techniques

Contrast agents

MR contrast imaging with conventional gadolinium chelates has proven useful in imaging gallbladder and hepatobiliary disease, particularly in cases of inflammation as may occur in cholecystitis and carcinoma [19]. The increased local blood flow and capillary leakage of inflammation effect greater enhancement on MR imaging [20]. Moreover, when combined with high-resolution fat-suppressed T1-weighted three-dimensional (3D) gradient echo imaging, gadolinium-enhanced evaluation of the biliary tree provides high spatial resolution evaluation with isotropic pixels that can be reconstructed in any plane [21]. Conventional gadolinium chelates, which are excreted renally, are nonspecific for the hepatobiliary system, and therefore, cannot offer assessment of biliary function [22].

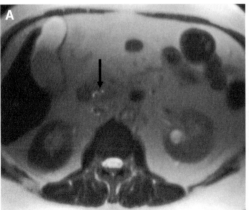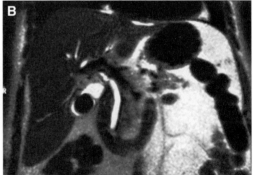

Fig. 1. (*A*) Axial T2-weighted single shot fast spin echo MR image shows through-plane flow artifact (*arrow*) mimicking choledocholithiasis. (*B*) Coronal T2-weighted single shot fast spin echo MR image reveals absence of biliary stone.

Newer contrast agents that are taken up by hepatocytes and excreted through the biliary system [23] offer a means of addressing some of the limitations of conventional MRC and conventional gadolinium enhancement. Agents, such as manganese dipyridoxyl diphosphate, the active component of mangafodipir trisodium (Teslascan, Amersham Biosciences, GE Healthcare Technologies, Chalfont St. Giles, United Kingdom); a manganese chelate, currently unavailable; and gadolinium chelates, such as gadobenate dimeglumine (MultiHance, Bracco, Milan, Italy) and gadolinium-ethoxybenzyl-diethylene-triamine-pentaacetic acid (Gd-EOB-DPTA, Eovist, Schering-AG, Berlin, Germany) shorten T1 and allow for improved visualization of the intrahepatic biliary system following their excretion approximately 15 minutes after IV injection [24]. Because obstructed or nonfunctional bile ducts lead to biliary stasis and reduced excretion, these contrast agents offer functional biliary information. Both of the gadolinium chelates have the advantage of being able to be given as rapid boluses and used to assess arterial and venous patency, whereas mangafodipir trisodium is limited to a slow injection over 1 minute [25]. Because these agents shorten T2, conventional T2-weighted MRC imaging should be performed before hepatobiliary contrast imaging so as to avoid decreased signal intensity of normal bile ducts [26].

Three-dimensional T2-weighted imaging

3D T2-weighted TSE is a promising technique; it offers improved anatomic accuracy, higher signal-to-noise ratio, and thinner sections without gaps between slices when compared with conventional two-dimensional (2D) imaging. As described by Wielopolski et al [27] and others [28,29], 3D MRC has been burdened by long acquisition times and poor anatomic coverage and resolution; however, the advent of recent improvements, such as parallel acquisition technique (PAT), which shortens data acquisition time while retaining spatial resolution and contrast of the base image [30], offer the possibility of realistically exploiting 3D T2 TSE in the clinical setting. Faster gradients and navigator-based respiratory triggering offer additional improvements for improved image quality. Our routine MRC protocol includes a commercially available navigator-based respiratory-triggered acquisition which uses PAT 3D fast spin echo to obtain 50 to 60 1-mm partitions in approximately 2 to 5 minutes (Fig. 2).

Patient preparation for MR cholangiography

Before MRC, patients optimally should fast for at least 4 hours. Oral contrast agents have been used to decrease signal from potentially distracting hyperintense bowel fluid. In the authors' experience, two cups of pineapple juice given 5 to 10 minutes before the examination effectively decreases gastric and duodenal signal as a result of the high manganese content of the fruit [31,32]. This has the advantage of affording improved visibility of the ducts. Other commercial agents, such as ferumoxsil (Gastromark, Mallinckrodt, Maryland Heights, Missouri) and the use of diluted IV contrast, gadopentetate dimeglumine (Magnevist, Berlex Laboratories, Wayne, New Jersey) as oral agents also have been used in this way [33]. Some researchers believe that a degree of high signal in the duodenum is valuable, however, and allows assessment of duodenal papillary tumor, pancreatic divisum, or anomalous pancreaticobiliary ductal union [34].

All MRC examinations, whether at 1.5 T or 3 T, should be performed with torso phased array coils for higher signal-to-noise ratios and improved image quality. Because many acquisitions require patients to suspend respiration, it is important to assess a subject's breath-holding capabilities before the study and to offer supplemental oxygen by way of nasal cannula, when needed.

Biliary anatomy

Normal anatomy

Couinaud classification divides the liver into eight segments, and their drainage pattern defines various patterns of biliary anatomy (see Fig. 2). An estimated 58% of the population has classic biliary anatomy [35]; the right hepatic duct drains right lobe segments V through VIII, the right posterior branch drains posterior segments VI and VII, and the right anterior duct drains segments V and VIII. The right posterior duct usually courses posterior to the right anterior duct and joins it from left and medially to create the right hepatic duct. The left hepatic duct drains segments II through IV. The common hepatic duct is formed by the usually short right hepatic duct and the left hepatic duct. The cystic duct generally meets the common hepatic duct below the biliary confluence to form the CBD [36].

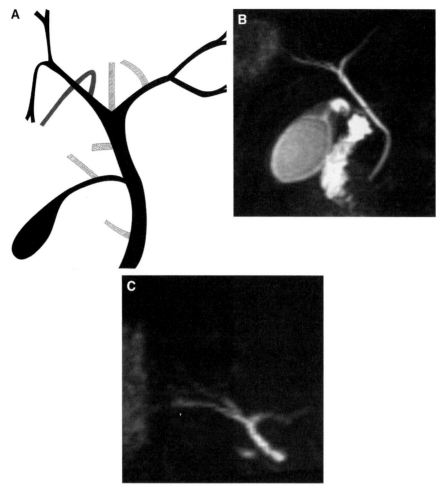

Fig. 2. (A) Classic biliary anatomy with variants. (B, C) Three-dimensional T2-weighted images of normal biliary anatomy. (A, Courtesy of M. Helmers, New York, NY.)

Anatomic variants

Variants of biliary anatomy are common (see Fig. 2A). Thirteen percent to 19% of the population has a right posterior duct which fuses with the left hepatic duct. The right posterior duct also may feed into the common hepatic, common bile, or cystic ducts. Another 11% have a triple confluence, in which the right posterior, right anterior, and left hepatic ducts empty into the common hepatic duct, which effectively obliterates the right hepatic duct. Accessory hepatic ducts also may be seen. The cystic duct also has many variants, including low cystic duct insertion, medial cystic duct insertion, and the parallel running of the cystic duct and common hepatic duct [35–37].

It is increasingly important to be able to image and thus anticipate variant biliary anatomy, not only for more established operations like cholecystectomy, but also for liver transplantation. The lack of available cadaveric livers has increased the number of living liver donors whose biliary anatomy must be evaluated carefully before operating [38], and in whom the risks of ERCP are unacceptable.

Living donors present a unique set of imaging difficulties, precisely because their healthy ducts tend to be small (1–2 mm) and unobstructed, which necessitates a higher spatial resolution than available through conventional MR imaging procedures [39–41]. In the authors' experience, 3D T2 MRC is one solution to this problem; it offers better visualization of the biliary tree and of third- and fourth-order biliary ducts than conventional thick-slab 2D TSE (Fig. 3).

In several small studies, mangafodipir trisodium also was shown to be particularly useful in visualizing small, nondilated ducts and duct variants and provided excellent contrast between biliary tree and background parenchyma and vasculature with improved resolution over conventional T2-weighted images [14,39,42,43]. Goldman et al [14], for example, showed that mangafodipir trisodium 3D MRCP identified 100% of anterior and posterior right intrahepatic bile ducts and 97% of medial and left lateral intrahepatic ducts as compared with thick-slab single-shot fast spin echo (35% and 0%, respectively) and thin-slice single-shot fast spin echo (12% and 0%, respectively). In a recent larger study, Lee et al [43] compared 3D mangafodipir trisodium–enhanced T1-weighted MRC with conventional T2-weighted MRC in 108 liver transplant donors. In 51 patients who subsequently underwent intraoperative cholangiography, mangafodipir trisodium–enhanced images had a significantly higher correct depiction of biliary anatomy than conventional MRC (92% versus 84%). Combined techniques resulted in a correct identification of biliary anatomy of 94%.

Results with the gadolinium chelates have been mixed. Gd-EOB-DTPA also was shown to improve biliary visualization significantly—albeit modestly; however, reviewers in one study preferred T2-MRCP to either Gd-EOB-MRC or

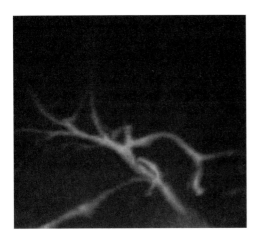

Fig. 3. Maximum intensity projection of a respiratory-triggered T2-weighted 3D fast spin echo MR image depicts right posterior duct draining into the left main biliary duct, a biliary tree variant.

combined technique [24]. Another group found results of thick-section MRCP with gadolinium chelate to be inconsistent; it demonstrated improved visualization of the pancreaticobiliary ducts in some patients, whereas it decreased the visualization in other patients, albeit less frequently. The investigators attributed these findings to susceptibility effect of gadolinium chelate in neighboring vessels, which may have interfered with visualization of the biliary tree [34].

CT cholangiography may provide more accuracy than MRC with contrast. In a small, eight-patient study, Yeh et al [44] showed that multidetector row CT cholangiography, with its higher spatial resolution, provided significantly better visualization of second-order biliary branching than conventional MRC or mangafodipir trisodium–enhanced MR, although the technique may have limitations in detecting branch variants when ducts run together closely. Unlike MRC, however, CT cholangiography involves the risk of radiation and iodinated contrast material.

Other reported means of improving biliary visualization include low-dose morphine administration as a means of improving biliary tree visualization. Morphine constricts the sphincter of Oddi, which causes increased pressure and distention of the biliary ducts and allows better visualization of the biliary and pancreatic ducts [45].

Gallbladder

Cholelithiasis

Gallstones tend to have low signal on T1- and T2-weighted images, but may be hyperintense on T1 [7]. Although earlier studies found that MR imaging was not useful in determining the chemical composition of gallstones, a recent study by Tsai et al [46] showed that 18 out of 20 pigment gallstones were hyperintense and all cholesterol gallstones were hypointense on 3D fast spoiled gradient T1-weighted imaging. The investigators also found T2-weighted imaging differences; the ratio of signal intensity of stone to bile averaged 3.36 ± 1.88 for pigment gallstone and 0.24 ± 0.10 for cholesterol gallstone. Another recent investigation of gallstones on MR imaging correlated signal intensity with chemical composition. T2-weighted high signal central intensity corresponded to fluid-filled clefts (Fig. 4), whereas central and peripheral high signal areas on T1-weighted images correspond to the fluid-clefts, as

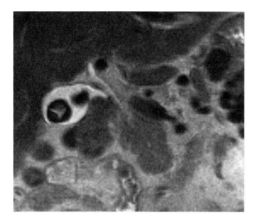

Fig. 4. "Mercedes-Benz" sign on coronal T2-weighted single shot fast spin echo MR image. The sign, classically appearing as radiolucent fissures on plain radiographs, arises from nitrogen gas which collects in the central fissures and corresponds to fluid-filled clefts on MR imaging.

well as regions that were high in copper content [47].

To assess biliary obstruction in the setting of stones, Inoue et al [48] suggest fatty-meal MRC as a means of evaluating gallbladder function. After drinking 250 mL of milk, 20 patients who had known gallstone disease were assessed every 10 minutes over the course of an hour with MRC. Postprandial changes in gallbladder volume and the diameter of the common duct were assessed as indicators of gallbladder contractility and biliary obstruction, respectively. Postprandial dilatation at 60 minutes was considered to be indicative of persistent biliary obstruction.

Cholecystitis

Cholecystitis occurs after obstruction from a gallstone 90% of the time. The remaining cases represent acalculous cholecystitis [7]. Ultrasonography and cholescintigraphy are standard methods of imaging suspected cholecystitis, whereas MR imaging usually is advocated only in the case of an ambiguous clinical picture [22]; however, MR is well-equipped to image the gallbladder. Typical MR findings include distention of the gallbladder, a thick gallbladder wall, and pericholecystic bright signal on T2-weighted MR imaging (sensitivity, 91%; specificity, 79%; positive predictive value, 87%; negative predictive value, 85%) [49], although it was noted that this study did not include patients who had liver disease and the potential confounders of hepatitis or ascites

[22]. Gadolinium enhancement of the acutely cholecystic gallbladder wall also has been well-described; Loud et al [50] found more than 80% contrast enhancement of the gallbladder wall in patients who had suspected acute cholecystitis. Park et al [51] showed that conventional MRC is not as sensitive, specific, or accurate as ultrasound for assessment of gallbladder wall thickening as a sign of inflammation. Hakansson [52] found that MR imaging was more sensitive than ultrasound (88% versus 65%) for diagnosing acute cholecystitis overall. Both studies agree that MRC is more sensitive than ultrasound for diagnosing cystic duct and gallbladder neck stones [51,52], and other literature supports the value of MRC in the diagnosis of Mirizzi syndrome—cystic duct stone impaction that impinges upon and obstructs the common hepatic duct (Fig. 5) [53]. MRC also is useful in imaging time-sensitive complications, such as perforation, which may be misread as contusion on CT (Fig. 6) [22,54].

Hepatobiliary contrast agents improve upon conventional MRC in evaluating acute cholecystitis. Kim et al [55] found that mangafodipir trisodium–enhanced MR imaging offers anatomic information and assessment of gallbladder function. In this study of 12 patients, 100% of the findings on manganese-enhanced 3D T1-weighted fat-saturated volumetric interpolated breath-hold images were consistent with scintigraphy as compared with only 58% on half-Fourier RARE MRCP. Fayad et al [56] also found that mangafodipir trisodium–enhanced 3D gradient echo

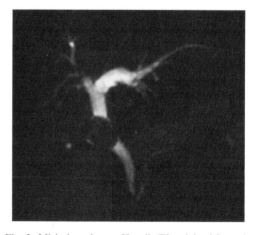

Fig. 5. Mirizzi syndrome. Heavily T2-weighted fast spin echo MR image shows large gallstone impacted in cystic duct and obstructing the common hepatic duct.

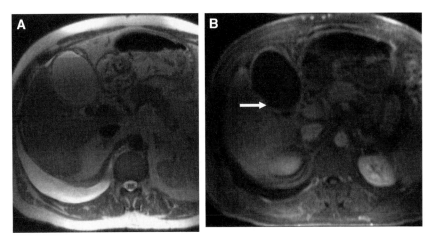

Fig. 6. (*A*) Axial T2-weighted single shot fast spin echo MR image shows markedly dilated and thick-walled gallbladder with stone (1 cm in diameter) impacted in gallbladder neck. (*B*) Axial fat-suppressed 3D gradient echo MR image clearly shows break in the perforated gallbladder wall (*arrow*).

functional MRC had a greater positive predictive value than conventional single-shot fast spin echo MRC (100% versus 33%) in acute cholecystitis. Combined techniques yielded a positive predictive value of 100%. The positive predictive value for chronic cholecystitis was not as strong for either technique (50% for mangafodipir trisodium versus 40% for conventional MRC).

Adenomyomatosis

Adenomyomatosis, a form of hyperplastic cholesterosis, is a common benign condition that is characterized by hyperplastic changes of the gallbladder wall, mucosal overgrowth, and thickening of the muscular wall. There are three forms of the disease: diffuse, segmental, and localized. Intramural diverticula or sinus tracts (Rokitansky-Aschoff sinuses) mark the condition and are seen easily on MR imaging—particularly T2-weighted MR imaging breath-hold sequences—as smoothly marginated cystic regions (Fig. 7) [56,57]. The sinuses are considered to be diagnostic [58]. Diffuse-type adenomyomatosis typically shows early mucosal enhancement and subsequent serosal enhancement. Localized adenomyomatosis exhibits

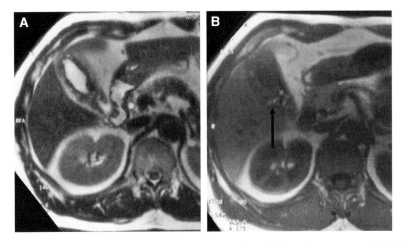

Fig. 7. (*A*) Axial T2-weighted single shot fast spin echo MR image shows diffuse adenomyomatosis with high signal foci in the gallbladder wall representing Rokitansky-Aschoff sinuses. (*B*) Axial T1-weighted image shows hyperintense regions consistent with proteinaceous fluid (*arrow*).

homogeneous enhancement and shows smooth continuity with the surrounding gallbladder epithelium [59].

Gallbladder carcinoma

Gallbladder carcinoma is the most common primary hepatobiliary carcinoma. It usually is detected in the late stages and prognosis is poor. Recent literature suggests that early diagnosis can improve the clinical outcome; this increases the importance of appropriate imaging [60]. On MR imaging, gallbladder carcinoma is hypointense to liver on T1-weighted images and hyperintense on T2-weighted MR images (Fig. 8). Associated findings may include stones (67% of cases), direct liver invasion (91%), and porcelain gallbladder with circumferential gallbladder wall calcification

surrounding tumor (3%) [61]. Schwartz et al [61] pointed out that the occurrence of porcelain gallbladder most likely is underestimated in MR imaging because the calcification may be too insubstantial to be visualized or may be hidden by the tumor mass.

Invasion into the bile duct and vascular involvement are key factors in evaluating the extent of disease and appropriate management strategies. One study advocated a combined approach, using MR imaging, MRCP, and contrast-enhanced dual phase 3D MR angiography to assess local tumor spread into visceral vessels, bile ducts, and organs [62]. The sensitivity, specificity, and diagnostic accuracy of this strategy were 100%, 89%, and 94%, respectively, for bile duct invasion, and 69%, 89%, and 77%,

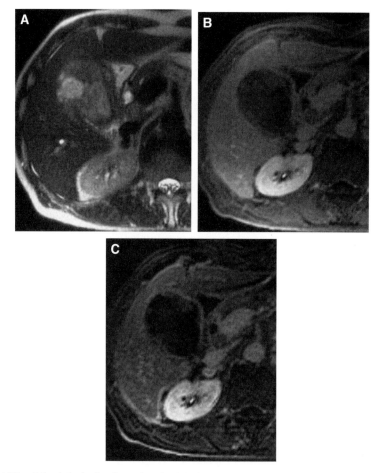

Fig. 8. (*A*) Axial T2-weighted single shot fast spin echo MR image shows heterogeneous mass in gallbladder. (*B*) Axial enhanced fat-suppressed 3D gradient echo MR image demonstrates mass. (*C*) Unenhanced fat-suppressed 3D gradient echo MR image subtracted from contrast-enhanced acquisition shows uneven enhancement of mass that is consistent with gallbladder carcinoma.

respectively, for hepatic invasion. For vascular invasion, MR imaging had 100% sensitivity and 87% specificity, whereas for lymph node metastases, MR imaging had a sensitivity of 56% and a specificity of 89% [62].

The thickened gallbladder wall with carcinoma is nonspecific and difficult to differentiate from that of chronic cholecystitis. Dynamic contrast-enhanced MR imaging may be useful in increasing contrast resolution and signal-to-noise of images. A study that compared 50 cases of chronic cholecystitis with 13 cases of gallbladder carcinoma using spoiled gradient recalled echo (SPGR) and fast SPGR pre- and postgadolinium enhancement found that all inflamed gallbladders had smoothly delineated enhancement (except for one case of adenomyomatosis), with inner wall early-phase enhancement and outer wall late- and delayed-phase enhancement. All carcinomas in the study, however, evidenced ill-defined enhancement in the early dynamic phase (see Fig. 8). Notably, dynamic MR imaging is limited in assessing tumors within mucosa or smooth muscle because mucosa and smooth muscle also are enhanced in the early-phase dynamic images [58,63].

Biliary system

Congenital

Conventional MRCP has been well-described as a means of evaluating a variety of congenital defects of the biliary system. Choledochal cysts—extrahepatic dilatations with occasional intrahepatic bile duct dilation—have high signal on T2-weighted images [19,64,65]. Eighty percent to 90% of choledochal cysts are classified as type 1 and involve the entire common hepatic and CBD. Type 2 involves isolated cysts which project from the CBD wall. Type 3 (choledochoceles) describes cysts in the intraduodenal portion of the CBD. Type 4A involves intra- and extrahepatic portions of the biliary tree (Fig. 9), whereas type 4B is composed of extrahepatic cysts. Type 5 cysts (Caroli's disease) involve dilated intrahepatic biliary radicles. Numerous cysts and strictures are present in this last case and lead to stasis, obstruction, and cholangitis [66]. MRC imaging of choledochal cysts has been reported widely and compares favorably to ERCP and conventional cholangiography [66,67]. In a study of 16 patients, Irie et al [68] found that MRCP better visualized the proximal biliary tree than did ERCP; however, MRCP missed two biliary defects in

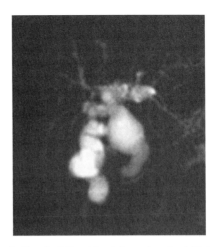

Fig. 9. Heavily T2-weighted fast spin echo MR image demonstrates ductal dilatations that are consistent with type 4A choledochal cyst that involves the common bile duct and left intrahepatic ductal system. The gallbladder is elongated and bulbous.

the distal CBD that were noted on ERCP as well as 6 out of 10 anomalous pancreaticobiliary junctions in pediatric patients.

Biliary atresia is an idiopathic congenital cholangiopathy that affects intra- and extrahepatic bile ducts. Early diagnosis is key because surgery leads to better outcome [69]. In a study of neonates who had cholestasis, MRCP had an accuracy of 82%, sensitivity of 90%, and specificity of 77% for depicting extrahepatic biliary atresia [70]. Another study of 12 infants and neonates who had biliary atresia showed that T2-weighted single-shot MR cholangiography can show a triangular area of high signal intensity in the porta hepatis which correlated with ultrasonographic and histopathologic findings and may represent cystic dilatation of the fetal bile duct [71].

Biliary calculi

Stones as small as 2 mm may be detected on MRC; they appear as areas of decreased signal on T2-weighted imaging [1,7]. MRC sensitivity, specificity, and accuracy ranges for choledocholithiasis compare favorably to ERCP, CT, and sonography and have been estimated at 85% to 100%, 90% to 99%, and 89% to 97%, respectively. Kim et al [72] used single-shot half-Fourier MRC in 121 patients who were referred for cholecystectomy for symptomatic gallstones to evaluate the accuracy of MRC in distinct patient populations. Patients were divided into high-, moderate-, and low-risk groups in terms of their likelihood of having stones. MRC proved to be highly accurate in the detection of CBD stones in all patients for all risk groups.

MRCP may be particularly effective in detecting intrahepatic calculi (Fig. 10), where stones proximal to strictures may be difficult to visualize by ERCP. In a retrospective study of 34 patients who had undergone MRCP and subsequent ERCP, MRCP showed a significantly higher sensitivity than ERCP (97% versus 59%) in the diagnosis of intrahepatic stones ($P < .001$), whereas no significant difference in sensitivity or specificity was found between MRCP and ERCP for detecting calculi in the common duct or gallbladder [73].

Diagnostic pitfalls, however, can occur in evaluating biliary calculi on MRC, including metal clips, blood clots, tumors, parasites. and air [7]. Postprocessing also may affect the diagnostic accuracy of MRC for biliary stones. Although suitable for presentation, MIP reconstructions are not as accurate as 2D source image review in the context of intraductal calculi and tumor [74].

Primary sclerosing cholangitis

Primary sclerosing cholangitis (PSC) is an idiopathic, chronic inflammation of the ducts that is characterized by intrahepatic and extrahepatic biliary stricture, thickened bile duct walls, and eventual liver failure. PSC often is associated with ulcerative colitis, and 10% to 15% of patients who have PSC develop cholangiocarcinoma [75]. On MR imaging, T1-weighted fat-suppressed spin-echo pulse sequences, with or without IV gadolinium, facilitates visualization of the bile duct wall. Peripheral wedge-shaped areas of high T2-weighted signal intensity in the liver parenchyma also may be observed in the disease [76,77]. MRC is sensitive for the strictures and obliterated ducts of PSC [75] and is an especially compelling alternative to ERCP given the higher rate of ERCP complication in patients who have PSC (Fig. 11) [78]. Vitellas et al [79], in a study of 20 patients and 19 volunteers, found that thick-slab MRCP had better visualization in a greater number of ducts than contrast cholangiography (84% versus 70%), and also showed a greater number of strictured ducts (47% versus 36%). Ferrara et al [80] found a sensitivity of 81%, specificity of 100%, positive predictive value of 100% and negative predictive value of 62% for detection of PSC in children using RARE and HASTE [80]; however, decreased detection of the initial stages of stenosis of PSC and overestimation of the extent of focal strictures has been reported [75]. Recently, a study that compared conventional MRCP to CT cholangiography in 16 patients who had PSC found that CT cholangiography offered significantly better imaging quality than MRCP and higher sensitivity (94% versus 63%) [81].

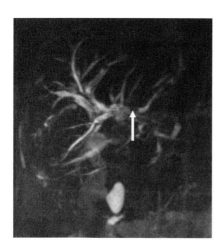

Fig. 10. Maximum intensity projection of a respiratory-triggered T2-weighted 3D fast spin echo demonstrates intrahepatic biliary stones (*arrow*).

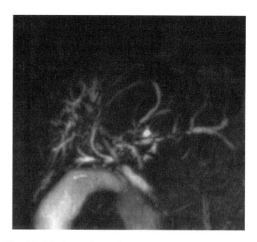

Fig. 11. Maximum intensity projection of a respiratory-triggered T2-weighted 3D fast spin echo MR image shows moderate and diffuse intrahepatic bile duct dilatation with irregularity and beading that are consistent with primary sclerosing cholangitis. Segmental dilatation of the common hepatic duct is observed.

Secondary cholangitis

Secondary cholangitis has multiple etiologies, including infection, ischemia, and chemotherapy. Signs of cholangitis on MR imaging include intrahepatic biliary dilatation, ductal stenosis or obstruction, and mild to moderate bile duct thickening. Pyogenic cholangitis or oriental cholangiohepatitis is marked by intrahepatic pigment stone formation that results in biliary obstruction with recurrent cholangitis, dilatation, and stricturing of the biliary tree (Fig. 12). The left hepatic duct, especially the left lateral segmental duct, usually is affected in the early course of the disease, although stones may be present in the right and left hepatic lobes and the extrahepatic biliary tree [82]. Gadolinium-enhanced images are useful for depicting bile duct thickening [20]. Nonspecific liver parenchyma hypointensities, or, less frequently, hyperintensities, may be observed on T1-weighted images; hyperintensities may be seen occasionally on T2-weighted images in cholangitis [20,52].

Obstruction

Obstruction of the biliary system may arise from stones, benign tumors, primary biliary tumors, lymphadenopathy, extension of malignancy from other regions of the gastrointestinal tract, intrapancreatic masses, metastases to the liver, and cholangiocarcinoma, among other causes. Differentiating benign from malignant biliary obstruction can be difficult on MR imaging, with estimates of accuracy ranging from 30% to 98%. Dynamic T2-weighted imaging has been used to differentiate true obstruction from closed ampulla. Kim et al [83] repeated 2D MRCP over time in 50 patients and looked at biliary peristalsis and intermittent opening of the ampulla to differentiate stricture from closed ampulla; they found a sensitivity of 88% and a specificity of 100% for the diagnosis of peri-ampullary lesions.

Benign biliary tumors

Benign biliary tumors are rare entities and include biliary cystadenoma, a rare multilocular cystic liver mass with origin in the bile duct that is seen more commonly in women. MR appearance is dependent upon the protein content of the cystic fluid and the existence of soft tissue [84]. Bile duct hamartomas (von Meyenburg complexes) are non-specific and appear hypointense on T1-weighted images and iso- or hyperintense on T2-weighted images (Fig. 13). Hamartomas usually can be distinguished from metastases or microabscesses by their appearance and the patient's clinical history. The lesions do not enhance with gadolinium contrast material. Bile duct adenomas also are nonspecific on MR imaging and are well-circumscribed masses that are made up of bile ductules and inflammatory reaction; this led to the suggestion that they actually are reactive entities [84].

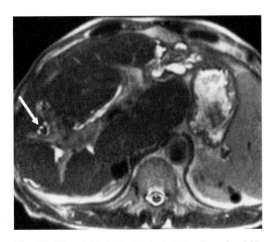

Fig. 12. T2-weighted single shot fast spin echo MR image shows biliary ductal dilatation and multiple filling defects that are consistent with calculi (*arrow*) in a patient who has oriental cholangiohepatitis.

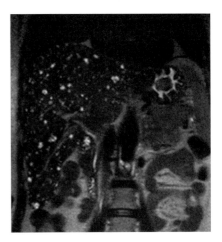

Fig. 13. Coronal T2-weighted single shot fast spin echo MR image shows numerous small cystic lesions that are consistent with hamartomas (von Meyenburg complexes).

Malignant biliary tumors: cholangiocarcinoma

Cholangiocarcinomas most frequently are adenocarcinomas of the biliary duct system and are classified as intrahepatic, extrahepatic (ie, perihilar), or distal extrahepatic [85,86]. Perihilar tumors, or Klatskin tumors, occur at the bifurcation of right and left hepatic ducts. Extrahepatic tumors often are found with biliary stricture, usually in the CBD (30%–36%), whereas Klatskin tumors (10%–26%) are associated with proximal bile duct dilatation [87,88]. Cholangiocarcinoma appears as an iso- to hypointense solid mass on T1-weighted images and as an iso- to mildly hyperintense mass on T2-weighted images (Fig. 14). Delayed enhancement in the center of the mass is due to fibrosis [85,89].

Gadolinium enhancement is useful in assessing cholangiocarcinoma, but optimal timing of acquisitions varies, depending upon tumor type. Worawattanakul et al [89], in a study of 15 patients, reported that on gadolinium-enhanced T1-weighted fat-suppressed spoiled gradient echo imaging, the degree of enhancement ranged from minimal to intense on immediate gadolinium-enhanced images. All tumors became more homogeneous in signal intensity on images that were obtained between 1 and 5 minutes following contrast administration.

HASTE MRCP is useful for observing the narrowing of the distal CBD and the dilation of the pancreatic duct which may occur with obstruction, and, unlike ERCP, allows visualization of the ducts above and below an obstructing mass [1,13].

One important diagnosis to consider in the setting of suspected cholangiocarcinoma is that of portal cavernomas of the solid type. Portal cavernomas develop following chronic portal vein occlusion and can cause biliary structure and obstruction. When of the solid type, these enhancing masses can mimic cholangiocarcinoma [90].

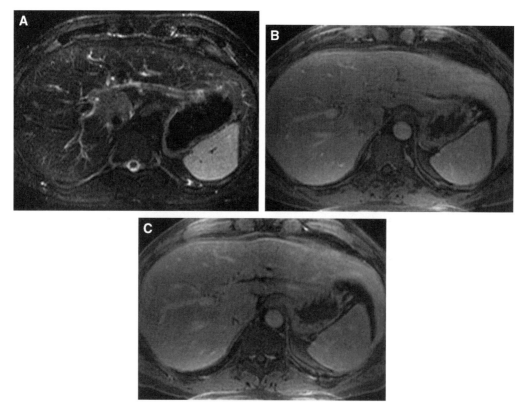

Fig. 14. Cholangiocarcinoma. (*A*) Axial T2-weighted short tau inversion recovery image shows slightly hyperintense mass infiltrating the caudate lobe in close proximity to the porta hepatis. (*B*) Axial portal venous phase contrast-enhanced fat-suppressed image shows that the mass is hypointense to the liver parenchyma. (*C*) Axial delayed contrast-enhanced imaging shows enhancement.

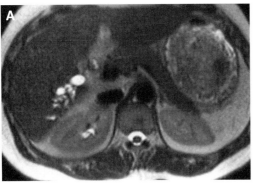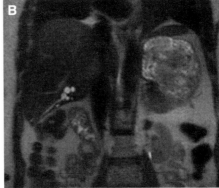

Fig. 15. Axial (*A*) and coronal (*B*) T2-weighted single shot fast spin echo MR images demonstrate inadvertently ligated right posterior duct with dilatation of obstructed ducts and resultant hepatic atrophy.

Postoperative complications

Small right hepatic duct size, edema at the anastomosis site, and adjacent dissection of the duct are conditions that lead to complications, such as bile leak, stricture, obstruction, and stones after liver transplantation and have been observed in 5.8% to 24.5% of adult liver recipients [91]. Bile duct complications after cholecystectomy include inadvertent hepatic duct transection and ligation (Fig. 15), bile leak at the cystic duct stump, liver abscess, and retained common duct stones and have been estimated to occur in 0% to 0.5% of cases in open cholecystectomy and 0% to 1.2% of cases in laparoscopic cholecystectomy [92–94].

MRC is the mode of choice for assessing postoperative complications of the biliary system [41,92]. A sensitivity of 93%, a specificity of 92%, a positive predictive value of 86%, and a negative predictive value of 96% have been reported for the detection of all posttransplant complications [95].

Bile duct leaks present, on average, several days after surgery. Forty-four percent of patients who have bile duct leaks may develop serious postoperative complications (peritonitis, sepsis, abscess, pulmonary infiltrates, death) [96]. Diagnosis typically involves a combination of modalities: ultrasonography, CT, scintigraphy, ERCP, percutaneous aspiration, percutaneous

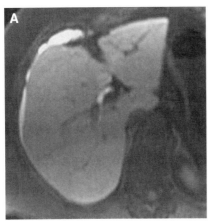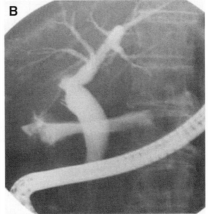

Fig. 16. (*A*) Fat-suppressed gradient echo image 1.5 hours after the administration of 10 mL of teslascan with extravasation of contrast agent from a right hepatic duct leak into the perihepatic space. (*B*) Endoscopic retrograde cholangiopancreatography image confirms contrast agent extravasating from a leak arising from the right hepatic duct. (*From* Vitellas K, El-Dieb A, Vaswani K, et al. Detection of bile duct leaks using MR cholangiography with mangfodipir trisodium (Teslascan). J Comput Assist Tomogr 2001;25:104; with permission.)

cholangiography, and conventional MRC. CT and sonography are nonspecific in terms of the nature of the fluid and must be followed up with an invasive means of fluid collection. Cholescintigraphy can help to characterize fluid as biliary in origin, but does not offer anatomic localization of a leak, nor does it offer information regarding extrabiliary structures [97]. ERCP is invasive, costly, and is prone to miss bile ducts that do not arise from the main biliary tree. MRC was shown to be useful in detecting leaks, particularly when there is high suspicion for a disconnected biliary segment which would not be visualized on ERC [98]; however, the static nature of conventional MRC implies only indirect evidence of a leak, which makes it difficult to distinguish a bile collection, such as a biliary leak, from a postoperative seroma [99].

Vitellas et al [100] described the use of mangafodipir trisodium contrast-enhanced MRC with fat-suppressed gradient echo-imaging as an all-in-one method of assessing bile leak that is capable of providing functional, cross-sectional, and anatomic information (Fig. 16) [100]. In a prospective study of 11 patients, Vitellas et al [97], using single-shot fast spin-echo and gradient-echo imaging, found one false-negative finding and one false-positive finding; this yielded a sensitivity of 86% and a specificity of 83% for the technique.

Bile duct strictures generally are late complications of hepatobiliary surgery [41]. Conventional MRC has a mean accuracy of 94% in the diagnosis of stricture with a sensitivity of 97%, specificity of 74%, positive predictive value of 86%, and negative predictive value of 96% reported, although the technique was shown to overestimate duct dilatation and stricture. Careful review of the source images is vital [101].

Summary

MR imaging is an established technique for the diagnosis of a spectrum of biliary and gallbladder pathologies and continues to improve with the advent of technologic advances, including new contrast agents and new sequences that are capable of improving upon the contrast resolution and signal-to-noise that are afforded by conventional MR imaging. These improvements already have shown promise for the increasing role of MRC as the initial modality in assessing living liver donors and evaluating postoperative hepato-biliary complications. Improved

spatial resolution and the added functional or physiologic information afforded by MR imaging promise ever expanding clinical applicability and usefulness.

References

[1] Van Epps K, Regan F. MR cholangiopancreatography using HASTE sequences. Clin Radiol 1999; 54:588–94.

[2] Fulcher AS, Turner MA. Benign diseases of the biliary tract: evaluation with MR cholangiography. Semin Ultrasound CT MR 1999;20:294–303.

[3] Baillie J, Paulson EK, Vitellas KM. Biliary imaging: a review. Gastroenterol Clin N Am 2003;124: 1686–99.

[4] Cotton P, Chong W. Complications of endoscopic retrograde cholangiography and therapy. In: Silvis S, Rohrmann C, Ansel H, editors. Endoscopic retrograde cholangiopancreatography. New York: Igaku-Shoin; 1995. p. 446–50.

[5] Sherman S, Lehman G. ERCP and endoscopic sphincterotomy-induced pancreatitis. Pancreas 1991;6:350–67.

[6] Wallner B, Schumacher K, Weidenmaier W, et al. Dilated biliary tract: evaluation with MR cholangiography with a T2-weighted contrast-enhanced fast sequence. Radiology 1991;181:805–8.

[7] Hartman EM, Barish MA. MR cholangiography. Magn Reson Imaging Clin N Am 2001;9:841–55.

[8] Fisher AR, Siegelman ES. Magnetic resonance imaging: techniques. Clin Liver Dis 2002;6:53–72.

[9] Morrin M, Farell R, McEntee G, et al. MR cholangiopancreatography of pancreaticobiliary diseases: comparison of single-shot RARE and multislice HASTE sequences. Clin Radiol 2000; 55:866–73.

[10] Watanabe Y, Dohke M, Takayoshi I, et al. Diagnostic pitfalls of MR cholangiopancreatography in the evaluation of the biliary tract and gallbladder. Radiographics 1999;19:415–29.

[11] Holzknecht N, Gauger J, Stehling M, et al. Choledocholithiasis after Billroth II surgery: MR cholangiographic diagnosis. Eur Radiol 1997;7:520–3.

[12] Regan F, Smith D, Khazan R, et al. MR cholangiography in biliary obstruction using half-Fourier acquisition. J Comput Assist Tomogr 1996;20: 627–32.

[13] Kim M-J, Mitchell DG, Ito K, et al. Biliary dilatation: differentiation of benign from malignant causes—value of adding conventional MR imaging to MR cholangiopancreatography. Radiology 2000; 214:173–81.

[14] Goldman J, Florman S, Varotti G, et al. Noninvasive preoperative evaluation of biliary anatomy in right-lobe living donors with mangafodipir trisodium-enhanced MR cholangiography. Transplant Proc 2003;35:1421–2.

[15] Soto JA, Barish MA, Alvarez O, et al. Detection of choledocholithiasis with MR cholangiography: comparison of three-dimensional fast spin echo and single- and multisection half-fourier rapid acquisition with relaxation enhancement sequences. Radiology 2000;215:737–45.

[16] Bridges MD, May GR, Harnois DM. Diagnosing biliary complications of orthotopic liver transplantations with mangafodipir trisodium-enhanced MR cholangiography: comparison with conventional MR cholangiography. AJR Am J Roentgenol 2004;182:1497–504.

[17] Watanabe Y, Dohke M, Ishimori T, et al. Pseudo-obstruction of the extrahepatic bile duct due to artifact from arterial pulsatile compression: a diagnostic pitfall of MR cholangiopancreatography. Radiology 2000;214:856–60.

[18] Sugita R, Sugimura E, Itoh M, et al. Pseudolesion of the bile duct caused by flow effect: a diagnostic pitfall of MR cholangiopancreatography. AJR Am J Roentgenol 2003;180:467–71.

[19] Kelekis N, Semelka R. MR imaging of the gallbladder. Top Magn Reson Imaging 1996;8:312–32.

[20] Bader TR, Braga L, Beavers KL, et al. MR imaging findings of infectious cholangitis. Magn Reson Imaging 2001;19:781–8.

[21] Rofsky N, Lee V, Laub G, et al. Abdominal MR imaging with a volumetric interpolated breath-hold examination. Radiology 1999;212:876–84.

[22] Adusumilli S, Siegelman E. MR imaging of the gallbladder. Magn Reson Imaging Clin N Am 2002;10:165–84.

[23] Reimer P, Schneider G, Schima W. Hepatobiliary contrast agents for contrast-enhanced MRI of the liver: properties, clinical development and applications. Eur Radiol 2004;14:559–78.

[24] Carlos RC, Hussain HK, Song JH, et al. Gadolinium-ethoxybenzyl-diethylenetriamine pentaacetic acid as an intrabiliary contrast agent: preliminary assessment. AJR Am J Roentgenol 2002;179:87–92.

[25] Carlos RC, Branam JD, Dong Q, et al. Biliary imaging with Gd-EOB-DTPA: is a 20-minute delay sufficient? Acad Radiol 2002;9:1322–5.

[26] Mitchell DG, Alam F. Mangafodipir trisodium: effects on T2- and T1-weighted MR cholangiography. J Magn Reson Imaging 1999;9:366–8.

[27] Wielopolski PA, Gaa J, Wielopolski DR, et al. Breath-hold MR cholangiopancreatography with three-dimensional, segmented, echo-planar imaging and volume rendering. Radiology 1999;210:247–52.

[28] Soto JA, Barish MA, Yucel E, et al. Pancreatic duct: MR cholangiopancreatography with a three-dimensional fast spin-echo technique. Radiology 1995;196:459–64.

[29] Barish M, Yucel E, Soto J, et al. MR cholangiopancreatography: efficacy of three-dimensional turbo

spin-echo technique. AJR Am J Roentgenol 1995;165:295–300.

[30] McKenzie CA, Lim D, Ransil BJ, et al. Shortening MR image acquisition time for volumetric interpolated breath-hold examination with a recently developed parallel imaging reconstruction technique: clinical feasibility. Radiology 2003;230:589–94.

[31] Hiraishi K, Narabayashi I, Fujita O, et al. Blueberry juice: preliminary evaluation as an oral contrast agent in gastrointestinal MR imaging. Radiology 1995;194:119–23.

[32] Schreyer AG, Herfarth H, Kikinis R, et al. 3D modeling and virtual endoscopy of the small bowel based on magnetic resonance imaging in patients with inflammatory bowel disease. Invest Radiol 2002;37:528–33.

[33] Chan JHM, Tsui EYK, Yuen MK, et al. Gadopentate dimeglumine as an oral negative gastrointestinal contrast agent for MRCP. Abdom Imaging 2000;25:405–8.

[34] Kanematsu M, Matsuo M, Shiratori Y, et al. Thick-section half-fourier rapid acquisition with relaxation MR cholangiopancreatography: effects of IV administration of gadolinium chelate. AJR Am J Roentgenol 2002;178:755–61.

[35] Puente S, Bannura G. Radiological anatomy of the biliary tract: variations and congenital abnormalities. World J Surg 1983;7:271–6.

[36] Mortele KJ, Ros PR. Anatomic variants of the biliary tree: MR cholangiographic findings and clinical applications. AJR Am J Roentgenol 2001;177:389–94.

[37] Taourel P, Bret P, Reinhold C, et al. Anatomic variations of the biliary tree: diagnosis with MR cholangiopancreatography. Radiology 1996;199:521–7.

[38] Bassignanni M, Fulcher A, Szucs R, et al. Living donor liver transplantation. Radiographics 2001;21:39–52.

[39] Lee VS, Rofsky NM, Morgan GR, et al. Volumetric mangafodipir trisodium–enhanced cholangiography to define intrahepatic biliary anatomy. AJR Am J Roentgenol 2001;176:906–8.

[40] Limanond P, Raman SS, Ghobrial RM, et al. The utility of MRCP in preoperative mapping of biliary anatomy in adult-to-adult living related liver transplant donors. J Magn Reson Imaging 2004;19:209–15.

[41] Fulcher AS, Turner MA, Ham JM. Late biliary complications in right lobe living donor transplantation recipients: imaging findings and therapeutic interventions. J Comput Assist Tomogr 2002;26:422–7.

[42] Kapoor V, Peterson MS, Baron RL, et al. Intrahepatic biliary anatomy of living adult liver donors: correlation of mangafodipir trisodium-enhanced MR cholangiography and intraoperative cholangiography. AJR Am J Roentgenol 2002;179:1281–6.

[43] Lee VS, Krinsky GA, Nazzaro CA, et al. Defining intrahepatic biliary anatomy in living liver

transplant donor candidates at mangafodipir trisodium-enhanced MR cholangiography versus conventional T2-weighted MR cholangiography.
Radiology 2004;23:659–66.

[44] Yeh BM, Breiman RS, Taouli B, et al. Biliary tract
depiction in living potential liver donors: comparison of conventional MR, mangafodipir trisodium-
enhanced excretory MR, and multi-detector row
CT cholangiography—initial experience. Radiology 2004;230:645–51.

[45] Silva AC, Friese JL, Hara AK, et al. MR cholangiopancreatography: improved ductal distention
with intravenous morphine administration. Radiographics 2004;24:677–87.

[46] Tsai H-M, Lin X-Z, Chen C-Y, et al. MRI of gallstones with different compositions. AJR Am J
Roentgenol 2004;182:1513–9.

[47] Ukaji M, Ebara M, Tsuchiya Y, et al. Diagnosis
of gallstone composition in magnetic resonance
imaging: in vitro analysis. Eur J Radiol 2002;
41:49–56.

[48] Inoue Y, Komatsu Y, Yoshikawa K, et al. Biliary
motor function in gallstone patients evaluated by
fatty-meal MR cholangiography. J Magn Reson
Imaging 2003;18:196–203.

[49] Regan F, Schaefer DC, Smith DP, et al. The diagnostic utility of HASTE MRI in the evaluation of
acute cholecystitis. J Comput Assist Tomogr
1998;22:638–42.

[50] Loud P, Semelka R, Kettritz U, et al. MRI of acute
cholecystitis: comparison with the normal gallbladder and other entities. Magn Reson Imaging 1996;
14:349–55.

[51] Park MS, Yu J-S, Kim YH, et al. Acute cholecystitis: comparison of MR cholangiography and US.
Radiology 1998;209:781–5.

[52] Hakansson K. MR characteristics of acute cholangitis. Acta Radiol 2002;43:175–9.

[53] Kim P, Outwater E, Mitchell D. Mirizzi syndrome:
evaluation by MRI imaging. Am J Gastroenterol
1999;94:2546–50.

[54] Sood B, Jain M, Khandelwal N, et al. MRI of perforated gall bladder. Australas Radiol 2002;46:
438–40.

[55] Kim KW, Park M-S, Yu J-S, et al. Acute cholecystitis at T2-weighted and manganese-enhanced T1-
weighted MR cholangiography: preliminary study.
Radiology 2003;227:580–4.

[56] Fayad LM, Holland GA, Bergin D, et al. Functional magnetic resonance cholangiography
(fMRC) of the gallbladder and biliary tree with
contrast-enhanced magnetic resonance cholangiography. J Magn Reson Imaging 2003;18:
449–60.

[57] Kim M, Oh Y, Park Y, et al. Gallbladder adenomyomatosis: findings on MRI. Abdom Imaging
1999;24:410–3.

[58] Yoshimitsu K, Honda H, Kaneko K, et al. Dynamic MR imaging of the gallbladder lesions: dif-

ferentiation of benign from malignant. J Magn
Reson Imaging 1997;7:696–701.

[59] Yoshimitsu K, Honda H, Jimi M. MR diagnosis of
adenomyomatosis of the gallbladder and differentiation from gallbladder carcinoma: importance of
showing Rokitansky-Aschoff sinuses. AJR Am J
Roentgenol 1999;172:1535–40.

[60] Rajagopalan V, Daines W, Grossbard M, et al.
Gallbladder and biliary tract carcinoma: a comprehensive update, Part 1. Oncology (Huntingt) 2004;
18:889–96.

[61] Schwartz L, Black J, Fong Y, et al. Gallbladder carcinoma: findings at MR imaging with MR cholangiopancreatography. J Comput Assist Tomogr
2002;26:405–10.

[62] Kim JH, Kim TK, Eun HW, et al. Preoperative
evaluation of gallbladder carcinoma: efficacy of
combined use of MR imaging, MR cholangiography, and contrast-enhanced dual-phase three-
dimensional MR angiography. J Magn Reson
Imaging 2002;16:676–84.

[63] Demachi H, Matsui O, Hoshiba K, et al. Dynamic
MRI using a surface coil in chronic cholecystitis
and gallbladder carcinoma: radiologic and histopathologic correlation. J Comput Assist Tomogr
1997;21:643–51.

[64] Kim SH, Lim JH, Yoon, et al. Choledochal cyst:
comparison of MR and conventional cholangiography. Clin Radiol 2000;55:378–83.

[65] Arshanskiy Y, Vyas P. Type IV choledochal cyst
presenting with obstructive jaundice: role of MR
cholangiography in preoperative evaluation. Am J
Roentgenol 1998;171:457–9.

[66] Krause D, Cercueil J, Dranssart M, et al. MRI for
evaluating congenital bile duct abnormalities.
J Comput Assist Tomogr 2002;24:541–52.

[67] De Backer A, Van den Abbeele K, De Schepper A,
et al. Choledochocele: diagnosis by magnetic resonance imaging. Abdom Imaging 2000;25:508–10.

[68] Irie H, Honda H, Jimi M, et al. Value of MR cholangiopancreatography in evaluating choledochal
cysts. AJR Am J Roentgenol 1998;171:1381–5.

[69] Kobayashi H, Stringer M. Biliary atresia. Semin
Neonatol 2003;8:383–91.

[70] Norton K, Glass R, Kogan D, et al. MR cholangiography in the evaluation of neonatal cholestasis:
initial results. Radiology 2002;222:687–91.

[71] Kim M, Park Y, Han S, et al. Biliary atresia in neonates and infants: triangular area of high signal intensity in the porta hepatis at T2-weighted MR
cholangiography with US and histopathologic correlation. Radiology 2000;215:395–401.

[72] Kim J, Kim M, Park S, et al. MR cholangiography
in symptomatic gallstones: diagnostic accuracy
according to clinical risk group. Radiology 2002;
224:410–6.

[73] Kim T, Kim B, Kim J, et al. Diagnosis of intrahepatic stones: superiority of MR cholangiopancreatography   over   endoscopic   retrograde

cholangiopancreatography. AJR Am J Roentgenol 2002;179:429–34.

[74] Cesari S, Liessi G, Balestreri L, et al. Raysum reconstruction algorithm in MR cholangiopancreatography. Magn Reson Imaging 2000;18:217–9.

[75] Vitellas KM, Keogan MT, Freed KS, et al. Radiologic manifestations of sclerosing cholangitis with emphasis on MR cholangiopancreatography. Radiographics 2000;20:959–75.

[76] Angulo P, Pearce D, Johnson C, et al. Magnetic resonance cholangiography in patients with biliary disease: its role in primary sclerosing cholangitis. J Hepatol 2000;33:520–7.

[77] Revelon G, Rashid A, Kawamoto S, et al. Primary sclerosing cholangitis: MR imaging findings with pathologic correlation. AJR Am J Roentgenol 1999;173:1037–42.

[78] Silverman W, Kaw M, Rabinovitz M, et al. Complication rate of endoscopic retrograde cholangiopancreatography (ERCP) in patients with primary sclerosing cholangitis (PSC): is it safe? Gastroenterology 1994;106:A359.

[79] Vitellas KM, Enns RA, Keogan MT, et al. Comparison of MR cholangiopancreatic techniques with contrast-enhanced cholangiography in the evaluation of sclerosing cholangitis. AJR Am J Roentgenol 2001;178:327–407.

[80] Ferrara C, Valeri G, Salvolini L, et al. Magnetic resonance cholangiopancreatography in primary sclerosing cholangitis in children. Pediatr Radiol 2002;32(6):413–7.

[81] Macchi V, Floreani A, Marchesi P, et al. Imaging of primary sclerosing cholangitis: preliminary results by two new non-invasive techniques. Dig Liver Dis 2004;36:614–21.

[82] Lim J. Oriental cholangiohepatitis: pathologic, clinical, and radiologic features. AJR Am J Roentgenol 1991;157:1–8.

[83] Kim J, Kim M, Park S, et al. Using kinematic MR cholangiopancreatography to evaluate biliary dilatation. AJR Am J Roentgenol 2002;178:909–14.

[84] Horton KM, Bluemke DA, Hruban RH, et al. CT and MR imaging of benign hepatic and biliary tumors. Radiographics 1999;19:431–51.

[85] Manfredi R, Barbaro B, Masselli G, et al. Magnetic resonance imaging of cholangiocarcinoma. Semin Liver Dis 2004;24:155–64.

[86] Brink J, Borrello J. MR imaging of the biliary system. Magn Reson Imaging Clin N Am 1995;3:143–60.

[87] Pavone P, Laghi A, Passariello R. MR cholangiopancreatography in malignant biliary obstruction. Semin Ultrasound CT MR 1999;20:317–23.

[88] Soto J, Alvarez O, Lopera J, et al. Biliary obstruction: findings at MR cholangiography and cross-sectional MR imaging. Radiographics 2000;20:353–66.

[89] Worawattanakul S, Semelka R, Noone T, et al. Cholangiocarcinoma: spectrum of appearances on MR images using current techniques. Magn Reson Imaging 1998;16:993–1003.

[90] Condat B, Vilgrain V, Asselah T, et al. Portal cavernoma-associated cholangiopathy: a clinical and MR cholangiography coupled with MR portography imaging study. Hepatology 2003;37:1302–8.

[91] Patkowski W, Nyckowski P, Zieniewicz K, et al. Biliary tract complications following liver transplantation. Transplant Proc 2003;35:2316–7.

[92] Khalid TR, Casillas VJ, Montalvo BM, et al. Using MR cholangiopancreatography to evaluate iatrogenic bile duct injury. AJR Am J Roentgenol 2001;177(6):1347–52.

[93] Richardson M, Bell G, Fullarton G. Incidence and nature of bile duct injuries following laparoscopic cholecystectomy: an audit of 5913 cases. West of Scotland Laparoscopic Cholecystectomy Audit Group. Br J Surg 1996;83:1356–60.

[94] Slanetz P, Boland G, Mueller P. Imaging and interventional radiology in laparoscopic injuries to the gallbladder and biliary system. Radiology 1996;201:595–603.

[95] Boraschi P, Braccini G, Gigoni R, et al. Detection of biliary complications after orthotopic liver transplantation with MR cholangiography. Magn Reson Imaging 2001;19:1097–105.

[96] Buanes T, Waage A, Mjaland O, et al. Bile leak after cholecystectomy significance and treatment: results from the National Norwegian Cholecystectomy Registry. Int Surg 1996;81:276–9.

[97] Vitellas KM, El-Dieb A, Vaswani KK, et al. Using contrast-enhanced MR cholangiography with IV mangafodipir trisodium (Teslascan) to evaluate bile duct leaks after cholecystectomy: a prospective study of 11 patients. AJR Am J Roentgenol 2002;179:409–16.

[98] Kalayci C, Aisen A, Canal D, et al. Magnetic resonance cholangiopancreatography documents bile site leak after cholecystectomy in patients with aberrant right hepatic duct where ERCP fails. Gastrointest Endosc 2000;52:277–81.

[99] Panharipande PV, Lee VS, Morgan GR, et al. Vascular and extravascular complications of liver transplantation: comprehensive evaluation with three-dimensional contrast-enhanced volumetric MR imaging and MR cholangiopancreatography. AJR Am J Roentgenol 2001;177:1101–7.

[100] Vitellas K, El-Dieb A, Vaswani K, et al. Detection of bile duct leaks using MR cholangiography with mangfodipir trisodium (Teslascan). J Comput Assist Tomogr 2001;25(1):102–5.

[101] Ward J, Sheridan M, Guthrie J, et al. Bile duct strictures after hepatobiliary surgery: assessment with MR cholangiography. Radiology 2004;231:101–8.

ELSEVIER
SAUNDERS

Magn Reson Imaging Clin N Am
13 (2005) 313–330

MAGNETIC
RESONANCE
IMAGING CLINICS
of North America

MR Imaging of the Pancreas

Ertan Pamuklar, MD, Richard C. Semelka, MD*

*Department of Radiology, University of North Carolina, 101 Manning Drive,
CB #7510, Chapel Hill, NC 27599-7510, USA*

MR imaging techniques

New MR imaging techniques that limit artifacts in the abdomen have increased the role of MR imaging to detect and characterize pancreatic disease. Breath-hold T1-weighted gradient echo sequences obtained as 2D- or 3D-gradient echo, fat-suppression techniques, and dynamic administration of gadolinium chelate have resulted in image quality of the pancreas sufficient to detect and characterize focal pancreatic mass lesions smaller than 1 cm in diameter and in the ability to evaluate diffuse pancreatic disease [1–4].

MR cholangiopancreatography (MRCP) permits good demonstration of the biliary and pancreatic ducts to assess ductal obstruction, dilatation, and abnormal duct pathways [2–4]. The combination of tissue-imaging sequences and MRCP provides comprehensive information to evaluate the full range of pancreatic disease.

MR imaging of the pancreas is optimal at high field (≥ 1.0 T) due to a good signal-to-noise ratio, which facilitates breath-hold imaging, and increased fat-water frequency shift, which facilitates chemically selective excitation-spoiling fat suppression. T1-weighted chemically selective fat suppression and T1-weighted, breath-hold gradient echo are effective techniques for imaging the pancreatic parenchyma. The normal pancreas is high in signal intensity on T1-weighted fat-suppressed images due to the presence of aqueous protein in the acini of the pancreas [1]. Normal pancreas is well shown using this technique [5,6]. In elderly patients, the signal intensity of the

pancreas may diminish and be lower than that of liver. This may reflect changes of fibrosis secondary to the aging process.

Our standard MR protocol includes T1-weighted, fat-suppressed gradient echo and post-gadolinium imaging in the capillary phase (immediate postcontrast) and interstitial phase (1–10 minutes postcontrast). There may be advantages in performing post-gadolinium gradient echo imaging as a 3D-gradient echo technique for the following reasons: (1) Thinner sections can be obtained (3 mm versus 5 mm for 2D-SGE) and (2) mirror artifacts, which are problematic on 2D-SGE from the aorta, are absent. T2-weighted echo-train spin-echo sequences, such as T2-weighted half-Fourier acquisition snapshot turbo spin-echo, provide a sharp anatomic display of the common bile duct on coronal plane images and of the pancreatic duct on transverse plane images. MRCP images can be acquired oriented in the plane of the pancreatic duct, in an oblique coronal projection, to delineate longer segments of the pancreatic duct in continuity [7]. T2-weighted fat-suppressed images are useful for demonstrating liver metastases and islet-cell tumors. T2-weighted images also provide information on the complexity of the fluid in pancreatic pseudocysts, which may reflect the presence of complications such as necrotic debris or infection. Regarding gadolinium enhancement, the pancreas demonstrates a uniform capillary blush on immediate postcontrast images, which renders it higher in signal intensity than liver, neighboring bowel, and adjacent fat. By 1 minute after contrast, the pancreas becomes approximately isointense with fat, and beyond 2 minutes, the pancreas is lower in signal intensity than background fat. Pancreatic head is readily distinguished from duodenum on

---

* Corresponding author.

E-mail address: richsem@med.unc.edu (R.C. Semelka).

1064-9689/05/$ - see front matter © 2005 Elsevier Inc. All rights reserved.
doi:10.1016/j.mric.2005.03.012

mri.theclinics.com

immediate postgadolinium images because the pancreas enhances substantially greater than bowel. MR imaging combining T1, T2, early and late postgadolinium images, MRCP, and MR angiography generates comprehensive information on the pancreas [8–11].

Recognition of the characteristic high signal intensity of normal pancreas on precontrast T1-weighted fat-suppressed, and immediate postgadolinium images is useful in circumstances of abnormalities of position. After left nephrectomy, the tail of the pancreas falls into the renal fossa, which can simulate recurrent disease on CT examination. Normal pancreas can be readily distinguished by its high signal intensity.

Acute pancreatitis

The signal-intensity features of the pancreas in uncomplicated mild acute pancreatitis resemble those of normal pancreatic tissue. The pancreas is high in signal intensity on precontrast T1-weighted

fat-suppressed images and enhances in a normal uniform fashion on immediate postgadolinium images reflecting a normal capillary blush. The diagnosis of acute pancreatitis on MR images is aided by the presence of morphologic changes [1]. The acutely inflamed pancreas shows focal or diffuse enlargement, which may be subtle (Fig. 1). Peripancreatic fluid is well shown on noncontrast or immediate postgadolinium gradient echo images and appears as low signal-intensity strands of fluid or fluid collections in a background of high signal intensity fat (Figs. 1 and 2). Single-shot, breathing-independent, T2-weighted images using fat suppression is the most sensitive technique at showing small-volume, high-signal fluid in a background of intermediate to low signal pancreas and low signal fat. MR imaging is sensitive for the detection of subtle changes of acute pancreatitis, particularly minor peripancreatic inflammatory changes. CT imaging examinations appear normal in 15% to 30% of patients with clinical features of acute pancreatitis [12]. The sensitivity of MR imaging exceeds that of CT imaging, suggesting a role for

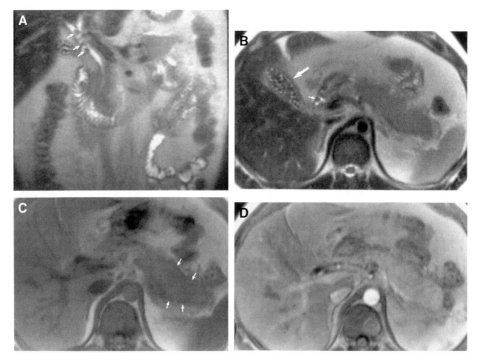

Fig. 1. Acute gallstone pancreatitis. Coronal (A) and transverse (B) T2-weighted SS-ETSE, T1-weighted gradient echo (C), and immediate postgadolinium T1-weighted gradient echo (D) images in a patient with acute gallstone pancreatitis demonstrate three stones in the CHD and common bile duct (A and B, *small arrows*). Multiple small stones are present in the gallbladder (B, *large arrow*). The pancreas is enlarged diffusely (C, *arrows*), with ill-defined margins and minimal volume of surrounding fluid.

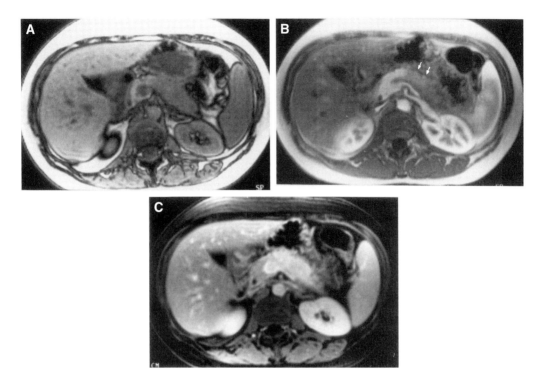

Fig. 2. Acute on chronic pancreatitis T1-weighted, out-of-phase gradient echo (*A*); immediate postgadolinium T1-weighted gradient echo (*B*); and 90-s postgadolinium, fat-suppressed, T1-weighted gradient echo (*C*). The body and tail of the pancreas are mildly enlarged, with minimal enhancement on immediate postgadolinium image (*B*), and show delayed increased enhancement (*C*). This pattern of enhancement is consistent with fibrosis. A thin layer of fluid around the pancreas appreciated on immediate postgadolinium image (*B*, *arrows*) is consistent with acute inflammation.

MR imaging in the evaluation of patients with suspected acute pancreatitis and negative CT imaging examination. As the extent of pancreatitis becomes more severe, the pancreas develops a heterogeneous appearance on precontrast T1-weighted fat-suppressed images and enhances in a more heterogeneous, diminished fashion on immediate postgadolinium images.

The percentage of pancreatic necrosis has been considered to be an important prognostic indicator in patients with acute pancreatitis [13,14]. Dynamic gadolinium-enhanced gradient echo images may be useful for this determination because MR imaging is sensitive for the demonstration of the presence or absence of gadolinium enhancement. Saifuddin et al [15] described comparable results for dynamic contrast-enhanced CT images and immediate postgadolinium gradient echo images for determining the presence of pancreatic necrosis. Complications of acute pancreatitis, such as hemorrhage, pseudocyst formation, or abscess, are clearly shown on MR imaging. Hemorrhagic fluid collections are high in signal intensity on T1-weighted fat-suppressed images, and depiction of hemorrhage is superior on MR images compared with CT images. Martin et al demonstrated a correlation between the extent of high signal on noncontrast T1-weighted fat-suppressed SGE and severity of acute pancreatitis, where high signal correlated with hemorrhagic changes. Simple pseudocysts are low in signal intensity or are signal void in a background of normal signal intensity pancreatic tissue on noncontrast T1-weighted fat-suppressed gradient echo images. Extrapancreatic pseudocysts are well shown on breath-hold gradient echo images due to high contrast with high signal intensity fat. Image acquisition in multiple planes permits the determination of pseudocyst location in relation to various organs and structures. Pseudocyst walls enhance minimally on early postgadolinium images and show progressively intense enhancement on 5-minute postcontrast images, consistent with the appearance of fibrous tissue. Simple pseudocysts are relatively homogeneous and high in signal intensity on T2-weighted images. Pseudocyst complicated by necrotic debris, hemorrhage, or infection is heterogeneous in signal intensity on T2-weighted images [15]. Proteinaceous fluid tends to layer in a gradation of concentration with low signal intensity, concentrated proteinaceous material in the dependent portion of the cyst. Necrotic material may appear as irregularly shaped regions of low signal intensity in the pseudocyst [16]. This information may provide therapeutic and prognostic information because pseudocysts that contain necrotic material may not respond to simple percutaneous drainage and thus may require open debridement. Breathing independent T2-weighted sequences, such as single-shot echo train spin echo, may be useful in evaluating these pseudocyst collections not only because they are the most effective at demonstrating the complexity of fluid but also because many of these patients are debilitated and unable to cooperate with breath-holding instructions.

Chronic pancreatitis

An analysis of patients with chronic pancreatitis imaged on dynamic contrast-enhanced CT images showed the following features: 66% had dilation of the main pancreatic duct, 54% had parenchymal atrophy, 50% had pancreatic calcifications, 34% had pseudocysts, 32% had focal pancreatic enlargement, 29% had biliary ductal dilatation, and 16% had densities in peripancreatic fat or fascia. No abnormalities were present in 7% of patients [17]. MR imaging may perform better than CT imaging at detecting changes of chronic pancreatitis because MR imaging detects not only morphologic findings but also the presence of fibrosis. Fibrosis is shown by diminished signal intensity on T1-weighted fat-suppressed images and diminished heterogeneous enhancement on immediate postgadolinium gradient echo images (Fig. 3) [18]. Low signal intensity on T1-weighted fat-suppressed images reflects loss of the aqueous

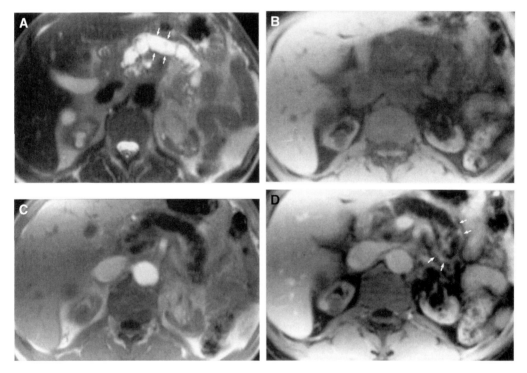

Fig. 3. Chronic pancreatitis. T2-weighted SS-ETSE (A); fat-suppressed, T1-weighted gradient echo (B); immediate postgadolinium T1-weighted gradient echo (C); and 90-s postgadolinium, fat-suppressed, T1-weighted gradient echo (D) images in a patient with chronic pancreatitis. A severely dilated pancreatic duct is demonstrated (A, arrows). The pancreas is atrophic and is low in signal intensity on pre-gadolinium fat-suppressed, T1-weighted gradient echo image (B). The atrophic pancreas enhances minimally on immediate postgadolinium image (C) and shows late enhancement (D, arrows), consistent with changes of fibrosis.

protein in the acini of the pancreas. Diminished enhancement on capillary-phase images reflects disruption of the normal capillary bed and increased chronic inflammation and fibrous tissue. Most cases of chronic pancreatitis show progressive parenchymal enhancement on 5-minute postcontrast images, reflecting the pattern of enhancement of fibrous tissue. A study that described MR imaging findings in 13 patients with chronic calcifying pancreatitis and nine patients with acute recurrent pancreatitis demonstrated differences between these groups on T1-weighted fat-suppressed images and immediate postgadolinium gradient echo images. All patients with pancreatic calcifications on CT examination had a diminished signal-intensity pancreas on T1-weighted fat-suppressed images and an abnormally low percentage of contrast enhancement on immediate postgadolinium gradient echo images. Patients with acute recurrent pancreatitis had signal intensity features of the pancreas comparable to normal pancreas.

Focal enlargement of the head of the pancreas with chronic pancreatitis may be difficult to distinguish from cancer on CT images. MR images permit the distinction between these two entities with greater reliability. Chronic pancreatitis and carcinoma show similar signal intensity changes of the enlarged region of pancreas on noncontrast T1-weighted fat-suppressed and T2-weighted images—generally mildly hypointense on T1-weighted images and heterogenous and mildly hyperintense on T2-weighted images. On immediate postgadolinium images, focal pancreatitis shows heterogeneous enhancement with the presence of signal-void cysts and calcifications without evidence of a marginated definable, minimally enhancing mass lesion. Demonstration of a definable, circumscribed mass lesion is most often diagnostic for tumor. In chronic pancreatitis, the focally enlarged portion of pancreas usually shows preservation of a glandular, feathery, or marbled texture similar to that of remaining pancreas. In contrast, in pancreatic cancer, the focally enlarged portion of pancreas loses its usual anatomic detail. Diffuse low signal intensity of the entire pancreas, similar to and including the area of focal enlargement, on T1-weighted fat-suppressed and immediate postgadolinium SGE images is typical for chronic pancreatitis. In the setting of pancreatic cancer, the enhancement of the tumor is less than adjacent pancreatic parenchyma. Rarely, chronic pancreatitis may involve only the focally enlarged portion of pancreas, with the remainder of the pancreas having no inflammatory changes. In these cases, the focus of chronic pancreatitis can simulate the appearance of pancreatic ductal adenocarcinoma. The inflammatory process may be sufficiently destructive that underlying stromal pattern is lost. In these rare cases, diagnosis can be established only by surgical resection and histopathologic examination confirming the absence of malignancy.

Pancreatic pseudocysts occur with an incidence of 10% in patients with chronic pancreatitis [19]. Small pseudocysts and cysts are well shown on gadolinium-enhanced, T1-weighted fat-suppressed images as nearly signal-void oval structures. Pseudocysts are generally high in signal intensity on T2-weighted images, but signal intensity varies considerably based on the presence of blood, protein, infection, and debris. Pseudocyst walls generally show minimal early post gadinolinium enhancement and progressive enhancement on 5-minute postcontrast images.

Pancreatic adenocarcinoma

Pancreatic ductal adenocarcinoma accounts for 95% of the malignant tumors of the pancreas. The tumor has a poor prognosis, with a 5-year survival of 5% [20].

Detection of carcinoma is best performed by immediate postgadolinium T1-weighted gradient echo images (Fig. 4) [1,4,21–23]. Pancreatic tissue is well delineated from tumors, and tumor margins are clearly shown using this sequence in all regions of the pancreas. Small tumors or tumors of the pancreatic tail are also well demonstrated on noncontrast T1-weighted fat-suppressed images. Larger tumors in the pancreatic head are revealed less consistently with noncontrast T1-weighted fat-suppressed images. Conventional spin-echo images are generally limited in the detection of pancreatic cancer [24]. Tumors are usually minimally hypointense relative to pancreas on T2-weighted images and are therefore difficult to visualize. One study evaluated MR imaging, including noncontrast T1-weighted fat-suppressed spin-echo, and immediate postgadolinium gradient echo, for the detection or exclusion of pancreatic cancer in 16 patients with findings indeterminate for cancer on spiral CT imaging [22]. Immediate postgadolinium gradient echo was found to be the most sensitive approach to detect pancreatic cancer, particularly in the head of the pancreas. Immediate postgadolinium gradient

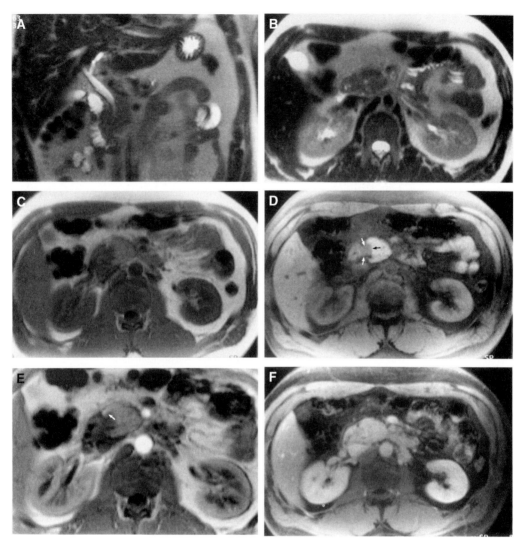

Fig. 4. Small pancreatic adenocarcinoma. Coronal (*A*) and transverse (*B*) T2-weighted SS-ETSE; T1-weighted gradient echo (*C*); fat-suppressed, T1-weighted gradient echo (*D*); immediate postgadolinium T1-weighted gradient echo (*E*); and 90-s postgadolinium, fat-suppressed T1-weighted gradient echo (*F*) images in a patient with pancreatic adenocarcinoma demonstrate a 1.5-cm mass arising in the pancreatic head. The tumor is most clearly appreciated on the pre-gadolinium fat-suppressed T1-weighted (*D, arrows*) and immediate postgadolinium T1-weighted gradient echo (*E*) images. Common bile duct obstruction and biliary dilation are best seen on T2-weighted images (*A, B*). The tumor invades the duodenal wall and gastroduodenal artery (*E, arrow*). Fat-suppressed T1-weighted gradient echo (*G*) and immediate postgadolinium T1-weighted gradient echo (*H*) images are shown in a second patient. On the fat-suppressed T1-weighted image, the tumor is low in signal intensity relative to background pancreas (*G, arrow*). On the immediate postgadolinium image, the tumor enhances less than the background pancreas (*H, arrow*).

echo and noncontrast T1-weighted fat-suppressed imaging performed well at excluding cancer, and both were significantly superior to spiral CT imaging. These findings are similar to those reported by Gabata et al [21], who compared these MR techniques to dynamic contrast-enhanced CT imaging.

Due to their abundant fibrous stroma and relatively sparse vascularity, pancreatic cancers enhance to a lesser extent than surrounding normal pancreatic tissue on early postcontrast images [21]. It is therefore critical to exploit this difference in vascularity on contrast-enhanced studies by imaging in the dynamic capillary phase

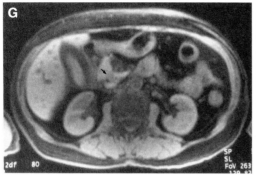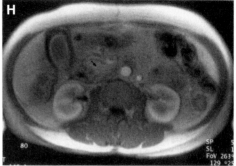

Fig. 4 (*continued*)

of enhancement (Fig. 4) [21,22]. Thin section acquisition is also helpful, but 8-mm thick sections may be sufficiently thin to detect even small (<1 cm) cancers due to the high contrast resolution on 2D-SGE images. An adequate signal-to-noise ratio may be achieved with section thickness of 5 mm by using a phased-array surface coil. On newer MR systems, 3D-gradient echo is a good technique to detect small pancreatic cancers. Although pancreatic cancers are lower in signal intensity than pancreas on immediate postgadolinium (capillary-phase) images, the appearance of cancers on ≥1-minute postgadolinium (interstitial-phase) images is variable [21]. The enhancement of cancer relative to pancreas on interstitial phase images reflects the volume of extracellular space and venous drainage of cancers compared with pancreatic tissue. In general, large pancreatic tumors tend to remain low in signal intensity on later images (Fig. 4), whereas smaller tumors may range from hypointense to hyperintense.

Pancreatic cancers appear as low signal-intensity masses on noncontrast T1-weighted fat-suppressed images and are clearly separated from normal pancreatic tissue, which is high in signal intensity [4,21,22]. Pancreatic tissue distal to pancreatic cancer is often lower in signal intensity than normal pancreatic tissue [21,22]. This finding may be explained by tumor-associated pancreatitis occurring distal to the tumor because of obstruction of the main pancreatic duct. With chronic inflammation of the pancreas, there is progressive fibrosis and glandular atrophy, and the proteinaceous fluid of the gland diminishes [21,25]. In these cases, depiction of cancer is poor on noncontrast T1-weighted fat-suppressed images [21,22]. Immediate postgadolinium gradient echo images are able to define the size and extent of cancers that obstruct the pancreatic duct

[21,22]. Demonstration of a rim of increased enhancement relative to surrounding pancreas is commonly observed in pancreatic cancers, particularly in those arising in the head. This is an important imaging feature that helps to establish the focal nature of the disease process. These tumors appear as low signal intensity mass lesions in a background of slightly greater enhancing chronically inflamed pancreas. Tumors are usually large when they cause changes of surrounding chronic pancreatitis, and in this setting, diagnosis is not problematic. In carcinomas involving the tail, uninvolved pancreatic parenchyma is proximal to the tumor and therefore usually is uninvolved and high in signal intensity on T1-weighted fat-suppressed images. This differs from carcinoma within the pancreatic head and reflects the fact that chronic pancreatitis occurs when a tumor obstructs the main pancreatic duct near its termination. An additional imaging feature that assists in the distinction between carcinoma and chronic pancreatitis is effacement of the fine, lobular contours of the gland by carcinoma. In contrast, in the setting of chronic pancreatitis, although there may be focal enlargement of the gland, the internal pancreatic architecture is generally preserved and retains the lobular, marbled, or feathery appearance on MR imaging. On immediate postgadolinium images, pancreatic carcinoma has diminished signal intensity without well-defined internal structure but with a mild heterogeneous morphology, whereas with chronic pancreatitis the architectural pattern is most often preserved, although enhancement is diminished.

Pancreatic carcinoma usually appears as a focal mass that is readily detected and characterized on immediate postgadolinium images. In these instances, the tumor is relatively well demarcated from adjacent uninvolved pancreas, which shows greater enhancement. Pancreatic cancer may occasionally be infiltrative in morphology with poorly defined margins. In this setting, tumors are ill defined and decreased in enhancement on immediate postgadolinium images and may show slightly increased enhancement on 2-minute postgadolinium fat-suppressed gradient echo images. This appearance is commonly observed in pancreatic cancer that has been treated with chemotherapy and radiation therapy (see below) but may also be seen at initial presentation. Features that may aid in the distinction from chronic pancreatitis are the relatively short history of clinical findings (eg, pain, jaundice) and the high-grade biliary or pancreatic ductal obstruction despite apparently small-volume disease.

Regarding tumor staging, local extension of cancer and lymphovascular involvement may be evaluated on nonsuppressed T1-weighted images [26,27]. A low signal intensity tumor is well shown in a background of high signal intensity fat. Gadolinium-enhanced fat-suppressed gradient echo images, acquired in the interstitial phase of enhancement (1–10 minutes postcontrast), demonstrate intermediate signal intensity tumor tissue extension into low signal intensity-suppressed fat. In comparison, noncontrast T1-weighted fat-suppressed images generally show minimal signal intensity difference between the tumor, which is low in signal intensity, and suppressed background fat [21]. When the tumor involves the body or tail of the pancreas, invasion of adjacent organs, such as the left adrenal gland, is well shown on a combination of sequences, including nonsuppressed T1-weighted images and interstitial-phase gadolinium-enhanced fat-suppressed T1-weighted images.

Vascular encasement by tumor is best shown using thin-section 3D-gradient echo images, which can be analyzed as source images in the transverse plane and reformatted images in the coronal plane. Coronal plane reformatted images are of value to determine the relationship between tumor and the portal vein as it enters the porta hepatis and tumor and the superior mesenteric vein along the medial margin of the head of pancreas. Immediate postgadolinium gradient echo images are useful for evaluating arterial patency, and immediate and 45-second postgadolinium gradient echo images are useful for evaluating venous patency.

When comparing approaches by CT and MR imaging, an interstitial-phase gadolinium-enhanced, fat-suppressed sequence is an effective technique to delineate peritoneal metastases and is superior to CT [28,29]. MR does not perform well at local staging if this technique is not used [30]. Peritoneal metastases appear as moderately high signal in a dark background of suppressed fat and are conspicuous even if peritoneal disease is of thin volume and is relatively linear. Demonstration of focal thickening or nodules increases the likelihood that peritoneal abnormalities represent a malignant process.

Lymph nodes are well shown on T2-weighted fat-suppressed images and interstitial-phase gadolinium-enhanced fat-suppressed T1-weighted images. Lymph nodes are moderately high in signal intensity in a background of low signal intensity suppressed fat using both of these techniques. T2-weighted, fat-suppressed imaging is useful for the demonstration of lymph nodes in close approximation to the liver due to the signal intensity difference between moderately high signal intensity nodes and moderately low signal intensity liver. Lymph nodes and liver appear moderately enhanced on the interstitial phase of gadolinium-enhanced, fat-suppressed, gradient echo technique, so lymph nodes are not as conspicuous in the region of the porta hepatis with this technique. To detect lymph nodes adjacent to liver, it is useful to identify suspicious foci of high signal on the T2-weighted fat-suppressed technique and confirm that they have the rounded morphology of lymph nodes on the gadolinium-enhanced fat-suppressed T1-weighted sequences. On nonsuppressed T1-weighted images, lymph nodes are conspicuous as low signal intensity focal masses in a background of high signal intensity fat [27], but this technique performs best in the detection of retroperitoneal nodes or mesenteric nodes in the setting of abundant fat in these locations. Coronal plane imaging provides adequate visualization of these locations.

Liver metastases from pancreatic cancers are generally irregular in shape and are low in signal intensity on conventional or fat-suppressed T1-weighted images; are minimally hyperintense on T2-weighted images; and demonstrate irregular rim enhancement on immediate postcontrast gradient echo images. The low signal intensity centers of metastatic lesions reflect the desmoplastic nature of the primary cancer [1]. The low fluid content and hypovascular nature of these metastases permits the distinction between these lesions and cysts and hemangiomas, respectively, even when lesions are 1 cm in diameter. Transient, ill-defined, increased perilesional enhancement in the hepatic parenchyma may be observed on immediate postgadolinium images. A similar appearance is observed more commonly for colon cancer metastases. Perilesional enhancement is more typically wedge-shaped with pancreatic cancer liver metastases than with colon cancer liver metastases and may have a dramatic appearance. Concomitant liver metastases in the setting of prominent wedge-shaped enhancement abnormalities are commonly small, hypervascular, and subcapsular in location. Small subcapsular hypervascular metastases are observed in over 80% of patients and may be the only pattern of liver metastases in up to 20% of patients [31].

Optimal uses of MR imaging in the investigation of pancreatic carcinoma occur in the following circumstances: (1) in the detection of small, noncontour-deforming tumors (due to the high contrast resolution of precontrast T1-weighted fat-suppressed and immediate postgadolinium gradient echo imaging), (2) in the determination of tumor location for imaging-guided biopsy, (3) in the evaluation of vascular involvement by tumor, (4) in the determination and characterization of associated liver lesions, and (5) in the evaluation of patients with diminished renal function or iodine contrast allergy. MR imaging may be particularly valuable in patients who have an enlarged pancreatic head with no definition of a mass on CT images.

Islet-cell tumors

In the MR imaging investigation for islet-cell tumors, precontrast T1-weighted fat-suppressed images; immediate postgadolinium gradient echo images; and T2-weighted fat-suppressed images or breath-hold T2-weighted images are useful [1,32–35]. Because many MR techniques independently demonstrate islet-cell tumors well, MR is particularly well suited for the investigation of these tumors. Tumors are low in signal intensity on T1-weighted fat-suppressed images; demonstrate homogeneous, ring, or diffuse heterogeneous enhancement on immediate postgadolinium gradient echo; and are high in signal intensity on T2-weighted fat-suppressed images [36]. In rare instances, islet-cell tumors may be desmoplastic, appear low in signal intensity on T2-weighted images, and demonstrate negligible contrast enhancement. In these cases, the tumors may mimic the appearance of pancreatic ductal adenocarcinoma. Large, noninsulinoma, islet-cell tumors commonly contain regions of necrosis [37].

Features that distinguish the majority of islet-cell tumors from ductal adenocarcinomas include high signal intensity on T2-weighted images, increased homogeneous enhancement on immediate postgadolinium images, and hypervascular liver metastases [34]. Because islet-cell tumors rarely obstruct the pancreatic duct, T1-weighted fat-suppressed images most often show high signal intensity of background pancreas, rendering clear depiction of low signal-intensity tumors in the majority of cases [33,34]. Lack of pancreatic ductal obstruction and vascular encasement by tumor are features that differentiate islet-cell tumor from pancreatic ductal adenocarcinoma. In contrast to the frequent occurrence of thrombosis in pancreatic ductal adenocarcinoma, thrombosis is rare in the setting of islet-cell tumors. Thromboses may rarely occur and may represent tumor thrombosis [38], unlike the circumstance with pancreatic ductal adenocarcinoma where the thrombus is usually bland. Peritoneal metastasis or regional lymph node enlargement, characteristic features of pancreatic ductal adenocarcinoma, are generally not present in islet-cell tumors.

Gastrinomas (G-cell tumors)

Gastrinomas occur most frequently in the region of the head of the pancreas, including the pancreatic head, the duodenum, the stomach, and the lymph nodes in a territory termed the gastrinoma triangle [39]. The anatomic boundaries of the triangle are the porta hepatis as the superior point of the triangle and the second and third parts of the duodenum forming the base. Although gastrinomas are usually solitary, multiple gastrinomas may occur, especially in the setting of multiple endocrine neoplasias, type 1. In this setting, patients have multiple pancreatic and duodenal islet-cell tumors [30,32,40].

Gastrinomas are not as frequently hypervascular as insulinomas. Mean size at presentation is 4 cm [37]. CT imaging is able to detect gastrinomas reliably when the tumors measure more than 3 cm in diameter but performs less well in the detection of smaller tumors [41]. Conventional spin-echo MR imaging also has been limited in the detection of gastrinomas [42,43]. MR imaging is effective at detecting tumors <1 cm in diameter.

Gastrinomas are low in signal intensity on T1-weighted fat-suppressed images and high in signal intensity on T2-weighted fat-suppressed images, demonstrating peripheral ring-like enhancement on immediate postgadolinium gradient echo images (Fig. 5) [33]. These imaging features are observed in the primary lesion and in hepatic metastases. Central low signal intensity on postgadolinium images reflects central hypovascularity. Occasionally, lesions are cystic. The enhancing rim of the primary tumor varies substantially in thickness, with the thickness of the rim reflecting the degree of hypervascularity of the tumor. If the enhancing rim is thin, it may be nearly imperceptible due to similar enhancement of the surrounding pancreatic parenchyma. Gastrinomas may occur outside the pancreas, and fat-suppressed T2-weighted images are particularly effective at detecting these high signal intensity tumors in a background of suppressed fat. Multiple gastrinomas may be scattered throughout the pancreas and frequently are small. T2-weighted breathing-independent echo train spin echo may be effective at demonstrating these tumors because breathing-averaged T2-weighted sequences may result in blurring, which may mask the presence of small tumors.

Gastrointestinal imaging findings that may be observed in gastrinomas include enlargement of the rugal folds of gastric mucosa (hypertrophic gastropathy) and intense mucosal enhancement on early postgadolinium gradient echo images, increased esophageal enhancement, and abnormal enhancement or thickness of proximal small bowel. These features are reflective of the inflammatory changes of peptic ulcer disease and gastric hyperplasia due to the effects of gastrin.

In general, islet-cell tumor metastases to the liver are well shown on MR images. Gastrinoma metastases frequently are relatively uniform in size and shape [34]. These metastases are generally hypervascular and possess uniform intense rim enhancement on immediate postgadolinium gradient echo images. Unlike pancreatic ductal cancer liver metastases, ill-defined perilesional enhancement is not observed with gastrinoma metastases, despite the substantial hepatic arterial blood supply of these tumors. Typically, lesions are high in signal intensity on T2-weighted fat-suppressed images and have well-defined margins.

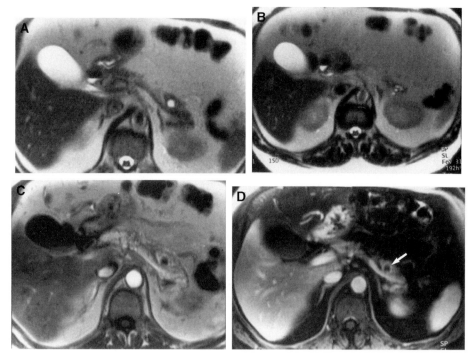

Fig. 5. Gastrinoma T2-weighted SS-ETSE (A, B); immediate postgadolinium T1-weighted gradient echo (C); and interstitial-phase, fat-suppressed, postgadolinium T1-weighted gradient echo (D) images in a patient with gastrinoma demonstrate multiple high signal intensity subcentimeter gastrinomas in the pancreatic tail. Ring enhancement is appreciated on the largest tumor (D, arrow).

This T2-weighted appearance may be confused with hemangiomas, which are also moderately high signal intensity and well defined. Islet-cell tumor liver metastases are differentiated from hemangiomas by their enhancement patterns. Islet-cell metastases have uniform ring enhancement on immediate postgadolinium images that fades with time [25], whereas hemangiomas have discontinuous peripheral nodular enhancement on immediate postgadolinium images with centripetal progression of enhancement. These appearances are better shown on MR than CT images due to the higher sensitivity of MR imaging to contrast enhancement, faster delivery of a compact bolus of intravenous contrast, and greater imaging temporal resolution [25]. The peripheral enhancing rim may be thin or thick, resulting in differences in the degree of vascularity. Occasionally, thick rim enhancement may have a peripheral-based, spoke-wheel enhancement. Centripetal enhancement of gastrinoma metastases may occur on serial postgadolinium images. Peripheral washout is commonly observed for hypervascular gastrinoma metastases.

Insulinomas

Insulinomas are low in signal intensity on T1-weighted images and high in signal intensity on T2-weighted images (Fig. 6). Insulinomas are well shown on T1-weighted fat-suppressed images [33]. Small insulinomas typically enhance homogeneously on immediate postgadolinium gradient echo images [34]. Larger tumors, which measure more than 2 cm in diameter, often show ring enhancement. Liver metastases from insulinomas typically have peripheral ring-like enhancement, although small metastases tend to enhance homogeneously. Enhancement of small metastases frequently occurs transiently in the capillary phase of enhancement and fades on images acquired at 1 minute after injection.

Glucagonomas, somatostatinomas, VIPomas, and ACTHomas

These islet-cell tumors are considerably less common than insulinomas or gastrinomas. They are usually malignant, with liver metastases present at the time of diagnosis [35,37,44–48]. The primary pancreatic tumors of glucagonoma and somatostatinoma are large and heterogeneous on MR images [45–48]. They are usually low in signal intensity on T1-weighted fat-suppressed images and high in signal intensity on T2-weighted fat-suppressed images, enhancing heterogeneously on immediate postgadolinium images [35]. Liver metastases are generally heterogeneous in size and shape, unlike gastrinoma metastases, which are typically uniform [34]. Metastases possess irregular peripheral rims of intense enhancement on immediate postgadolinium gradient echo images. Peripheral spoke-wheel enhancement may be observed in liver metastases on immediate postgadolinium images. Hypervascular liver metastases are best shown on immediate postgadolinium gradient echo images, which are superior to spiral CT images for this determination [35]. Splenic metastases are not uncommon. ACTHoma may present with a large heterogeneous enhancing primary tumor and small hypervascular liver metastases. Their appearance may resemble glucagonomas and somatostatinomas.

VIPoma may have a characteristic appearance of a small primary tumor despite large and extensive liver metastases (Fig. 7). Case reports have described ostensibly primary VIPoma of the liver without visualization of a pancreatic primary. The possibility exists that the primary pancreatic tumor may have been too small to detect.

Islet-cell tumors, untyped or uncategorized

Tumors are generally large at presentation because they are clinically silent. The imaging appearance of these tumors resembles glucagonomas and somatostatinomas. Liver metastases are generally present at the time of diagnosis.

Carcinoid tumors

Carcinoid tumors are generally large at presentation, with coexistent liver metastases. Focal and diffuse involvements of the pancreas have been observed. Tumors are generally mildly hypointense on T1, moderately hyperintense on T2, and show diffuse heterogeneous enhancement on immediate postgadolinium images [36]. Enhancement of the primary tumor may be mild despite extensive enhancement of liver metastases. Liver metastases are variable in size and often exhibit intense enhancement, similar to glucagonoma and somatostatinoma liver metastases.

Cystic pancreatic neoplasm

Serous cystadenoma (microcystic serous cystadenoma)

On MR images, the tumors are well defined and do not demonstrate invasion of fat or

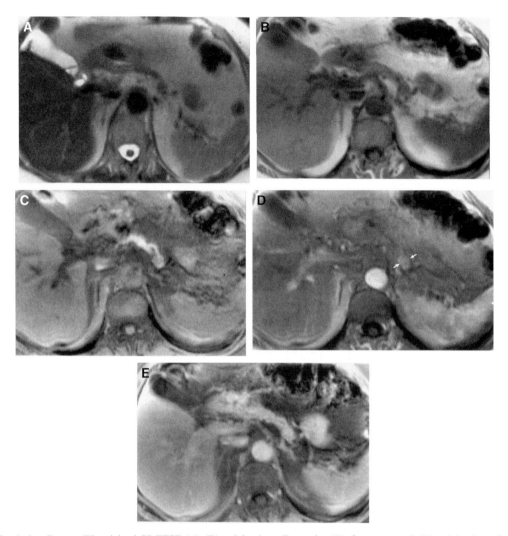

Fig. 6. Insulinoma. T2-weighted SS-ETSE (*A*); T1-weighted gradient echo (*B*); fat-suppressed, T1-weighted gradient echo (*C*); immediate postgadolinium T1-weighted gradient echo (*D*); and interstitial-phase, fat-suppressed, T1-weighted gradient echo (*E*) images demonstrate a small tumor arising in the body of the pancreas. The tumor is isointense on T2-weighted (*A*) and T1-weighted (*B*) images and shows low signal on the fat-suppressed T1-weighted image (*C*). The tumor enhances intensely and homogenously on the immediate postgadolinium image (*D, arrows*) and fades to mild hyperintensity isointensity (*E*).

adjacent organs [49]. On T2-weighted images, the small cysts and intervening septations may be well shown as a cluster of small grape-like, high signal intensity cysts. This appearance is more clearly shown on breath hold or breathing-independent sequences, such as single-shot echo train-spin echo, because the thin septations blur using longer-duration, nonbreath-hold sequences. Cystic pancreatic masses that contain cysts measuring <1 cm in diameter may represent microcystic cystadenoma or side-branch type intraductal papillary mucinous tumor (IPMT), which can be difficult to distinguish. Definition of communication with the pancreatic duct on MRCP images establishes the diagnosis of side-branch IPMT. Uncommonly, serous cystadenomas may be macrocystic (cysts measuring from 1–8 cm) and oligo- or unilocular. Macrocystic or unilocular serous cystadenomas exhibit distinctly different macroscopic features from microcystic lesions and may

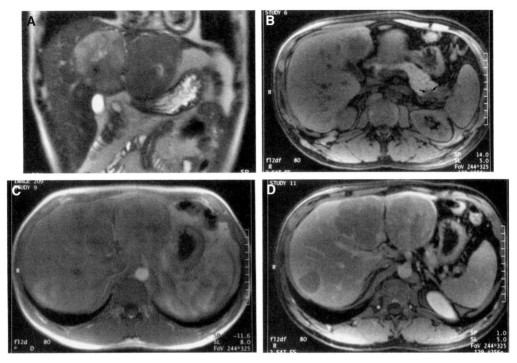

Fig. 7. VIPoma. Coronal T2-weighted SS-ETSE (*A*); fat-suppressed, T1-weighted gradient echo (*B*); immediate postgadolinium T1-weighted gradient echo (*C*); and 90-s postgadolinium fat-suppressed, T1-weighted gradient echo (*D*) images demonstrate a small tumor arising from the pancreatic tail (*B, arrows*). Multiple hypervascular metastases are appreciated in the liver (*C*).

pose diagnostic difficulties for the radiologist and the pathologist. A CT study evaluating these tumors misinterpreted all five cases to be mucinous cystic neoplasms or pseudocysts. Microcystic and macrocystic serous tumors represent morphologic variants of the same benign pancreatic neoplasm, namely serous cystadenoma [49]. Relatively thin uniform septations and the absence of infiltration of adjacent organs and structures are features that distinguish serous cystadenoma from serous cystadenocarcinoma (Fig. 8). Tumor septations usually enhance minimally with gadolinium on early and late postcontrast images, although moderate enhancement on early postcontrast images may occur. Delayed enhancement of the central scar may occasionally be observed (Fig. 8) [1] and is more typical of large tumors. Delayed enhancement of the central scar on postgadolinium images is apparent in larger tumors, and this enhancement pattern is typical for fibrous tissue in general. The central scar may represent compressed contiguous cyst walls of centrally located cysts. The presence of a central

scar is a distinguishing feature from side-branch IPMT, which does not exhibit this finding.

Mucinous cystadenoma/cystadenocarcinoma

On gadolinium-enhanced T1-weighted fat-suppressed images, large, irregular cystic spaces separated by thick septa are demonstrated [1]. Mucinous cystadenomas are well circumscribed and show no evidence of metastases or invasion of adjacent tissues (Fig. 9). Mucinous cystadenomas, described pathologically as having borderline malignant potential, may be large but may not show imaging or gross evidence of metastases or local invasion (Fig. 9). Histopathologically, these tumors show moderate epithelial dysplasia. Mucinous cystadenocarcinoma may be locally aggressive malignancies with extensive invasion of adjacent tissues and organs. The absence of demonstration of tumor invasion into surrounding tissue does not exclude malignancy. The higher inherent soft-tissue contrast of MR imaging compared with CT imaging results in superior

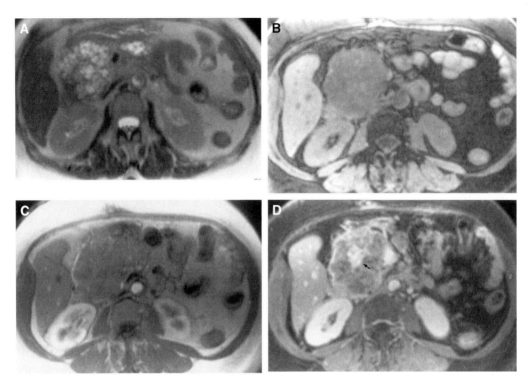

Fig. 8. Microcystic serous cystadenoma. T2-weighted SS-ETSE (*A*); fat-suppressed T1-weighted gradient echo (*B*); immediate postgadolinium T1-weighted gradient echo (*C*); and 90-s postgadolinium fat-suppressed T1-weighted gradient echo (*D*) images demonstrate multiple tiny, clustered cysts in the pancreatic head (*A*). There is a central scar, which is typical for serous cystadenoma, that enhances on late images (*D*, *arrow*), consistent with fibrosis.

differentiation between microcystic and macro-cystic adenomas because of the sharp definition of cysts, which permits evaluation of cyst size and margins [50]. Breathing-independent T2-weighted images are effective at defining the cysts.

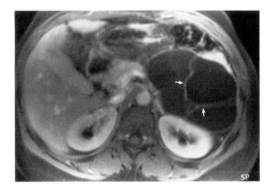

Fig. 9. Mucinous cystadenoma. 90-s postgadolinium fat-suppressed, T1-weighted gradient echo image. A well-defined cystic mass arises from the body and tail of the pancreas and demonstrates enhancement of septations (*arrows*). No evidence of tumor nodules, invasion of adjacent tissue, or liver metastases is appreciated.

Mucin produced by these tumors may result in high signal intensity on T1- and T2-weighted images of the primary tumor and liver metastases. Liver metastases are generally hypervascular and have intense ring enhancement on immediate gadolinium images. Metastases are commonly cystic and may contain mucin, which results in mixed low and high signal intensity on T1- and T2-weighted images.

Intraductal papillary mucinous tumors

Main-branch type

On MR images, a greatly expanded main pancreatic duct is demonstrated on T2-weighted images or MRCP images. Irregular enhancing tissue along the ductal epithelium is appreciated on postgadolinium images, confirming that underlying tumor is the cause of the ductal dilatation.

Side-branch type

Septations are generally present, creating a cluster of grapes appearance. Side-branch type

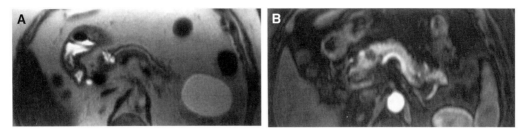

Fig. 10. IPMT, side-branch type. T2-weighted SS-ETSE (*A*) and immediate postgadolinium fat-suppressed T1-weighted gradient echo (*B*) images in a patient with side-branch IPMT demonstrate multiple small, clustered cysts (*A*) in the pancreatic head.

IPMT is usually a benign process that appears as a localized cystic parenchymal lesion. The majority of side-branch IPMT tumors are located in the head of the pancreas (Fig. 10). MRCP images show communication of the cystic tumor with the main pancreatic duct in the majority of cases [51–56]. A distinguishing feature from microcystic cystadenoma is that central compacted septations are not present (Fig. 10).

Metastases

Metastases are low in signal intensity on T1-weighted images and high in signal intensity on T2-weighted images. Small metastases (<1 cm in diameter) enhance uniformly on immediate postgadolinium gradient echo images, and larger metastases enhance in a ring fashion. This appearance is analogous to the appearance of hypervascular metastases to the liver and reflects the

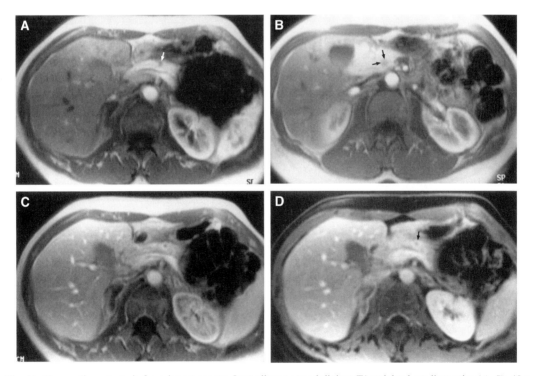

Fig. 11. Pancreatic metastasis from breast cancer. Immediate postgadolinium T1-weighted gradient echo (*A, B*); 45-s postgadolinium T1-weighted gradient echo (*C*); and 90-s postgadolinium fat-suppressed, T1-weighted gradient echo (*D*) images demonstrate multiple small metastases (*A, B, arrow*) in the pancreatic head and body. Metastases show ring enhancement on postgadolinium images (*D, arrow*).

pathophysiology of parasitization of host blood supply by metastatic disease. Renal cancer metastases resemble the appearance of islet-cell tumors. Clinical history of renal cancer, even if remote, is essential to establish the correct diagnosis. Metastases from other primary tumors generally appear as focal pancreatic masses that are mildly hypointense on T1-weighted images; moderately hypointense on T1-weighted fat-suppressed images; and mildly hyperintense on T2-weighted images. Metastases to the pancreas often enhance in a ring fashion (Fig. 11), as observed with liver metastases, and their extent of enhancement generally varies with the angiogenic properties of the primary neoplasms. Ductal obstruction is uncommon even with larger tumors, which is an important distinguishing feature from pancreatic ductal adenocarcinoma. The lack of ductal obstruction explains why metastases are generally well seen on noncontrast T1-weighted fat-suppressed images. Chronic pancreatitis that arises secondary to ductal obstruction is not present, and therefore the background pancreas is shown with moderately high signal intensity, creating sharp contrast with hypointense tumors.

Melanoma metastases may be high in signal intensity on T1-weighted images due to the paramagnetic properties of melanin pigment [1]. Metastatic deposits tend to be focal, well-defined masses.

Summary

MR imaging is a valuable tool in the assessment of the full spectrum of pancreatic diseases. MR imaging techniques are sensitive for the evaluation of pancreatic disorders in the following settings: (1) T1-weighted fat-suppressed and dynamic gadolinium-enhanced SGE imaging for the detection of chronic pancreatitis, ductal adenocarcinoma, and islet-cell tumors; (2) T2-weighted fat-suppressed imaging and T2-weighted breathhold imaging for the detection of islet-cell tumors; and (3) precontrast breath-hold SGE imaging for the detection of acute pancreatitis. Relatively specific morphologic and signal intensity features permit characterization of acute pancreatitis, chronic pancreatitis, ductal adenocarcinoma, insulinoma, gastrinoma, glucagonoma, microcystic cystadenoma, macrocystic cystadenoma, and solid and papillary epithelial neoplasm. MR imaging is effective as a problem-solving modality because it distinguishes chronic pancreatitis from normal

pancreas and chronic pancreatitis with focal enlargement from pancreatic cancer in the majority of cases.

MR imaging studies should be considered in the following settings: (1) in patients with elevated serum creatinine, allergy to iodine contrast, or other contraindications for iodine contrast administration; (2) in patients with prior CT imaging who have focal enlargement of the pancreas with no definable mass; (3) in patients in whom clinical history is worrisome for malignancy and in whom findings on CT imaging are equivocal or difficult to interpret; and (4) in situations requiring distinction between chronic pancreatitis with focal enlargement and pancreatic cancer. Patients with biochemical evidence of islet-cell tumors should be examined by MR imaging as the first-line imaging modality because of the high sensitivity of MR imaging for detecting the presence of islet-cell tumors and determining the presence of metastatic disease.

References

[1] Semelka RC, Ascher SM. MRI of the pancreas: state of the art. Radiology 1993;188:593–602.

[2] Winston CB, Mitchell DG, Outwater EK, et al. Pancreatic signal intensity on T1-weighted fat satuation MR images: clinical correlation. J Magn Reson Imaging 1995;5:267–71.

[3] Mitchell DG, Vinitski S, Saponaro S, et al. Liver and pancreas: improved spin-echo T1 contrast by shorter echo time and fat suppression at 1.5 T. Radiology 1991;178:67–71.

[4] Semelka RC, Kroeker MA, Shoenut JP, et al. Pancreatic disease: prospective comparison of CT, ERCP, and 1.5 T MR imaging with dynamic gadolinium enhancement and fat suppression. Radiology 1991;181:785–91.

[5] Takehara Y, Ichijo K, Tooyama N, et al. Breathhold MR cholangiopancreatography with a long-echo-time fast spin-echo sequence and a surface coil in chronic pancreatitis. Radiology 1994;192: 73–8.

[6] Bret PM, Reinhold C, Taourel P, et al. Pancreas divisum: evaluation with MR cholangiopancreatography. Radiology 1996;199:99–103.

[7] Soto JA, Barish MA, Yucel EK, et al. Pancreatic duct: MR cholangiopancreatography with a three-dimensional fast spin-echo technique. Radiology 1995;196:459–64.

[8] Semelka RC, Simm FC, Recht M, et al. MRI of the pancreas at high field strength: a comparison of six sequences. J Comput Assist Tomogr 1991;15: 966–71.

[9] Mitchell DG, Winston CB, Outwater EK, et al. Delineation of pancreas with MR imaging: multi-

observer comparison of five pulse sequences. J Magn Reson Imaging 1995;5:193–9.

[10] Fulcher AS, Turner MA. MR pancreatography: a useful tool for evaluating pancreatic disorders. Radiographics 1999;19:5–24.

[11] Catalano C, Pavone P, Laghi A, et al. Pancreatic adenocarcinoma: combination of MR imaging, MR angiography and MR cholangiopancreatography for the diagnosis and assessment of respectability. Eur Radiol 1998;8:428–34.

[12] Balthazar E. CT diagnosis and staging of acute pancreatitis. Radiol Clin North Am 1989;27: 19–37.

[13] Balthazar EJ, Robinson DL, Megibow AJ, et al. Acute pancreatitis: value of CT in establishing prognosis. Radiology 1990;174:331–6.

[14] Johnson CD, Stephens DH, Sarr MG. CT of acute pancreatitis: correlation between lack of contrast enhancement and pancreatic necrosis. AJR Am J Roentgenol 1991;156:93.

[15] Saifuddin A, Ward J, Ridgway J, et al. Comparison of MR and CT scanning in severe acute pancreatitis: initial experiences. Clin Radiol 1993;48:111–6.

[16] Morgan DE, Baron TH, Smith JK, et al. Pancreatic fluid collections prior to intervention: evaluation with MR imaging compared with CT and US. Radiology 1997;203:773–8.

[17] Luetmer PH, Stephens DH, Ward EM. Chronic pancreatitis reassessment with current CT. Radiology 1989;171:353–7.

[18] Semelka RC, Shoenut JP, Kroeker MA, et al. Chronic pancreatitis: MR imaging features before and after administration of gadopentetate dimeglumine. J Mag Reson Imaging 1993;3:79–82.

[19] Steer ML, Waxman I, Freedman S. Chronic pancreatitis. N Engl J Med 1995;332:1482–90.

[20] Warshaw AL, Fernandez-del Castillo C. Pancreatic carcinoma. N Engl J Med 1992;326:455–65.

[21] Gabata T, Matsui O, Kadoya M, et al. Small pancreatic adenocarcinomas: efficacy of MR imaging with fat suppression and gadolinium enhancement. Radiology 1994;193:683–8.

[22] Semelka RC, Kelekis NL, Molina PL, et al. Pancreatic masses with inconclusive findings on spiral CR: is there a role for MRI? J Magn Reson Imaging 1996;6:585–8.

[23] Birchard KR, Hyslop WB, Brown A, et al. Suspected pancreatic cancer: evaluation by dynamic gadolinium-enhanced 3D-gradient echo MRI. AJR Am J Roentgenol, in press.

[24] Steiner E, Stark DD, Hahn PF, et al. Imaging of pancreatic neoplasms: comparison of MR and CT. AJR Am J Roentgenol 1989;152:487–91.

[25] Sarles H, Sahel J. Pathology of chronic calcifying pancreatitis. Am J Gastroenterol 1976;66:117–39.

[26] Vellet AD, Romano W, Bach DB, et al. Adenocarcinoma of the pancreatic ducts: comparative evaluation with CT and MR imaging at 1.5 T. Radiology 1992;183:87–95.

[27] Pavone P, Occhiato R, Michelini O, et al. Magnetic resonance imaging of pancreatic carcinoma. Eur Radiol 1991;1:124–30.

[28] Low RN, Semelka RC, Worawattanakul S, et al. Extrahepatic abdominal imaging in patients with malignancy: comparison of MR imaging and helical CT in 164 patients. J Magn Reson Imaging 2000; 12:269–77.

[29] Low RN, Semelka RC, Worawattanakul S, et al. Extrahepatic abdominal imaging in patients with malignancy: comparison of MR imaging and helical CT, with subsequent surgical correlation. Radiology 1999;210:625–32.

[30] Nishiharu T, Yamashita Y, Abe Y, et al. Local extension of pancreatic carcinoma: assessment with thin-section helical CT versus with breath-hold fast MR imaging—ROC analysis. Radiology 1999;212: 445–52.

[31] Danet IM, Semelka RC, Nagase LL, et al. Liver metastases from pancreatic adenocarcinoma: MR imaging characteristics. J Magn Reson Imaging 2003; 18:181–8.

[32] Mitchell DG, Cruvella M, Eschelman DJ, et al. MRI of pancreatic gastrinomas. J Comput Assist Tomogr 1992;16:583–5.

[33] Kraus BB, Ros PR. Insulinoma: diagnosis with fat-suppressed MR imaging. AJR Am J Roentgenol 1994;162:69–70.

[34] Semelka RC, Cummings M, Shoenut JP, et al. Islet cell tumors: a comparison of detection by dynamic contrast-enhanced CT and MR imaging with dynamic gadolinium enhancement and fat suppression. Radiology 1993;186:799–802.

[35] Kelekis NL, Semelka RC, Molina PL, et al. ACTH-secreting islet cell tumor: appearances on dynamic gadolinium-enhanced MRI. Magn Reson Imaging 1995;13:641–4.

[36] Semelka RC, Custodio CM, Balci C, et al. Neuroendocrine tumors of the pancreas: spectrum of appearances on MRI. Magn Res Imaging 2000;11:141–8.

[37] Buetow PC, Parrino TV, Buck JL, et al. Islet cell tumors of the pancreas: pathologic-imaging correlation among six, necrosis and cysts, calcification, malignant behavior, and functional status. AJR Am J Roentgenol 1995;165:1175–9.

[38] Smith TM, Semelka RC, Noone TC, et al. Islet cell tumor of the pancreas associated with tumor thrombus in the portal vein. Magn Reson Imaging 1999;17: 1093–6.

[39] Wittenberg J, Simeone JF, Ferrucci JT Jr, et al. Non-focal enlargement in pancreatic carcinoma. Radiology 1982;144:131–5.

[40] Pipeleers-Marichal M, Donow C, Heitz PU, et al. Pathologic aspects of gastrinomas in patients with Zollinger-Ellison syndrome with and without multiple endocrine neoplasia type I. World J Surg 1993; 17:481–8.

[41] Wank SA, Doppman JL, Miller DL, et al. Prospective study of the ability of computed axial

tomography to localize gastrinomas in patients with Zollinger-Ellison syndrome. Gastroenterology 1987; 92:905–12.

[42] Frucht H, Doppman JL, Norten JA, et al. Gastrinomas comparison of MR imaging with CT, angiography, and US. Radiology 1989;171:713–7.

[43] Muller MF, Meyenberger C, Bertschinger P, et al. Pancreatic tumors: evaluation with endoscopic US, CT, and MR imaging. Radiology 1994;190:745–51.

[44] Mozell E, Stenzel P, Woltering EA, et al. Functional endocrine tumors of the pancreas: clinical presentation, diagnosis, and treatment. Curr Probl Surg 1990;27:304–85.

[45] Tjon A, Tham RTO, Jansen JBMJ, et al. MR, CT, and ultrasound findings of metastatic vipoma in pancreas. J Comput Assist Tomogr 1989;13:142–4.

[46] Carlson B, Johnson CD, Stephens DH, et al. MRI of pancreatic islet cell carcinoma. J Comput Assist Tomogr 1993;17:735–40.

[47] Tjon A, Tham RTO, Jansen JBMJ, et al. Imaging features of somatostatinoma: MR, CT, US, and angiography. J Comp Assist Tomogr 1994;18:427–31.

[48] Doppman JL, Nieman LK, Cutler GB Jr, et al. Adrenocorticotropic hormone-secreting islet cell tumors: are they always malignant? Radiology 1994;190:59–64.

[49] Lewandrowski K, Warshaw A, Compton C. Macrocystic serous cystadenoma of the pancreas: a mor-phologic variant differing from microcystic adenoma. Hum Pathol 1992;23:871–5.

[50] Minami M, Itai Y, Ohtomo K, et al. Cystic neoplasms of the pancreas: comparison of MR imaging with CT. Radiology 1989;171:53–6.

[51] Buetow PC, Rao P, Thompson LDR. From the archives of the AFIP: mucinous cystic neoplasm of the pancreas: radiologic-pathologic correlation. Radiographics 1998;18:433–49.

[52] Procacci C, Megibow AJ, Carbognin G, et al. Intraductal papillary mucinous tumor of the pancreas: a pictorial essay. Radiographics 1999;19:1447–63.

[53] Koito K, Namieno T, Ichimura T, et al. Mucin-producing pancreatic tumors: comparison of MR cholangiopancreatography with endoscopy retrograde cholangiopancreatography. Radiology 1998; 208:231–7.

[54] Onaya H, Itai Y, Niitsu M, et al. Ductectatic mucinous cyst neoplasm of pancreas: evaluation with MR cholangiopancreatography. AJR 1998;171: 171–7.

[55] Irie H, Honda H, Aibe H, et al. MR cholangiopancreatography differentiation of benign and malignant intraductal mucin-producing tumors of the pancreas. AJR 2000;174:1403–8.

[56] Kelekis NL, Semelka RC, Siegelman ES. MRI of pancreatic metastases from renal cancer. J Comp Assist Tomogr 1996;20:249–53.

ELSEVIER
SAUNDERS

Magn Reson Imaging Clin N Am
13 (2005) 331–348

MAGNETIC
RESONANCE
IMAGING CLINICS
of North America

Small Bowel

Andrea Laghi, MD[a],*, Pasquale Paolantonio, MD[b],
Roberto Passariello, MD[b]

[a]*Department of Radiological Sciences, University of Rome "La Sapienza," "Polo Didattico Pontino" - I.C.O.T.,
Latina, Via Franco Faggiana 34, 04100 Latina, Italy*
[b]*Department of Radiological Sciences, University of Rome "La Sapienza," Policlinico Umberto I,
Viale Regina Elena 324, 00161 Rome, Italy*

MR imaging of the small bowel has been an unexplored field of application for several years—often confined to advanced and selected research centers—without any real clinical impact. The first experimental studies were published in 1985 [1,2] followed by a limited number of contributions until 1997 [3–28]. It was only in 1998 that the number of publications started to increase (Fig. 1) [29–34]. The reason was not lack of interest, but the technical inadequacy of MR scanners to perform motion-free examinations. Developments in hardware (gradients, multichannel coils) and software (fast and ultrafast sequences) enabled breath-held studies, reezing voluntary (respiratory) and involuntary (peristaltic) motion artifacts [33,34], and opening the access to modern abdominal MR imaging.

High soft tissue contrast resolution; acquisition of multiplanar images, particularly in the coronal plane; and the possibility to obtain functional information make MR an interesting imaging technique for the evaluation of the small bowel. The absence of ionizing radiation is another important feature because inflammatory diseases are studied most frequently, in particular, Crohn's disease; this disease is prevalent among pediatric patients and young adults [35].

The major advantage of MR imaging, compared with conventional barium radiograph studies, is direct visualization of small bowel wall. This feature dramatically changes the image interpretation process; radiologists must shift their attention from analysis of mucosal profile and lumen caliber to direct evaluation of bowel wall thickness and parietal inflammatory changes. The outcome of this cultural radiologic challenge may alter radically the management of patients who have suspected small bowel disease in the next few years.

Imaging protocols

Sequences

Fast sequences that are able to acquire T1- and T2-weighted images within a single breath-hold are essential requisites for MR imaging evaluation of the small bowel. With regards to T2-weighted images, several studies [29,33,34,36] support the validity of single-shot sequences (including half-Fourier single-shot turbo spin-echo [HASTE] and single-shot fast spin-echo). These sequences, based on the half-Fourier reconstruction technique, have extremely fast acquisition times (on the order of approximately 1 second per image), and therefore, are capable of freezing motion artifacts, even peristaltic ones. Single-shot sequences differ from each other by the value of the echo time (TE). When extremely long TEs (eg, ~600 milliseconds) are used, selective images of fluids with complete cancellation of surrounding organs (similar to MR cholangiography) are obtained (Fig. 2); with shorter TEs (on the order of 60–90 milliseconds), simultaneous evaluation of fluids, intestinal wall, and surrounding structures can be obtained (Fig. 3).

---

* Corresponding author.

E-mail address: andrea.laghi@uniroma1.it
(A. Laghi).

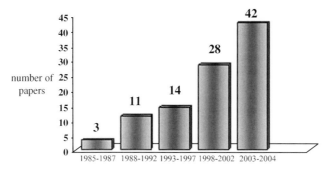

Fig. 1. The exponential growth in the number of publications on small bowel magnetic resonance imaging from 1985 to 2004. (Source: Medline; Keywords: small bowel, MT imaging.)

The major drawback of T2-weighted single-shot sequences, which are more relevant at extremely long TEs, comes from the evidence of "flow void" artifacts within the luminal fluid that possibly simulate an intraluminal lesion. These artifacts are generated by propulsive intestinal movements (peristaltic motion) and can be minimized by the administration of an antiperistaltic drug immediately before the examination (Fig. 4).

A useful complement to the acquisition of T2-weighted sequences is the use of fat saturation pulses. Fat saturation causes an increase in contrast between the intestinal wall and the surrounding fat tissue. This is particularly useful in the assessment of bowel wall inflammation and

in the identification of inflammatory changes in peritoneal fat tissue [37,38].

More recently, the "balanced" or "hybrid" gradient-echo sequence has been introduced in clinical practice. This sequence, known as "true fast imaging with steady-state precession" (true-FISP) [39], presents an intermediate contrast

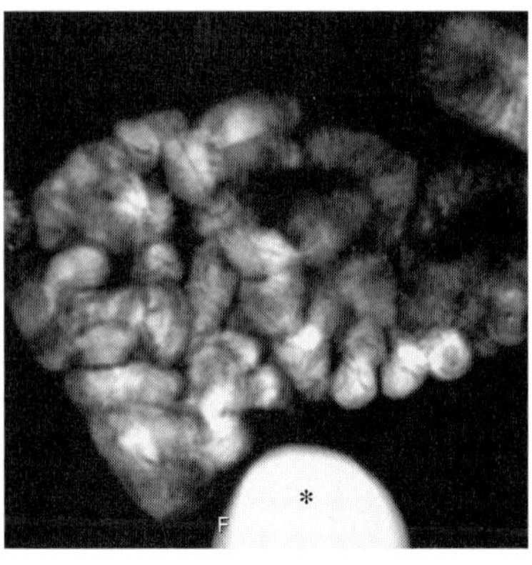

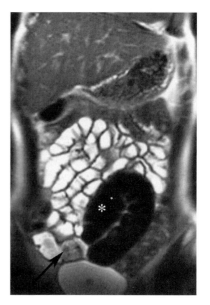

Fig. 3. Single-shot T2-weighted turbo spin-echo (HASTE) sequence acquired on coronal plane optimally shows small bowel loops morphology. Small intestine is distended by oral contrast material. The bowel wall is hypointense compared with the hyperintensity of the lumen content. Residual air bubbles within the small bowel loops (*arrow*) and the presence of air within the sigmoid colon (*asterisk*) do not cause significant artifacts.

Fig. 2. Single-shot T2-weighted turbo spin-echo (HASTE) sequence, acquired with long TE, showing distension of small bowel loops. Using this technical approach, a unique image that shows static fluids within the bowel loops and the urinary bladder (*asterisk*) is obtained.

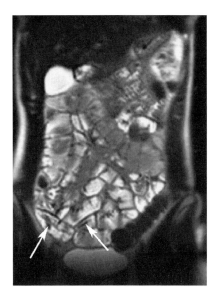

Fig. 4. Typical artifacts of single-shot T2-weighted turbo spin-echo (HASTE) sequence due to peristaltic motion of intestinal content (*arrows*); such artifacts can simulate the presence of endoluminal lesions.

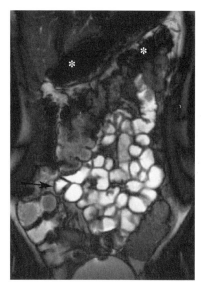

Fig. 5. Balanced gradient-echo sequence, known as true-FISP. Stationary fluids are markedly hyperintense, and allow for an optimal evaluation of bowel lumen distended by oral contrast material. The relative thickening of the bowel wall is noted; this is due to "chemical shift" artifact, a hypointense band (*arrow*) which is evident in the frequency-encoding direction. This sequence is not sensitive to peristaltic artifacts because of the mixing of oral contrast medium within the loops (no false filling defects are seen along the entire small bowel). Conversely, this sequence is more sensitive to susceptibility artifacts than HASTE sequence because of the residual air within stomach or colon (*asterisks*).

between T1- and T2-weighted images and a technical configuration which renders it particularly suitable for MR imaging of the small bowel. Short repetition times (TR) are used (<3 milliseconds) and the acquisition time is short; therefore, respiratory and peristaltic motion artifacts are reduced. This sequence seems to be useful in the study of children or uncooperative patients who are unable to maintain the required breath-hold. Compared with single-shot turbo spin echo (TSE) sequences, "balanced" gradient-echo—although it provides a high signal from fluids (it also is a "water sensitive" sequence)—does not suffer from "flow voids" that are due to peristaltic motion.

T1 and T2 hybrid signals also enable optimal visualization of intestinal wall, mesenteric fat tissue, and main vascular structures (because it is a gradient-echo sequence, mesenteric vessels appear hyperintense because of the phenomenon of paradoxic enhancement). One possible drawback, however, might be the chemical shift artifact which clearly is evident on the intestinal wall as an hypointense band along the direction of the frequency encoding gradient. This artifact causes a possible overestimation of the bowel wall thickness, although the relative hypointensity of band artifact compared with real intestinal wall and the observer's experience may offer a concrete solution to this problem (Fig. 5).

T1-weighted images are obtained with fast spoiled-gradient-echo sequences, using two-dimensional or three-dimensional acquisition [40]. The acquisition time is on the order of 15 to 20 seconds. T1-weighted sequences generally are used following intravenous injection of contrast material to evaluate parietal enhancement, a useful parameter to assess disease activity. Similar to T2-weighted sequences, T1-weighted images benefit from the use of fat saturation; it increases the contrast between wall and mesenteric fat tissue and improves the detection of even minimal parietal enhancement (Fig. 6).

The latest technical development to speed up the acquisition process is parallel imaging, based on simultaneous acquisition of spatial harmonics, or sensitivity encoding techniques [41]. Parallel imaging enables a reduction in the number of phase encodings to be acquired per TR. Consequently, the spatial resolution—while maintaining

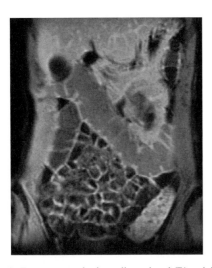

Fig. 6. Fat-suppressed, three-dimensional T1-weighted spoiled gradient-echo sequence obtained during a single breath-hold. The sequence usually is acquired following intravenous injection of contrast material, which is necessary for the optimal visualization of the wall. In this case, normal parietal enhancement is noted.

an acquisition time that is compatible with a single breath-hold—or the number of scans to be acquired—which allows a larger volume coverage—can be increased; alternatively the acquisition time can be reduced drastically. The downside of the use of parallel imaging is the reduction of signal-to-noise ratio (SNR) and the need to perform a calibration of the equipment immediately before image acquisition [42].

Coils

The development of phased-array coils [43] has enabled one of the main limitations of fast and ultrafast sequences to be overcome—the intrinsically low SNR. The use of phased-array coils increases SNR by a factor of two, with benefits in terms of temporal, spatial, or contrast resolution. The problem of a small field of view that does not cover the entire small bowel loops has been solved, thanks to new selective multichannel coils that allow imaging of abdomen and pelvis in a single examination [44].

Small bowel distension

Bowel distension is a fundamental requisite for any imaging method of the small intestine, as revealed by decades of experience with barium radiograph studies. A collapsed bowel loop can

hide lesions or simulate pathologic wall thickenings. The presence of a lesion that generates small bowel obstruction creates a natural distension of the lumen and the possibility of examining the patient without the need for any previous preparation (Fig. 7) [17,34,45]. In contrast, the relative collapse of bowel loops, in standard conditions and in different nonobstructive pathologies, has led researchers to study a variety of methods of luminal distension.

There are two main approaches to MR imaging of the small bowel: (1) study following oral administration of contrast material ("MR small bowel follow through"); and (2) study with distension of the lumen obtained with contrast material that is introduced through a naso-jejunal tube ("MR enteroclysis"). Before going into details of the two techniques, a brief review of major contrast agents for small bowel study is provided.

Oral contrast agents for small bowel MR imaging

Oral contrast agents can be classified into positive, negative, and biphasic categories according to their action on the signal intensity of bowel lumen. A positive oral contrast agent is a paramagnetic substance that produces high signal intensity on T1-weighted sequences. At the concentrations that are used in clinical practice, they reduce T1 relaxation time without, or by only minimally, influencing T2 relaxation time. For this reason and because of the water content of the contrast solution, they also result in high signal intensity on T2-weighted images (Fig. 8). Positive contrast materials include paramagnetic substances, such as gadolinium chelates and ferrous and manganese ions [5,14,18,20,30,47,48]. A T1 effect also has been reported for special substances, such as oil emulsions [8] and nutritional supports [16]. The use of positive contrast agents has been abandoned almost completely because of the difficult image interpretation (an hyperintense lumen does not enable a clear differentiation with inflammatory parietal enhancement).

A negative oral contrast agent is a substance that produces low signal intensity on T1- and T2-weighted sequences. These substances, which have paramagnetic effects, induce local inhomogeneity in the magnetic field that affect T1 and T2 relaxation times (Fig. 9). T2 effects predominate and are caused by spin dephasing with a consequent loss of signal intensity. Negative contrast materials include perfluoroctylbromide [19], iron oxides [9,21], and oral magnetic particles [15]. Barium sulfate, if used at high concentrations, can

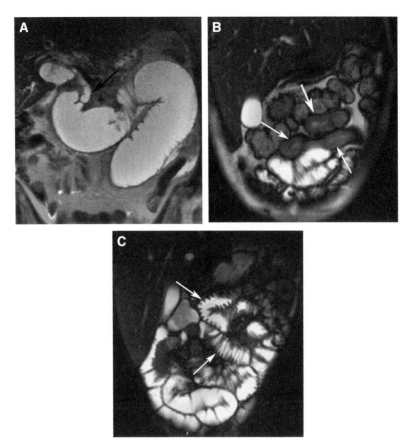

Fig. 7. (*A*) In a case of proximal jejunal obstruction, no patient preparation is needed because the obstructive process generates fluid accumulation and distension of proximal bowel loops. Proximal jejunal obstruction and dilation of the common bile duct (*arrow*) that are due to an increase in endoluminal duodenal pressure are noted. Conversely, with patient preparation by means of oral contrast agent, obtaining a complete and homogeneous intestinal distension may be considered a challenge that requires multiple acquisition of the same sequence during the oral contrast media transit through the small bowel. For example, in a delayed true-FISP image (*B*), collapsed jejunal loops easily may be misinterpreted as multiple strictures (*arrows*). A few minutes before (*C*), the same loops (*arrows*) that are well-distended from the contrast medium show normal caliber and wall thickness with the regular appearance of mucosal jejunal folds.

be considered a negative contrast agent [12]. Negative contrast agents are more favorable if hyperintense signal of the bowel wall and the surrounding fat tissue—signs of acute inflammation—have to be detected on T2-weighted sequences [38]; however, magnetic susceptibility artifacts that are induced by ferrous oxide on gradient echo sequences may alter image quality on breath-held T1-weighted images.

The term "biphasic" recently was introduced to define those substances that show different signal intensities depending on different sequences [46]. In essence they show a hyperintense signal on T1-weighted images and a hypointense signal on T2-weighted images, and the opposite situation,

a hypointense signal on T1 and a hyperintense signal on T2. The first group (hyperintensity on T1 and hypointensity on T2) includes manganese and substances that contain manganese, and gadolinium chelates, which can act as biphasic contrast agents if administered at high concentrations (Fig. 10) [13,49]. The second group (hypointensity on T1 and hyperintensity on T2) includes water, hyperosmolar and isosmolar watery solutions, and barium sulfate.

Although water is the safest and cheapest agent, it suffers the limitation of intestinal absorption, which compromises an adequate distension of the distal ileum in many patients [50,51]. To obviate this problem, hyperosmolar solutions,

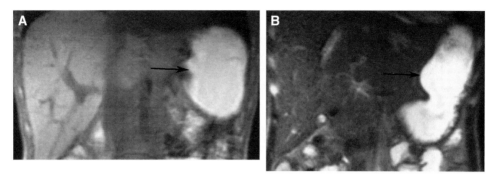

Fig. 8. Positive contrast material (gadolinium chelate water solution). The contrast material presents a hyperintense signal (*arrow*) on T1-weighted sequences (*A*) and T2-weighted sequences (*B*).

such as mannitol-based solutions, have been tested; mannitol reduces water absorption and facilitates the distension of the distal ileal loops. Major drawbacks are the undesirable side effects, such as diarrhea, meteorism, and abdominal cramps, which are limited when low-concentration solutions are used (mannitol 2.5%) [52].

In the attempt to reduce undesirable side effects, isosmolar watery solutions, such as polyethylene glycol (PEG) 4000, also have been tested [53,54]. PEG has the same signal properties as water, but it is not absorbed through the intestinal wall because of the molecule's size; thus, better distension of the distal ileum is obtained (Fig. 11).

No more than 600 mL to 700 mL can be administered orally because larger volumes trigger catharsis [53,54].

Recently, Lauenstein et al [55] proposed the use of a water mixture based on low concentration mannitol and locust bean gum (LBG). LBG is known for its thickening properties and is used in ice creams, dairy gels, and canned products. The properties of LBG seem to reduce side effects that are related to high osmolarity of mannitol; this ensures optimal intestinal distension with reasonable transit time (see Fig. 11).

A new oral mixture with biphasic properties, which is made of low concentration barium sulfate and sorbitol, that is designed for CT and

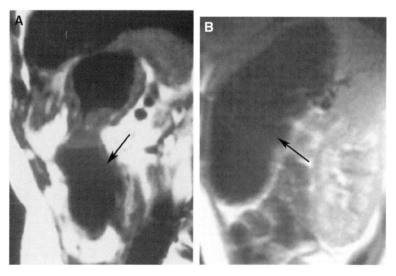

Fig. 9. Negative contrast material (iron oxide water solution). The contrast material presents a low signal intensity (*arrow*) on T1-weighted images (*A*) and T2-weighted images (*B*).

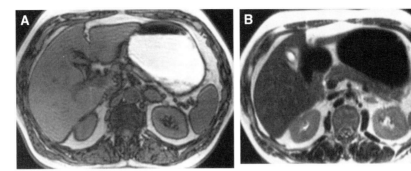

Fig. 10. Biphasic contrast material (highly-concentrated gadolinium chelate water solution). The contrast agent that fills the stomach presents high signal intensity on T1-weighted sequences (*A*) and low signal intensity on T2-weighted sequences (*B*).

MR studies of the bowel recently was approved by the U.S. Food and Drug Administration (Volumen; E-Z-EM, Lake Success, New York). On the basis of the authors' preliminary personal experience, Volumen has a signal intensity profile that is similar to other biphasic contrast agents with excellent patient compliance, especially in the pediatric population, because of the high palatability of this mixture. It is similar to other hyperosmolar oral contrast agents in terms of intestinal distension, with reduced side effects (Fig. 12).

MR small bowel follow through: technique

The study technique is based on the oral ingestion of an adequate amount of contrast agent (~600–1000 mL) and the following acquisition of serial sequences. The patient is asked to drink the oral agent continuously beginning approximately 15 to 20 minutes before the examination; the final two cups of agent are drunk inside the scanner room before lying on the table. A spasmolytic agent is administered intravenously immediately before the examination. T2-weighted and T1/T2 hybrid sequences are acquired serially on coronal and axial planes, until the terminal ileum is distended completely [54,56–58]. If needed, contrast-enhanced T1-weighted images on coronal and axial planes are acquired, using a starting delay of 50 seconds.

MR enteroclysis: technique

In MR enteroclysis, small bowel distension is obtained with the administration of a contrast agent through a prepositioned naso-jejunal tube [59–61]. The placement of the tube is performed under fluoroscopic guidance to avoid a time-consuming procedure inside the MR scanner. It also is advisable to use a tube with an antireflux balloon to prevent duodeno-gastric reflux.

The use of negative [31,62] and positive [30,63] contrast agents has been abandoned in favor of biphasic agents. Similar to radiograph enteroclysis, methylcellulose can be administered; it is not absorbed and provides optimal luminal distension, with the known inconvenience of the emetic effect in case of duodeno-gastric reflux [59]. For this reason it is now replaced by other biphasic agents (isosmotic or hyperosmotic watery solutions).

Volume and infusion rate are crucial for the success of the examination, as in the case of conventional enteroclysis. Volume is variable among different subjects, and ranges between 1500 mL and 3000 mL. Infusion rate (the use of a peristaltic pump is good practice) varies between 80 mL/min and 150 mL/min. The use of spasmolytics is controversial; higher infusion rates (on the order of 200 mL/min) induce natural small bowel reflexive atony [62] without the need for any pharmaceutical agent.

Major advantages of MR enteroclysis are better bowel distension compared with the oral approach and the possible use of "MR fluoroscopy," based on ultrafast imaging techniques. MR fluoroscopy offers a real-time evaluation of the small bowel and provides functional information (identification of nonobstructive or partially obstructive lesions) of the intestinal lumen; this may compensate for the lack of compression maneuvers (Fig. 13). Excessive distension of the bowel loops can worsen the assessment of the mesenteric structures as a result of compression

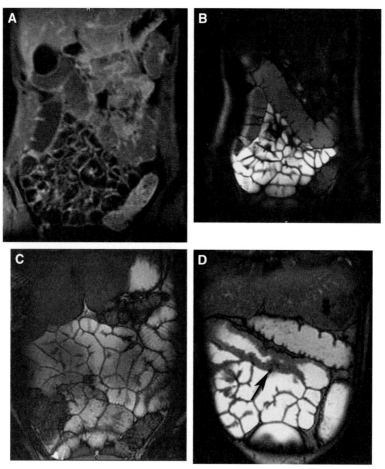

Fig. 11. (*A, B*) Biphasic contrast material (PEG—isosmotic solution). The contrast material presents low signal intensity on T1-weighted sequences (*A*) and high signal intensity on T2-weighted sequences (*B*). These signal intensity properties are useful and lead to optimal contrast resolution between the enhancing small bowel wall on contrast-enhanced T1-weighted images (*A*) and the hypointense lumen which is filled with contrast medium. Using water-sensitive sequences (eg, true-FISP or HASTE T2-weighted) analogous optimal contrast resolution is obtained between the hyperintense lumen and the hypointense small bowel wall (*B*). (*C, D*) A new biphasic oral contrast agent, LBG mixture, with similar signal intensity properties offers optimal results in terms of intestinal distension and lumen-wall contrast resolution with excellent identification of Crohn's disease lesions also in the proximal small intestine (*D, arrow*). (*D,* Courtesy of T. Lauenstein, MD, Essen, Germany.)

by the loops. Analogous to conventional radiograph enteroclysis, MR approach lacks evaluation of the duodenum, a possible site of involvement of Crohn's disease.

Clinical indications

Inflammatory bowel disease (Crohn's disease)

Chronic inflammatory bowel disease, and in particular, Crohn's disease, represents the most common application of MR imaging of the small bowel [22,29–32,36,64–67].

Spectrum of findings

In patients who have proved or suspected Crohn's disease, cross-sectional images should be analyzed specifically for identification and characterization of pathologically altered bowel segment. The normal wall thickness of the small intestine is between 1 mm and 3 mm, when the lumen is distended [68]. Any portion of the bowel wall that exceeds 4 mm to 5 mm is considered abnormal

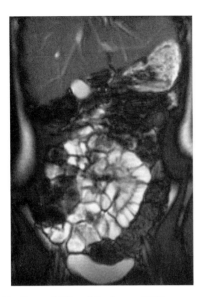

Fig. 12. Coronal T2-weighted true-FISP sequence acquired in a 6-year-old child following oral administration of 200 mL of Volumen. The image shows a good and homogeneous small bowel distension with optimal luminal-to-wall contrast resolution.

(Fig. 14). An adequate intestinal distension is mandatory because collapsed loops or spastic intestinal segments may mimic wall thickening.

Small bowel wall thickening is a sensitive, but not pathognomonic, sign of Crohn's disease because it is observed in several other intestinal diseases (eg, infections, ischemic disorders, graft-versus-host disease). Although superficial mucosal

lesions are missed easily as a result of inadequate spatial resolution, MR imaging is able to detect early inflammatory changes of the bowel wall, based on enhancement following intravenous injection of contrast medium.

There are two patterns of enhancement of a pathologic bowel segment: "homogeneous" and "stratified". Homogeneous enhancement is a diffuse transmural enhancement with no recognition of different bowel layers. A stratification of the bowel wall (the so-called "target" or "double halo" appearance) is related to mucosal enhancement with a hypoenhancing outer layer.

If T2-weighted and contrast-enhanced T1-weighted images are considered simultaneously, two different patterns can be recognized:

Stratification on T2-weighted images (slightly hyperintense mucosa and submucosa and hypointense muscular layer) associated with transmural enhancement (no stratification) on T1-weighted images. This pattern is associated more frequently with early stages of Crohn's disease and is common in pediatric patients and young adults (Fig. 15).

Absence of stratification on T2-weighted images, where the bowel wall is diffusely hypointense, that is due to fibrosis and associated with stratified enhancement pattern on T1-weighted images. This is typical of long-standing Crohn's disease, with fibrosis, or of patients following intense medical treatment (Fig. 16).

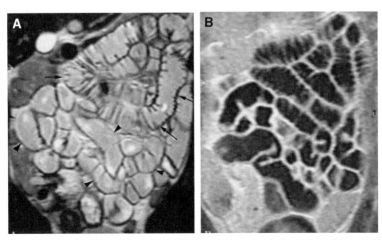

Fig. 13. MR enteroclysis. (A) On T2-weighted HASTE sequence, optimal distension of the entire small bowel is depicted, with typical differentiation between jejunum (*arrows*) and ileum (*arrowheads*). (B) Similar to the study with oral contrast material, in MR enteroclysis, contrast-enhanced T1-weighted images show typical normal parietal enhancement. (Courtesy of L. Broglia, MD, Rome, Italy.)

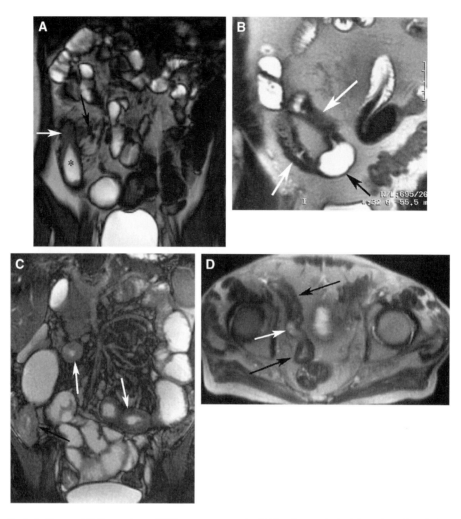

Fig. 14. Crohn's disease. (*A*) Coronal true-FISP sequence acquired following oral administration of PEG shows a long tract of terminal ileum with an abnormal parietal thickening (*white arrow*) that induced severe grade stricture and dilatation of prestenotic loop (*asterisk*). Some enlarged lymph nodes also are visible (*black arrow*). (*B*) Coronal T2-weighted HASTE image showing typical segmental involvement of Crohn's disease of the terminal ileum; two adjacent intestinal segments show increased wall thickness and reduction of luminal caliber (*white arrows*). Distended nonaffected segment is visible between them (*black arrow*). (*C*) Patient following ileocecal resection. Coronal true-FISP image showing recurrence of Crohn's disease at the level of the neo-terminal ileum (*black arrow*) and in two different proximal segments (*white arrows*). (*D, E*) Elderly patient who has long-standing history of Crohn's disease. (*D*) Axial T2-weighted HASTE image showing a long tract of terminal ileum with an increased bowel wall thickness composed of two different segments that are affected by Crohn's disease (*black arrows*) with a small skip segment (*white arrow*). (*E*) Gd-enhanced fat-suppressed T1-weighted image showing pathologic enhancement of the thickened bowel wall as a sign of mild activity of disease and a stratified pattern of the bowel wall that is due to an hypoenhancing fibrous tissue (*asterisks*) in the outer layer and hyperenhancing inner layers (*arrows*).

The recognition of a stricture is easy, considering that the normal lumen of the small intestine is approximately 2.5 cm in diameter. The presence of a prestenotic dilatation may help in the diagnosis (Fig. 17). MR is able to identify long-standing fibrotic strictures (with a thick hypointense bowel wall without a significant contrast enhancement), that would not benefit from medical treatment; however, in most cases, the choice between surgery or medical therapy is related

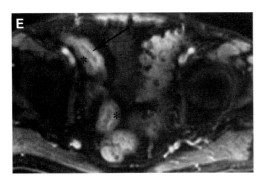

Fig. 14 (*continued*)

primarily to the number and severity of episodes of intestinal occlusions or subocclusions.

Extramural abnormalities include fibro-fatty proliferation, vascular engorgement on the mesenteric side of the bowel, and mesenteric lymphadenopathy. From a pathologic point of view, Crohn's disease is a chronic granulomatous inflammation that affects the bowel wall and extends to the perivisceral mesenteric fatty tissue. The chronic inflammation of the mesenteric fatty tissue also induces proliferation of the fat tissue itself, together with a fibrotic component. On MR imaging, the fibro-fatty proliferation may demonstrate a pseudo-mass with prevalent fibrous or fatty components (Fig. 18).

The "comb sign," a sign of active inflammation, arises from the combination of vascular engorgement of vasa recta and fibro-fatty proliferation and is demonstrated as multiple tubular, tortuous opacities on the mesenteric side of the ileum, aligned as the teeth of a comb (Fig. 19) [69,70]. Other typical findings of active Crohn's disease are the presence of deep ulcers that penetrate the small bowel wall (Fig. 20) and lead to the cobblestone appearance of the mucosal profile (see Fig. 19).

Mesenteric lymphadenopathies that range in size from 3 mm to 8 mm are well-depicted using true-FISP or T2-weighted turbo spin-echo sequences [6,16,28]. When lymph nodes are multiple and larger than 10 mm, lymphoma and carcinoma should be excluded (Fig. 21).

Common complications of Crohn's disease include fistulas, abscesses, and phlegmons. The reported sensitivity of MR imaging for depicting fistulous sinus tracts is 50% to 75% when compared with conventional enteroclysis [62]. Even if direct visualization of fistulous tracts is not possible with MR imaging, indirect signs can be recognized (Fig. 22). The finding shown in Fig. 22 often is associated with inhomogeneity and enhancement of the mesenteric fat around the sinus tract. MR imaging is a suitable technique in the evaluation of a patient who, after surgery, has been found to have a recurrence of Crohn's disease (Fig. 23).

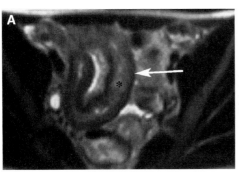

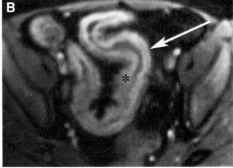

Fig. 15. (*A, B*) Seven-year-old child who has active Crohn's disease. (*A*) Axial T2-weighted HASTE image showing a long segment of terminal ileum (*arrow*) with increased wall thickness and luminal narrowing. Signal intensity differences between a slightly hyperintense inner layer (inflamed mucosa and submucosa; *asterisk*) and the hypointense, inflamed muscular layer are preserved, which leads to a stratification of bowel wall layer. (*B*) Axial contrast-enhanced T1-weighted image showing strong enhancement of the affected bowel wall (*arrow*); enhancement pattern is homogenous (*asterisk*) and is a sign of active transmural disease. These findings may be considered a sign of active inflammatory changes of the bowel wall without fibrotic modification and are more frequent in young patients who never underwent medical treatment.

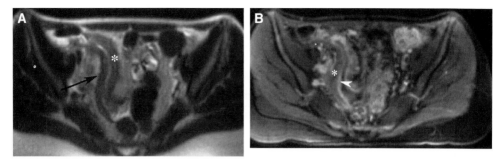

Fig. 16. (*A, B*) Twenty-five-year-old patient who has active Crohn's disease. (*A*) Axial T2-weighted HASTE image showing a long segment of terminal ileum (*arrow*) with increased wall thickness and luminal narrowing; signal intensity is homogeneous along the bowel wall (*asterisk*) with loss of signal intensity differences between muscular layer and inner layer. (*B*) Axial contrast-enhanced T1-weighted image showing strong enhancement of the inner layer (*arrowhead*) with a hypoenhancement of outer layer (*asterisk*), the so called "stratified" contrast enhancement pattern. This pattern of unstratified pattern on T2-weighted images (*A*) and stratified contrast-enhancement pattern on T1-weighted images (*B*) may be considered a sign of active inflammatory changes of the bowel wall with fibrotic modification and is more frequent in patients who have long-standing active Crohn's disease and in recurrence of disease following medical treatment.

Assessment of disease activity

The assessment of disease activity is extremely important, given its influence on the choice of therapy (choice of drug and adequate dose) and its ability to provide an assessment of the patient's clinical course. In several studies, MR imaging was used to evaluate disease activity [25,37,38,57,58,71,72]. Based on different experiences [73], contrast-enhanced fat-suppressed T1-weighted images offer the best correlation between MR findings and Crohn's Disease Activity Index (CDAI), although a correlation that used fat-suppressed T2-weighted images also was demonstrated [38].

In a recent article, Koh et al [74] found that contrast-enhanced MR imaging and CDAI demonstrated a similar sensitivity, but MR imaging had a higher specificity. Given the lower cost of

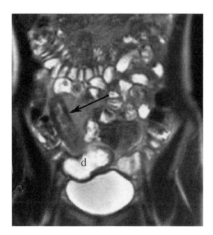

Fig. 17. Bowel stricture secondary to marked fibrotic thickening of the bowel wall (*arrow*). The evidence of a prestenotic dilated loop (*d*) is indicative of a severe stenosis, which possibly causes episode of intestinal subocclusions.

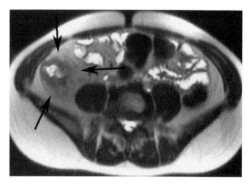

Fig. 18. Fibro-fatty proliferation visible on T2-weighted axial HASTE sequence as a volumetric growth of the fatty tissue that surrounds the affected intestinal loop. The peritoneum that encompasses this tissue is thickened (*arrows*). The fatty tissue also presents an inhomogeneous appearance which is typical of inflammatory changes.

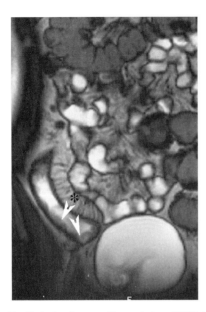

Fig. 19. Crohn's disease. Coronal true-FISP image showing wall thickening of a long tract of terminal ileum; several deep ulcers (*arrowheads*) lead to the so-called "cobblestone pattern" of the mucosal profile. The same bowel loop presents an enlargement of vasa recta (vascular engorgement) on the mesenteric side ("comb sign"; *asterisk*).

CDAI and the limited organizational and economic possibility of performing MR imaging in all patients, the investigators concluded that MR imaging can play a useful role in the diagnostic algorithm of Crohn's disease, particularly when CDAI score is equivocal.

A correlation between contrast-enhanced MR imaging and CDAI and the findings of distal ileoscopy was demonstrated in the authors' study on a pediatric population of patients [58].

Malabsorption syndromes

Malabsorption syndromes, in general, and celiac disease, in particular, are other possible indications for MR study of the small bowel. Celiac disease is a chronic inflammatory pathology that involves the gastrointestinal tract in genetically predisposed individuals. It is common in European countries, with a prevalence of approximately 1 in 250 to 300. The role of diagnostic imaging in the assessment of the disease is limited, given that diagnosis is obtained by way of jejunal biopsy. Nonetheless, approximately 75% of patients have radiologically identifiable alterations that are represented by intestinal atonia; changes in mucosal fold pattern (ileal jejunalization and the so-called "reversal fold pattern"); and complications, such as intussusception [75].

Intestinal atonia is a nonspecific sign of intestinal disease; it presents as diffuse dilatation (greater than 3 cm) of the small intestine without the evidence of any obstructing lesion (Fig. 24). The most specific signs of celiac disease are the alterations of fold pattern—a decrease in the number of mucosal jejunal folds (less than three per inch) and an increase of ileal mucosal folds

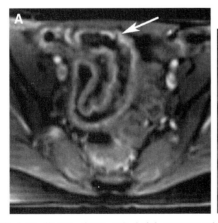
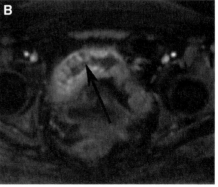

Fig. 20. Crohn's disease ulcers. (*A*) Axial contrast-enhanced fat-suppressed T1-weighted image showing a deep penetrating ulcer (*arrow*). (*B*) In a different case, the same sequence shows multiple penetrating ulcers (*arrow*).

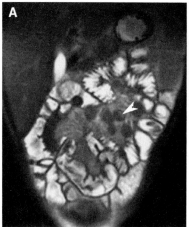
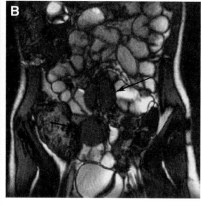

Fig. 21. Lymph node enlargement. (*A*) Coronal T2-weighted HASTE sequence demonstrates multiple mesenteric adenopathies, some of them with central necrotic areas (*arrowhead*) secondary to intestinal infection. (*B*) Pediatric patient affected by lymphoma. When the lymph node enlargement exceeds 10 mm, malignancy should be excluded. In this patient, true-FISP image shows multiple bulky lymph node masses (*arrows*) along mesenteric vessels. These cause the so-called "sandwich sign" which is typical of lymphoma.

(more than four per inch; so-called "ileal jejuniza-tion"). A smooth appearance of jejuna mucosal profile together with ileal jejunization is known as "reversal fold" pattern (Fig. 25).

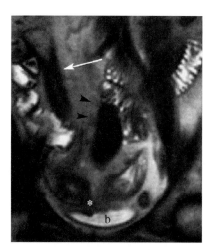

Fig. 22. Crohn's disease fistula. Direct visualization of fistulous tracts is not always possible using cross-sectional imaging. On coronal T2-weighted HASTE image, a distortion of an affected bowel (*asterisk*) which converges to the urinary bladder (*b*) is strongly suggestive of a fistula between the ileal loop and urinary bladder. The terminal ileum also is affected (*arrow*) and multiple enlarged lymph nodes are visible along the mesenteric tissue (*arrowheads*).

Complications of celiac disease are represented by transient intestinal intussusception secondary to intestinal atonia. MR appearance is the so-called "double halo" or "target" sign, with different stratified layers representing bowel wall and peritoneal fat tissue [75].

An extraintestinal finding of patients who have celiac disease is represented by mesenteric adeno-pathies. The evaluation and follow-up of enlarged nodes in these patients who do not respond to gluten-free diet is a radiologic challenge considering that a few patients might develop lymphoma.

Other pathologic conditions

A still mostly unexplored field of application of MR of the small bowel is in the study of neoplasms (adenocarcinomas; lymphomas; and to a lesser extent, metastatic localizations). The accuracy of the technique in cases of nonocclu-sive tumors of the lumen is not known, given the lack of large case series (because of the rarity of the lesions and the recent advent of MR studies) [24].

Other pathologic disorders are represented by intestinal infections, ischemic disorders, vasculitis, and graft-versus-host disease. All of them may induce alterations of bowel wall thickness and enhancement pattern (Fig. 26).

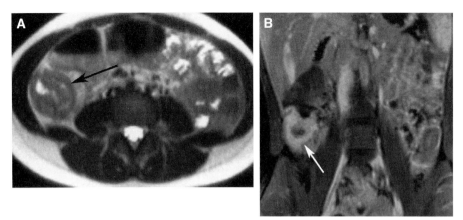

Fig. 23. (*A, B*) Recurrence of Crohn's disease 1 year after surgery (ileocecal resection). (*A*) Axial T2-weighted HASTE image demonstrates thickening of the cecal wall (*arrow*). (*B*) On coronal contrast-enhanced T1-weighted image, strong pathologic enhancement of the cecal wall (*arrow*) is indicative of disease activity.

Summary

MR imaging, using modern equipment and a rigorous technical approach, can offer detailed morphologic information and functional data on the small bowel. The optimal study technique is debatable, although the oral administration of contrast material as a first-line approach is less expensive, faster, easier to perform, and better tolerated by patients. MR enteroclysis might be reserved for selected cases as a second-line study.

The major clinical indication is the evaluation of patients who have suspected or known Crohn's disease. The absence of ionizing radiation, considering the young age of most of the patients and the frequency of the examinations, is an important advantage over other techniques (radiograph and CT enteroclysis).

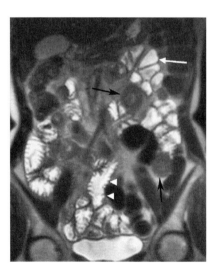

Fig. 25. Coronal T2-weighted HASTE image in a patient who has severe celiac disease. A jejuno-ileal fold pattern reversal is observed. Note a decreased number of jejunal folds (*white arrow*) and an increased number of ileal folds (*arrowheads*) in a dilated ileum. This image also clearly also dilatation of small bowel loops without the evidence of stenosis and two jejunal intussusceptions which are demonstrated by the so-called "target sign" (*black arrows*).

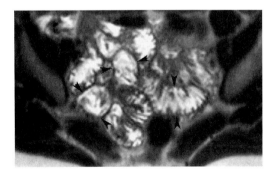

Fig. 24. Intestinal atonia. Axial T2-weighted HASTE sequence showing an increased and diffuse small bowel loops caliber (>2.5 cm) without bowel wall alterations. The boundary of three different luminal bowel loops can be seen (*arrowheads*). This is an aspecific sign of intestinal disease, sometimes the only one to be observed in patients who have malabsorption syndromes.

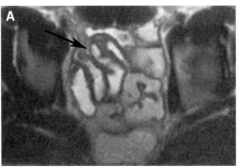 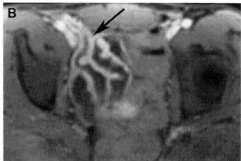

Fig. 26. (*A, B*) Intestinal manifestations of Henock-Schonlein purpura. (*A*) Axial T2-weighted HASTE image showing mild bowel wall thickening of some distal ileal loops (*arrow*). (*B*) On contrast-enhanced T1-weighted image, pathologic enhancement is seen (*arrow*).

References

[1] Runge VM, Foster MA, Clanton JA, et al. Particulate oral NMR contrast agents. Int J Nucl Med Biol 1985;12:37–42.

[2] Wesbey GE, Brasch RC, Goldberg HI, et al. Dilute oral iron solutions as gastrointestinal contrast agents for magnetic resonance imaging; initial clinical experience. Magn Reson Imaging 1985;3:57–64.

[3] Hahn PF, Stark DD, Saini S, et al. Ferrite particles for bowel contrast in MR imaging: design issues and feasibility studies. Radiology 1987;164:37–41.

[4] Widder DJ, Edelman RR, Grief WL, et al. Magnetite albumin suspension: a superparamagnetic oral MR contrast agent. AJR 1987;149:839–43.

[5] Laniado M, Kornmesser W, Hamm B, et al. MR imaging of the gastrointestinal tract: value of Gd-DTPA. AJR 1988;150:817–21.

[6] Bisset GS III. Evaluation of potential practical oral contrast agents for pediatric magnetic resonance imaging. Preliminary observations. Pediatr Radiol 1989;20:61–6.

[7] Lonnemark M, Hemmingsson A, Bach-Gansmo T, et al. Effect of superparamagnetic particles as oral contrast medium at magnetic resonance imaging. A phase I clinical study. Acta Radiol 1989;30:193–6.

[8] Li KC, Ang PG, Tart RP, et al. Paramagnetic oil emulsions as oral magnetic resonance imaging contrast agents. Magn Reson Imaging 1990;8:589–98.

[9] Hahn PF, Stark DD, Lewis JM, et al. First clinical trial of a new superparamagnetic iron oxide for use as an oral gastrointestinal contrast agent in MR imaging. Radiology 1990;175:695–700.

[10] Tart RP, Li KC, Storm BL, et al. Enteric MRI contrast agents: comparative study of five potential agents in humans. Magn Reson Imaging 1991;9:559–68.

[11] Rubin DL, Muller HH, Young SW. Methods for the systematic investigation of gastrointestinal contrast media for MRI: evaluation of intestinal distribution by radiographic monitoring. Magn Reson Imaging 1991;9:285–93.

[12] Li KC, Tart RP, Fitzsimmons JR, et al. Barium sulphate suspension as a negative oral MRI contrast agent: in vitro and human optimization studies. Magn Reson Imaging 1991;9:141–50.

[13] Ros PR, Steinman RM, Torres GM, et al. The value of barium as a gastrointestinal contrast agent in MR imaging: a comparison study in normal volunteers. AJR Am J Roentgenol 1991;157:761–7.

[14] Patten RM, Moss AA, Fenton TA, et al. OMR, a positive bowel contrast agent for abdominal and pelvic MR imaging: safety and imaging characteristics. J Magn Reson Imaging 1992;2:25–34.

[15] Van Beers B, Grandin C, Jamart J, et al. Magnetic resonance imaging of lower abdominal and pelvic lesions: assessment of oral magnetic particles as an intestinal contrast agent. Eur J Radiol 1992;14:252–7.

[16] Mirowitz SA, Susman N. Use of nutritional support formula as a gastrointestinal contrast agent for MRI. J Comput Assist Tomogr 1992;16:908–15.

[17] Chou CK, Liu GC, Chen LT, et al. The use of MRI in bowel obstruction. Abdom Imaging 1993;18:131–5.

[18] Hirohashi S, Uchida H, Yoshikawa K, et al. Large scale clinical evaluation of bowel contrast agent containing ferric ammonium citrate in MRI. Magn Reson Imaging 1994;12:837–46.

[19] Anderson CM, Brown JJ, Balfe DM, et al. MR imaging of Crohn disease: use of perflubron as a gastrointestinal contrast agent. J Magn Reson Imaging 1994;4:491–6.

[20] Bernardino ME, Weinreb JC, Mitchell DG, et al. Safety and optimum concentration of a manganese chloride-based oral MR contrast agent. J Magn Reson Imaging 1994;4:872–6.

[21] Haldemann Heusler RC, Wight E, Marincek B. Oral superparamagnetic contrast agent (ferumoxsil): tolerance and efficacy in MR imaging of gynaecologic diseases. J Magn Reson Imaging 1995;5:385–91.

[22] Rollandi GA, Martinoli C, Conzi R, et al. Magnetic resonance imaging of the small intestine and colon in Crohn's disease. Radiol Med 1996;91:81–5.

[23] Van Beers BE, Grandin C, De Greef D, et al. Ferristene as intestinal MR contrast agent. Distribution and safety of a fast ingestion procedure with oral metoclopramide. Acta Radiol 1996;37:676–9.

[24] Semelka RC, John G, Kelekis NL, et al. Small bowel neoplastic disease: demonstration by MRI. J Magn Reson Imaging 1996;6:855–60.

[25] Madsen SM, Thomsen HS, Munkholm P, et al. Magnetic resonance imaging of Crohn disease: early recognition of treatment response and relapse. Abdom Imaging 1997;22:164–6.

[26] Faber SC, Stehling MK, Holzknecht N, et al. Pathologic conditions in the small bowel: findings at fat-suppressed gadolinium-enhanced MR imaging with an optimized suspension of oral magnetic particles. Radiology 1997;205:278–82.

[27] Aschoff AJ, Zeitler H, Merkle EM, et al. MR enteroclysis for nuclear spin tomographic diagnosis of inflammatory bowel diseases with contrast enhancement. Rofo 1997;167:387–91.

[28] Paley MR, Ros PR. MRI of the gastrointestinal tract. Eur Radiol 1997;7:1387–97.

[29] Ernst O, Asselah T, Cablan X, et al. Breath-hold fast spin-echo MR imaging of Crohn's disease. AJR Am J Roentgenol 1998;170:127–8.

[30] Rieber A, Wruk D, Nussle K, et al. MRI of the abdomen combined with enteroclysis in Crohn disease using oral and intravenous Gd-DTPA. Radiologe 1998;38:23–8.

[31] Holzknecht N, Helmberger T, von Ritter C, et al. MRI of the small intestine with rapid MRI sequences in Crohn disease after enteroclysis with oral iron particles. Radiologe 1998;38:29–36.

[32] Ha HK, Lee EH, Lim CH, et al. Application of MRI for small intestinal diseases. J Magn Reson Imaging 1998;8:375–83.

[33] Lee JK, Marcos HB, Semelka RC. MR imaging of the small bowel using the HASTE sequence. AJR Am J Roentgenol 1998;170:1457–63.

[34] Regan F, Beall DP, Bohlman ME, et al. Fast MR imaging and the detection of small-bowel obstruction. AJR Am J Roentgenol 1998;170:1465–9.

[35] Adamek HE, Breer H, Karschkes T, et al. Magnetic resonance imaging in gastroenterology: time to say good-bye to all that endoscopy? Endoscopy 2000;32:406–10.

[36] Marcos HB, Semelka RC. Evaluation of Crohn's disease using half-fourier RARE and gadolinium-enhanced SGE sequences: initial results. Magn Reson Imaging 2000;18:263–8.

[37] Durno CA, Sherman P, Williams T, et al. Magnetic resonance imaging to distinguish the type and severity of pediatric inflammatory bowel diseases. J Pediatr Gastroenterol Nutr 2000;30:170–4.

[38] Maccioni F, Viscido A, Broglia L, et al. Evaluation of Crohn disease activity with magnetic resonance imaging. Abdom Imaging 2000;25:219–28.

[39] Gourtsoyiannis N, Papanikolaou N, Grammatikakis J, et al. MR enteroclysis protocol optimization: comparison between 3D FLASH with fat saturation after intravenous gadolinium injection and true FISP sequences. Eur Radiol 2001;11:908–13.

[40] Rofsky NM, Lee VS, Laub G, et al. Abdominal MR imaging with a volumetric interpolated breath-hold examination. Radiology 1999;212:876–84.

[41] Sodickson DK, Manning WJ. Simultaneous acquisition of spatial harmonics (SMASH): fast imaging with radiofrequency coil arrays. Magn Reson Med 1997;38:591–603.

[42] Lomas DJ. Techniques for magnetic resonance imaging of the bowel. Topics in MRI 2002;13:379–88.

[43] Roemer PB, Edelstein WA, Hayes CE, et al. The NMR phased array. Magn Reson Med 1990;16:192–225.

[44] Barkhausen J, Quick HH, Lauenstein T, et al. Whole-body MR imaging in 30 seconds with real-time true FISP and a continuously rolling table platform: feasibility study. Radiology 2001;220:252–6.

[45] Beall DP, Fortman BJ, Lawler BC, et al. Imaging bowel obstruction: a comparison between fast magnetic resonance imaging and helical computed tomography. Clin Radiol 2002;57:719–24.

[46] Debatin JF, Patak MA. MRI of the small and large bowel. Eur Radiol 1999;9:1523–34.

[47] Rieber A, Nussle K, Reinshagen M, et al. MRI of the abdomen with positive oral contrast agents for the diagnosis of inflammatory small bowel disease. Abdom Imaging 2002;27:394–9.

[48] Malcolm PN, Brown JJ, Hahn PF, et al. The clinical value of ferric ammonium citrate: a positive oral contrast agent for T1-weighted MR imaging of the upper abdomen. J Magn Reson Imaging 2000;12:702–7.

[49] Laghi A, Paolantonio P, Iafrate F, et al. Oral contrast agent for MRI of the bowel. Topics in MRI 2002;13:389–96.

[50] Lomas DJ, Graves MJ. Small bowel MRI using water as a contrast medium. Br J Radiol 1999;72:994–7.

[51] Minowa O, Ozaki Y, Kyogoku S, et al. MR imaging of the small bowel using water as a contrast agent in a preliminary study with healthy volunteers. AJR Am J Roentgenol 1999;173:581–2.

[52] Schunk K. Small bowel magnetic resonance imaging for inflammatory bowel disease. Topics in MRI 2002;13:409–26.

[53] Sood RR, Joubert I, Franklin H, et al. Small bowel MRI: comparison of a polyethylene glycol preparation and water as oral contrast media. J Magn Reson Imaging 2002;15:401–8.

[54] Laghi A, Carbone I, Catalano C, et al. Polyethylene glycol solution as an oral contrast agent for MR imaging of the small bowel. AJR Am J Roentgenol 2001;177:1333–4.

[55] Lauenstein TC, Schneemann H, Vogt FM, et al. Optimization of oral contrast agents for MR imaging of the small bowel. Radiology 2003;228(1):279–83.

[56] Patak MA, Froehlich JM, von Weymarn C, et al. Non-invasive distension of the small bowel for magnetic-resonance imaging. Lancet 2001;358:987–8.

[57] Schunk K, Kern A, Oberholzer K, et al. Hydro-MRI in Crohn's disease: appraisal of disease activity. Invest Radiol 2000;35:431–7.

[58] Laghi A, Borrelli O, Paolantonio P, et al. Contrast-enhanced magnetic resonance imaging of the terminal ileum in children with Crohn's disease. Gut 2002;52:393–7.

[59] D'Arienzo A, Scaglione G, Bennato R, et al. The prognostic value, in active ulcerative colitis, of an increased intensity of colonic perivisceral fat signal on magnetic resonance imaging with ferumoxil. Am J Gastroenterol 2001;96:481–6.

[60] Umschaden HW, Szolar D, Gasser J, et al. Small-bowel disease: comparison of MR enteroclysis images with conventional enteroclysis and surgical findings. Radiology 2000;215:717–25.

[61] Maglinte DD, Siegelman ES, Kelvin FM. MR enteroclysis: the future of small-bowel imaging? Radiology 2000;215:639–41.

[62] Gourtsoyiannis N, Papanikolaou N, Grammatikakis J, et al. MR enteroclysis: technical considerations and clinical applications. Eur Radiol 2002;12:2651–82.

[63] Rieber A, Aschoff A, Nussle K, et al. MRI in the diagnosis of small bowel disease: use of positive and negative oral contrast media in combination with enteroclysis. Eur Radiol 2000;10:1377–82.

[64] Gourtsoyiannis N, Papanikolaou N, Grammatikakis J, et al. MR imaging of the small bowel with a true-FISP sequence after enteroclysis with water solution. Invest Radiol 2000;35:707–11.

[65] Papanikolaou N, Prassopoulos P, Grammatikakis J, et al. Optimization of a contrast medium suitable for conventional enteroclysis, MR enteroclysis, and virtual MR enteroscopy. Abdom Imaging 2002;27:517–22.

[66] Prassopoulos P, Papanikolaou N, Grammatikakis J, et al. MR enteroclysis imaging of Crohn disease. Radiographics 2001;21:161–72.

[67] Rieber A, Wruk D, Potthast S, et al. Diagnostic imaging in Crohn's disease: comparison of magnetic resonance imaging and conventional imaging methods. Int J Colorectal Dis 2000;15:176–81.

[68] Laghi A, Carbone I, Catalano C, et al. Polyethylene glycol solution as an oral contrast agent for MR imaging of the small bowel. AJR Am J Roentgenol 2001;177(6):1333–4.

[69] Madureira AJ. The comb sign. Radiology 2004;230:783–4.

[70] Gore RM, Balthazar EJ, Ghahremani GG, et al. CT features of ulcerative colitis and Crohn's disease. AJR Am J Roentgenol 1996;167:3–15.

[71] Madsen SM, Thomsen HS, Schlichting P, et al. Evaluation of treatment response in active Crohn's disease by low-field magnetic resonance imaging. Abdom Imaging 1999;24:232–9.

[72] Shoenut JP, Semelka RC, Magro CM, et al. Comparison of magnetic resonance imaging and endoscopy in distinguishing the type and severity of inflammatory bowel disease. J Clin Gastroenterol 1994;19:31–5.

[73] Low RN, Sebrechts CP, Politoske DA, et al. Crohn disease with endoscopic correlation: single-shot fast spin-echo and gadolinium-enhanced fat-suppressed spoiled gradient-echo MR imaging. Radiology 2002;222:652–60.

[74] Koh DM, Miao Y, Chinn RJ, et al. MR imaging evaluation of the activity of Crohn's disease. Am J Roentgenol 2001;177:1325–32.

[75] Laghi A, Paolantonio P, Catalano C, et al. MR imaging of the small bowel using polyethylene glycol solution as an oral contrast agent in adults and children with celiac disease. Preliminary Observations. Am J Roentgenol 2003;180:191–4.

ELSEVIER
SAUNDERS

Magn Reson Imaging Clin N Am
13 (2005) 349–358

MAGNETIC
RESONANCE
IMAGING CLINICS
of North America

MR Imaging of the Large Bowel

Thomas C. Lauenstein, MD*, Christiane A. Kuehle, MD, Waleed Ajaj, MD

Department of Diagnostic and Interventional Radiology and Neuroradiology, University Hospital Essen, Hufelandstrasse 55, 45122 Essen, Germany

Conventional colonoscopy has a high accuracy for the detection of colorectal masses or inflammatory bowel disease (IBD). Poor patient acceptance, which reflects considerable procedural pain, has limited the use of colonoscopy as a screening method for colorectal cancer [1,2]. In addition, anticipation of an endoscopic study of the colon frequently is associated with unpleasant expectations that focus on disco mfort and the risk of complications, such as perforations [3]. This generally leads to poor patient participation [4]. The presence of stenoses or elongated bowel segments may result in an inability to visualize the entire colon and the ileocecal valve in a considerable number of patients [5]. This has motivated investigators to develop alternative concepts to assess the colon. Main efforts have focused on virtual endoscopy that is based on the acquisition of cross-sectional images; this can be accomplished by using CT or MR imaging. Recent studies have shown that CT and MR colonography (MRC) are effective in the detection of clinically relevant diseases [6–9]. In a study that included more than 100 patients who underwent virtual and conventional endoscopy, virtual endoscopy was favored by 82% of the patients [10]. Similar results were obtained by Angtuaco et al [11]; 77% of 400 potential screening patients preferred virtual endoscopy over conventional colonoscopy. Virtual colonoscopy that is based on the acquisition of CT data sets is associated with considerable doses of ionizing radiation, however [12,13]. This issue plays a mayor role

because patients who have IBD often are young. Also, screening examinations for colorectal cancer should be repeated every 3 to 5 years. Therefore, it seems preferable to use MR imaging for virtual colonography.

Technique

Three main requirements need to be fulfilled for MRC:

1. The use of an appropriate hardware system: because data acquisition must be performed under breath-hold conditions, the use of new 1.0 or 1.5 tesla scanners that are equipped with strong gradient systems is mandatory. Whether MRC is possible is determined largely by the minimum repetition time. If it exceeds 5 milliseconds, collection of a three-dimensional (3D) data set that contains the entire colon will take more than 30 seconds—too long for a comfortable breathhold.
2. Distension of the colonic bowel loops: in their physiologic state, parts of the large bowel are collapsed and cannot be assessed properly. Thus, the colon needs to be distended by administering liquid or gasiform-distending media rectally.
3. A high contrast between the bowel wall and the bowel lumen: this feature, which allows the accurate display of the colonic wall, strongly depends on the MR sequences that are applied and the use of intravenous (IV) and rectal contrast agents.

Before the MR examination, patients need to undergo bowel cleansing in a manner which is similar to that required for conventional

* Corresponding author.
E-mail address: thomas.lauenstein@uni-essen.de
(T.C. Lauenstein).

colonoscopy. To avoid unnecessary patient discomfort, MRC should be performed in the morning. Administration of sedative or analgesics is not required. Before the examination, patients have to be screened for possible contraindications to MR imaging, such as metallic implants or severe claustrophobia. The presence of hip prosthesis, which generally is not regarded as a contraindication to MR imaging, may lead to avid artifacts in the region of the rectum and sigmoid colon. Hence, these patients should not be examined.

For data acquisition, a combination of two large "flex surface coils" should be used for signal reception to assure the coverage of the entire colon (Fig. 1). To obviate bowel spasms and minimize artifacts that are due to bowel motion, a spasmolytic agent (eg, scopolamine, 20 mg, IV; glucagon, 1 mg, IV) has to be administered. Following the placement of a rectal tube (Fig. 2), the colon is filled, while the patient is in the prone position, with approximately 2000 mL to 2500 mL of tap water using hydrostatic pressure. The filling procedure should be stopped after the application of the entire amount of water or whenever the patient complains about discomfort. Other investigators propose the acquisition of monitoring sequences during the filling process (eg, nonslice select sequences that provide an update image every 1–2 seconds).

Different 3D sequence types can be acquired. For T1-weighted MR imaging (dark-lumen MRC), the IV administration of gadolinium is mandatory. After a first "precontrast" T1-weighted 3D gradient echo data set, paramagnetic

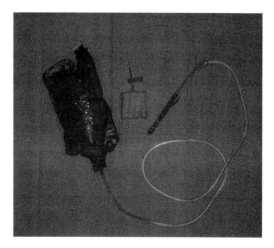

Fig. 2. The water-containing enema bag is connected by way of a catheter with a rectal tube. The tube may be blocked at its tip with a balloon.

contrast should be administered IV at a dosage of 0.2 mmol/kg using an automatic injector. The paramagnetic contrast application should be followed by rapid injection of normal saline. After a delay of 75 seconds, the "precontrast" 3D acquisition has to be repeated (Fig. 3). Imaging parameters are listed in Table 1. In case of insufficient image quality (eg, due to patient's movement or technical problems), the postcontrast scan can be repeated over a long time period after contrast injection because of a stable contrast enhancement of the colonic wall. Furthermore, T1-weighted data should be amplified by 3D fast imaging with steady-state precession sequences. Different vendor-specific names for these sequences have been introduced: FIESTA (General Electric Medical Systems, Milwaukee, Wisconsin), TrueFISP (Siemens Medical Solutions, Erlangen, Germany), and Balanced Fast Field Echo (Philips Medical Systems, Best, The Netherlands). Image features are characterized by a mixture of T1- and T2-contrast which leads to a homogenous bright signal of the colonic lumen filled with water (bright-lumen MRC). The colonic wall and masses that arise from are seen as dark filling defects (Fig. 4). After data acquisition, the enema bag is placed on the floor for draining the water and the patient is removed from the scanner.

Data interpretation

All 3D data sets should be transferred to a postprocessing workstation. A special software

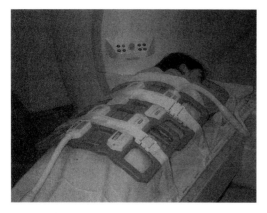

Fig. 1. Clinical setup for MRC. The patient is placed in a prone position on the scanner table. A combination of two surface coils is used to permit coverage of the entire abdomen.

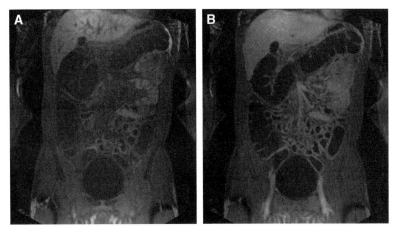

Fig. 3. Pre- (A) and postcontrast (B) T1-weighted sequence. The colonic lumen is rendered dark because of the water enema. An avid contrast enhancement leads to a high signal of the colonic wall on the postcontrast scan.

tool should be used to enable the perception of the MR source data as well as virtual endoscopic views of the colon (Fig. 5). Initially, however, MRC should be interpreted in the multiplanar reformation mode by scrolling through the T1-weighted contrast-enhanced 3D data set in all three orthogonal planes. Whenever a mass that arises from the colonic wall is detected, the identical part of the colon should be analyzed on the precontrast scan. Thus, a contrast enhancement value can be determined by measuring signal intensities of the mass in native and postcontrast scans. This method assures a reliable discrimination between residual stool particles and real colorectal masses. Although residual stool does not show any contrast enhancement (Fig. 6), colorectal lesions always do (Fig. 7). Scar tissue (eg, after appendectomy) may mimic polypoid lesions (Fig. 8).

In addition, MR data should be evaluated based on virtual endoscopic renderings. A virtual endoscopic fly-through facilitates the depiction of

small lesions. In addition, the 3D depth perception allows the evaluation of haustral fold morphology, which enhances the observer's ability to distinguish polyps from haustra. To visualize both sides of haustral folds and to minimize the risk of missing relevant lesions, the virtual fly-through should be performed in an antegrade and a retrograde direction.

Because the quality of fast imaging with steady-state precession data is superior as a result of the high contrast and relative motion

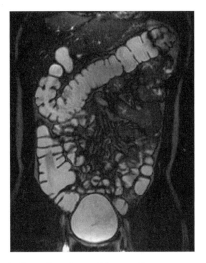

Fig. 4. Fast imaging with steady-state precession sequence of the colon. The contrast mechanism is different compared with the T1-weighted images; the colonic lumen is rendered bright, whereas the colonic wall is seen as a dark filling defect.

Table 1
Sequence parameters of T1-weighted gradient echo data for MR colonography

Repetition time (ms)	3.1
Echo time (ms)	1.1
Flip (degrees)	12
Slice thickness (mm)	1.8
No. of slices	96
Matrix	180 × 256
Acquisition time (s)	22
Acquisition plane	Coronal

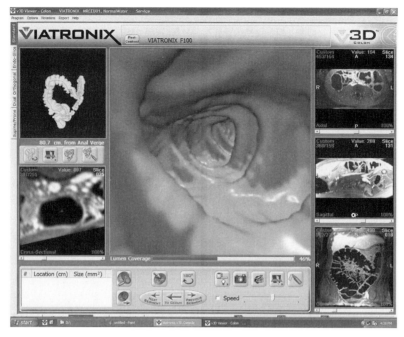

Fig. 5. Software platform for the evaluation of MR colonography. The T1-weighted data sets are displayed simultaneously in different manners: a virtual endoscopic view, the coronal source data, and axial and sagittal reconstructions are shown (Viatronix, Stony Brook, NY).

insensitivity, the analysis should be repeated with these data sets as well (Fig. 9). No information about perfusion of the bowel wall is available, however, which may complicate the differentiation between polyps and residual fecal material in these sequences.

Indications of MR colonography

Detection of colorectal masses

Most colorectal cancers develop over a period of several years from adenomatous polyps [14].

This pathogenesis makes colorectal cancer preventable to a large extent. Detection and removal of polyps eliminates the risk of subsequent malignant degeneration. Thus, implementation of screening programs can reduce the incidence of colorectal cancer by more than 80% [15,16].

Ajaj et al [17] evaluated the impact of MRC for the detection of colorectal polyps in a high-risk population. One hundred and twenty-two subjects who had suspected colorectal diseases were studied. A contrast-enhanced T1-weighted 3D volumetric interpolated breath-hold examination

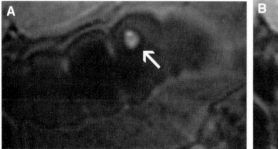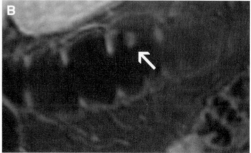

Fig. 6. The acquisition of pre- (A) and postcontrast-enhanced (B) T1-weighted data allows a reliable differentiation between residual stool and polyps, because stool particles (arrow) already are of high signal intensity on the native scan and do not show any contrast uptake.

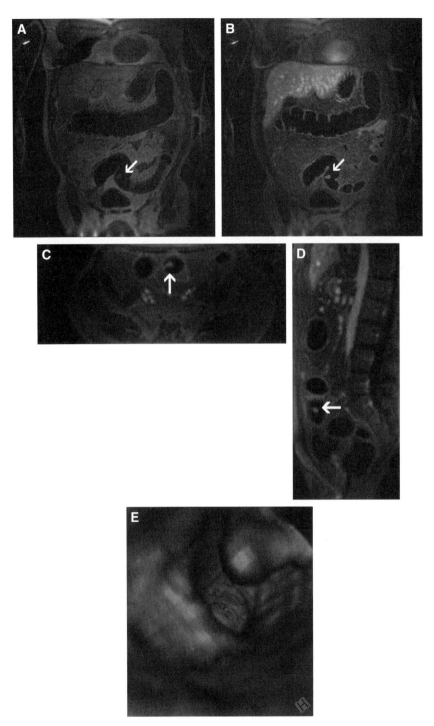

Fig. 7. Colorectal lesions (*arrow*) always show a contrast enhancement when comparing the native (*A*) and postcontrast scan (*B*). Furthermore, pathologies (*arrow*) can be displayed in an axial (*C*) or sagittal (*D*) reformation or as a virtual endoscopic view (*E*).

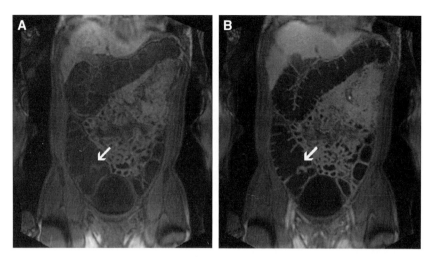

Fig. 8. (*A, B*) Scar tissue after appendectomy may mimic a colorectal mass (*arrow*) by showing a contrast enhancement.

(VIBE) sequence was collected after the rectal administration of water. The presence of colorectal masses was documented. Results were compared with those of a subsequently performed colonoscopy. None of the polyps that measured less than 5 mm that were detected by colonoscopy was identified based on MRC images. In the size group that ranged between 5 mm and 10 mm, MRC correctly detected 16 of 18 lesions and two polyps that were larger than 10 mm also were seen correctly on MRC images. Two of three patients who had documented polyposis coli were diagnosed correctly on MRC (Fig. 10). Furthermore,

all nine colorectal carcinomas were seen correctly on MRC images.

Thus, one major concern relates to the inability of the MR technique to identify colorectal lesions that are smaller than 5 mm. The significance of this limitation is equivocal because of the direct observational data on growth rates which indicate that small polyps (<10 mm) tend to remain stable over a time range of 36 to 48 months. Furthermore, these small lesions are not prone to malignant degeneration [18]. Nevertheless, small colorectal lesions probably will become detectable by MRC as technical refinements, including

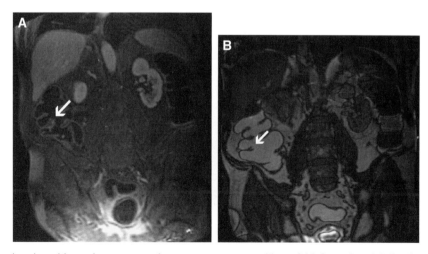

Fig. 9. Fast imaging with steady-state precession sequences may provide useful information. (*A*) On the T1-weighted image, a thickened haustral fold is shown (*arrow*). (*B*) This turns out to be a motion artifact (*arrow*), because the TrueFISP scan shows no abnormality.

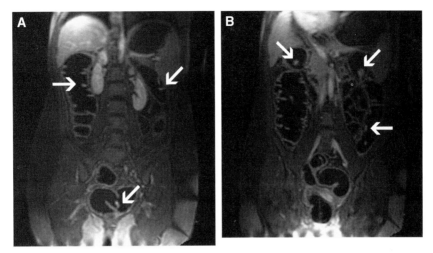

Fig. 10. (*A, B*) Patient who has polyposis coli. Multiple colorectal polyps (*arrows*) are shown on the contrast-enhanced T1-weighted data sets.

parallel acquisition techniques, are implemented [19]. Flat adenomas, however, are likely to remain elusive.

In another trial, the diagnostic accuracy of contrast-enhanced T1-weighted data was compared with 3D fast imaging with steady-state precession sequences [20]. Thirty-seven patients who had suspected colorectal lesions were included. MRC was performed as described earlier. The detection rate of colorectal masses and inflammatory lesions was determined for T1-weighted data and TrueFISP sequences separately. Image quality also was assessed. All patients underwent conventional colonoscopy as the standard of reference. Sensitivity of dark lumen T1-weighted MRC was 78.9%. There were no false positive results; residual stool could be differentiated from colorectal masses. The TrueFISP-based MRC, however, failed to detect two polyps which resulted in a sensitivity of 68.4%. Furthermore, false positive results were seen in five patients; however, image quality of TrueFISP was rated superior to that of dark lumen MRC because of less motion artifacts.

Detection of bowel inflammation

Crohn's disease and ulcerative colitis are the most frequent specific IBDs, with a prevalence of approximately 1 in 500 [21–23]. Diagnostic procedures in IBD serve to validate the diagnosis and to optimize treatment. Endoscopic biopsy is considered the gold standard for the detection and quantification of IBDs [24,25]. Several studies reported on the ability of MR imaging to detect

IBD [26,27]. Ajaj et al [28] examined 15 normal subjects and 23 patients who had suspected IBD of the large bowel by means of MR imaging. The presence of inflammatory changes was documented based on four criteria: bowel wall thickness, bowel wall contrast enhancement, loss of haustral folds, and presence of perifocal lymph nodes. All results were quantified relative to data that were obtained from normal subjects and summarized in a single score. This MRC-based score was compared with endoscopic and histopathologic data. MRC correctly identified 93% of the segments that were found to reveal IBD changes by histopathology. All severely inflamed segments were identified correctly and there were no false positive findings. Thus, MRC may be used for monitoring IBD activity or assessing therapeutic effectiveness.

Patients who have incomplete colonoscopy

The diagnostic impact of conventional colonoscopy is linked with the ability to reach the ileocecal valve; however, incomplete conventional colonoscopy can be observed in 5% to 26% of colonoscopic examinations that are performed, even by experienced endoscopists [29,30]. There are several reasons for incomplete colonoscopy, including severe procedure-related abdominal discomfort and technical challenges that are due to elongated bowel segments or the presence of intraluminal stenosis. In patients who have known IBD or colorectal carcinoma, the failure rate of conventional colonoscopy may reach 50% [31]. Virtual colonography is associated with significantly higher completion rates; considerably less abdominal pain enhances patient compliance and only a high-grade stenosis prohibits the passage of water that is required for distending prestenotic segments. Furthermore, bowel elongation does not harm the visualization of colonic segments.

In a recent study, 37 subjects who had an incomplete endoscopy underwent MRC [32]. Contrast-enhanced T1-weighted 3D VIBE images were acquired, and the presence of colorectal pathologies was assessed on a segmental basis. Conventional colonoscopy failed to evaluate almost 50% of the potentially visible colonic segments, whereas 96% of the bowel segments were assessable by means of MR imaging. Beyond stenoses and poststenotic lesions, MR-based assessment of prestenotic segments revealed two carcinoma-suspected lesions, five polyps, and four colitis-affected segments.

Extraintestinal findings

In contrast to a conventional colonoscopic analysis, virtual colonoscopy is not limited to endoscopic viewing. Analysis of the acquired source data allows the simultaneous depiction of the colon and all surrounding abdominal structures. Especially in the case of patients who have a suspected colorectal tumor, imaging of the liver is a benefit. Because of the acquisition of pre- and postcontrast T1-weighted data and TrueFISP sequences, MRC is reliable for the identification and characterization of hepatic lesions, including metastases, hepatocellular carcinoma, and hemangiomas. Other relevant pathologies also can be detected, such as bone metastases, renal cell cancer, or aortic aneurysms. Similarly, MR imaging may provide useful additional information in patients who have IBD. Beyond the depiction of inflammatory processes in the bowel wall, extramural abscesses can be seen. Furthermore, pathologies, such as interintestinal fistulae or conglomerate tumor formations, can be detected easily by means of MR imaging, whereas most of these extraintestinal findings often are not suspected by endoscopy.

Further developments

Fecal tagging

MRC still requires bowel purgation, which negatively impacts patient acceptance. One can overcome bowel cleansing by modulating the signal characteristics of fecal material (fecal tagging). By adding contrast agents to regular meals, the signal intensity of stool can be adapted to the signal properties of the rectal enema.

For dark lumen MRC without bowel cleansing, a highly concentrated, barium sulfate–containing contrast agent has been proposed for fecal tagging [33,34]. Barium sulfate is administered in a volume of 200 mL with each of four principle meals beginning 36 hours before MRC. Barium sulfate has an excellent safety profile; it is not absorbed, it mixes well with stool, and allergic reactions after the ingestion are not known. The barium-based approach of fecal tagging was applied successfully in a volunteer study [33]. Ingestion of barium sulfate before the MR examination leads to a decreasing signal of stool on heavily T1-weighted 3D gradient echo images; this renders fecal material virtually indistinguishable from the administered water enema. Although the concept of fecal tagging with barium sulfate resulted in diagnostic image quality for dark lumen MRC, a recent study revealed that patient acceptance was not increased [35]; ingestion of the barium sulfate compound was considered almost as unpleasant as the bowel-cleansing protocols. A new approach is based on the administration of oral or rectal stool softener; their effect on the signal intensity of fecal material was assessed in another volunteer study [36]. Oral administration of lactulose before the MRC, in combination with a rectal enema that contained ducosate sodium, resulted in low signal intensity values of feces and high image quality (Fig. 11A). In addition, the ingestion of lactulose or the rectal enema that contained ducosate sodium did not impact patients' acceptance negatively. This combination of oral and rectal stool softener may evolve as a promising technique for dark lumen MRC without bowel cleansing; however, data analysis of simultaneous bright lumen MRC is limited (Fig. 11B).

Combined small and large bowel MR imaging

MRC is a reliable method for the assessment of inflammatory diseases of the large bowel; however, IBD often affects the small and large bowel at the same time. Therefore, new approaches have focused on displaying the small bowel and colon simultaneously. An initial study included 18 patients who had IBD [37]. In addition to the rectal administration of water, patients ingested 1.5 L of a hydro solution that contained mannitol before the MR examination. The latter resulted in

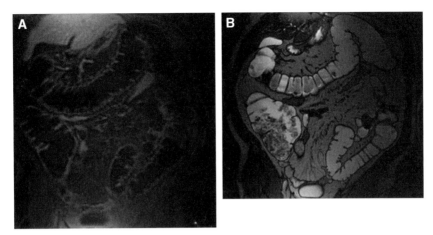

Fig. 11. Using a combination of oral and rectal stool softener, signal intensity of fecal material can be adapted to the low signal of the rectal enema on the T1-weighted sequences (*A*). Thus, stool becomes virtual invisible and a diagnostic image quality can be achieved; however, diagnostic accuracy of TrueFISP images is limited because stool impresses as dark-filling defects on the bright colonic lumen (*B*).

a good distension of small bowel loops, whereas the rectal administration of water allowed the visualization of the colon at the same time. Thus, inflammatory lesions in the colon and terminal ileum and affected bowel segments in the upper small bowel could be detected.

References

[1] Lieberman D. Colon cancer screening: beyond efficacy. Gastroenterology 1994;106:803–7.

[2] Frommer DJ. What's new in colorectal cancer screening? J Gastroenterol Hepatol 1998;13:528–33.

[3] Gatto NM, Frucht H, Sundararajan V, et al. Risk of perforation after colonoscopy and sigmoidoscopy: a population-based study. J Natl Cancer Inst 2003; 95:230–6.

[4] Rex DK, Rahmani EY, Haseman JH, et al. Relative sensitivity of colonoscopy and barium enema for detection of colorectal cancer in clinical practice. Gastroenterology 1997;112:17–23.

[5] Bowles CJ, Leicester R, Romaya C, et al. A prospective study of colonoscopy practice in the UK today: are we adequately prepared for national colorectal cancer screening tomorrow? Gut 2004;53:277–83.

[6] Pickhardt PJ, Choi JR, Hwang I, et al. Computed tomographic virtual colonoscopy to screen for colorectal neoplasia in asymptomatic adults. N Engl J Med 2003;349:2191–200.

[7] Furukawa A, Saotome T, Yamasaki M, et al. Cross-sectional imaging in Crohn disease. Radiographics 2004;24:689–702.

[8] Saar B, Rosch T, Rummeny EJ. Colorectal cancer screening: a challenge for magnetic resonance colonography. Top Magn Reson Imaging 2002;13: 427–34.

[9] Schreyer AG, Furst A, Agha A, et al. Magnetic resonance imaging based colonography for diagnosis and assessment of diverticulosis and diverticulitis. Int J Colorectal Dis 2004;19:474–80.

[10] Svensson MH, Svensson E, Lasson A, et al. Patient acceptance of CT colonography and conventional colonoscopy: prospective comparative study in patients with or suspected of having colorectal disease. Radiology 2002;222:337–45.

[11] Angtuaco TL, Banaad-Omiotek GD, Howden CW. Differing attitudes toward virtual and conventional colonoscopy for colorectal cancer screening: surveys among primary care physicians and potential patients. Am J Gastroenterol 2001;96: 887–93.

[12] Hara AK, Johnson CD, Reed JE, et al. Reducing data size and radiation dose for CT colonography. AJR 1997;168:1181–4.

[13] Sosna J, Morrin MM, Copel L, et al. Computed tomography colonography (virtual colonoscopy): update on technique, applications, and future developments. Surg Technol Int 2003;11:102–10.

[14] Stryker SJ, Wolff BG, Culp CE, et al. Natural history of untreated colonic polyps. Gastroenterology 1987;93:1009–13.

[15] Winawer SJ, Zauber AG, O'Brien MJ, et al. The National Polyp Study. Design, methods, and characteristics of patients with newly diagnosed polyps. The National Polyp Study Workgroup. Cancer 1992; 70:1236–45.

[16] Winkleman BJ, Matthews DE, Wiebke EA. Colorectal cancer screening at a Veterans Affairs hospital. Am J Surg 2003;186:468–71.

[17] Ajaj W, Pelster G, Treichel U, et al. Dark lumen magnetic resonance colonography: comparison with conventional colonoscopy for the detection of colorectal pathology. Gut 2003;52:1738–43.

[18] Villavicencio RT, Rex DK. Colonic adenomas: prevalence and incidence rates, growth rates, and miss rates at colonoscopy. Semin Gastrointest Dis 2000;11:185–93.

[19] Steidle G, Schafer J, Schlemmer HP, et al. Two-dimensional parallel acquisition technique in 3D MR colonography. Rofo 2004;176:1100–5.

[20] Lauenstein TC, Ajaj W, Kuehle CA, et al. Magnetic resonance colonography: comparison of contrast-enhanced three-dimensional vibe with two-dimensional FISP sequences: preliminary experience. Invest Radiol 2005;40(2):89–96.

[21] Ochsenkuhn T, Sackmann M, Goke B. Inflammatory bowel diseases (IBD): critical discussion of etiology, pathogenesis, diagnostics, and therapy. Radiologe 2003;1:1–8.

[22] Schneider W. Epidemiology of chronic inflammatory intestinal diseases. Z Gesamte Inn Med 1981; 3:228–30.

[23] Karlinger K, Gyorke T, Mako E, et al. The epidemiology and the pathogenesis of inflammatory bowel disease. Eur J Radiol 2000;3:154–67.

[24] Fiocca R, Ceppa P. The diagnostic reliability of endoscopic biopsies in diagnosis colitis. J Clin Pathol 2003;56:321–2.

[25] Nahon S, Bouhnik Y, Lavergne-Slove A, et al. Colonoscopy accurately predicts the anatomical severity of colonic Crohn's disease attacks: correlation with findings from colectomy specimens. Am J Gastroenterol 2002;12:3102–7.

[26] Kettritz U, Isaacs K, Warshauer DM, et al. Crohn's disease. Pilot study comparing MRI of the abdomen with clinical evaluation. J Clin Gastroenterol 1995;3: 249–53.

[27] Koh DM, Miao Y, Chinn RJ, et al. MR imaging evaluation of the activity of Crohn's disease. AJR Am J Roentgenol 2001;6:1325–32.

[28] Ajaj W, Lauenstein TC, Pelster G, et al. Magnetic resonance colonography for the detection of inflammatory diseases of the large bowel: quantifying the inflammatory activity. Gut 2005;54(2): 257–63.

[29] Cirocco WC, Rusin LC. Factors that predict incomplete colonoscopy. Dis Colon Rectum 1995;389: 964–8.

[30] Marshall JB, Barthel JS. The frequency of total colonoscopy and terminal ileal intubation in the 1990s. Gastrointest Endosc 1993;39:518–20.

[31] Rottgen R, Schroder RJ, Lorenz M, et al. CT-colonography with the 16-slice CT for the diagnostic evaluation of colorectal neoplasms and inflammatory colon diseases. Rofo 2003;175:1384–91.

[32] Ajaj W, Lauenstein TC, Pelster G, et al. MR colonography in patients with incomplete conventional colonoscopy. Radiology 2005;234(2):452–9.

[33] Lauenstein T, Holtmann G, Schoenfelder D, et al. MR colonography without colonic cleansing: a new strategy to improve patient acceptance. AJR Am J Roentgenol 2001;177:823–7.

[34] Lauenstein TC, Goehde SC, Ruehm SG, et al. MR colonography with barium-based fecal tagging: initial clinical experience. Radiology 2002; 223:248–54.

[35] Goehde SC, Descher E, Boekstegers A, et al. Dark lumen MR colonography based on fecal tagging for detection of colorectal masses: accuracy and patient acceptance. Abdom Imaging, in press.

[36] Ajaj W, Goehde SC, Ruehm SG, et al. MR colonography without bowel cleansing: impact of an oral and rectal softener. Presented at the 12th Scientific Meeting of the International Society for Magnetic Resonance in Medicine. Kyoto (Japan), May 15–21, 2004.

[37] Narin B, Ajaj W, Gohde S, et al. Combined small and large bowel MR imaging in patients with Crohn's disease: a feasibility study. Eur Radiol 2004;14:1535–42.

ELSEVIER
SAUNDERS

Magn Reson Imaging Clin N Am
13 (2005) 359–380

MAGNETIC
RESONANCE
IMAGING CLINICS
of North America

Three-Dimensional Contrast-Enhanced MR Angiography of the Thoraco-Abdominal Vessels

Kambiz Nael, MD[a],*, Gerhard Laub, PhD[b], J. Paul Finn, MD[a]

[a]Department of Radiological Sciences, David Geffen School of Medicine University of California Los Angeles,
10945 Le Conte Avenue, Suite #3371, Los Angeles, CA 90095-7206, USA
[b]Siemens Medical Solutions, 10945 Le Conte Avenue, Suite 3371, Los Angeles, CA 90095-7206, USA

Within a decade after its initial description by Prince et al [1], three-dimensional (3D) contrast-enhanced MR angiography (CEMRA) has become established as an accurate, noninvasive tool for the diagnostic assessment of almost all vascular territories. CEMRA has advantages over alternative modalities in that it uses non-nephrotoxic contrast agents and does not involve ionizing radiation.

Over the past decade, advances in scanner hardware and software have steadily improved the quality, speed, and reliability of CEMRA, and it is now widely practiced and accepted. This article reviews existing state-of-the-art 3D CEMRA techniques for the assessment of the thoraco-abdominal vasculature and summarizes current applications and clinical experience. It also highlights evolving techniques that are likely to enhance the future impact of CEMRA.

Contrast-enhanced MR angiography techniques

CEMRA relies on the T1 shortening effect of paramagnetic contrast agents on the blood during the image acquisition [1]. Paramagnetic contrast agents shorten the T1 relaxation time of blood and elevate the vessel to background contrast-to-noise ratio. CEMRA uses a T1-weighted, fast, spoiled 3D gradient-echo (GRE) pulse sequence. Spoiling is used to remove the residual magnetization after each echo and isolates the T1

weighting from potential contamination by unwanted coherent echoes. To perform CEMRA, the sequence parameters and the contrast administration should be fine-tuned to balance the available signal-to-noise ratio (SNR) with the required spatial and temporal resolution.

Recent technical advances have played an important role in the evolution of CEMRA. High-performance gradients are available with slew rates of up to 200 mT/m/s and gradient amplitudes up to 45 mT/m. With fast gradients, 3D GRE sequences with repetition time (TR) <3 milliseconds and echo time (TE) ~1 millisecond can generate high-resolution images in a comfortable breath-hold. Pulse sequence attributes, such as asymmetrical echoes and varying k-space trajectories, have increased the flexibility and performance of CEMRA. Asymmetric k-space sampling in-plane and through-plane can further reduce the acquisition time required for each 3D data set. An important recent advance in MRI, with specific applications to CEMRA, was the introduction of parallel imaging.

Well-timed and controlled contrast administration is a prerequisite for successful CEMRA. For optimal results, the low spatial frequency k-space data, which are principally responsible for image contrast, should be aligned with peak vascular enhancement [2,3]. Premature acquisition results in lower SNR and may result in visualization of only the vessel edges [4], whereas late acquisition results in diminished vascular contrast and possible venous overlay. Accurate timing can be achieved by using a test bolus or automated bolus detection. The bolus timing method chosen often depends on the specific scanner type, the

---

* Corresponding author.
E-mail address: nkambiz@mednet.ucla.edu
(K. Nael).

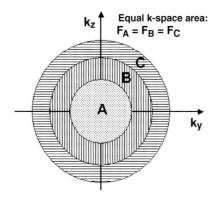

Fig. 1. The k-space area in the k_y-k_z plane is divided into three segments, labeled A, B, and C. For simplicity, the readout direction is omitted in this diagram. Each segment contains the same number of readout lines.

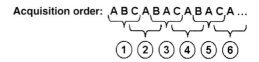

Fig. 2. The acquisition order in the TREAT sequence shows a shorter temporal distance between scanning of the center segment. The outer segments, B and C, are used in two subsequent 3D data sets.

software and equipment available, and the preferences of the operator. k-Space acquisition is another important factor for time adjustment. Traditionally, k-space is acquired linearly (also termed sequentially), with the central k-space data being obtained about a third of the way through the imaging period. With real-time triggering algorithms, the low spatial frequency k-space data (center of k-space) are acquired at the beginning of the imaging period [5]. Contrast doses between 0.1 and 0.2 mmol/kg body weight Gd-based contrast agent have been reported to be sufficient for most single-station MR angiography examinations [6,7].

With CEMRA, the vascular signal is relatively immune to flow-related artifacts, such as signal loss from spin saturation or slow flow, that can degrade flow-based MRA techniques [8–10]. This is a clear advantage over time-of-flight and phase-contrast MRA, which exploit the inherent motion of blood flow to generate vascular signal [10,11]. 3D MRA can quickly provide high spatial resolution 3D angiographic data sets that can be projected in views similar to those of conventional x-ray angiograms. In addition, 3D MRA is tomographic and benefits from various 3D visualization techniques, such as maximum intensity

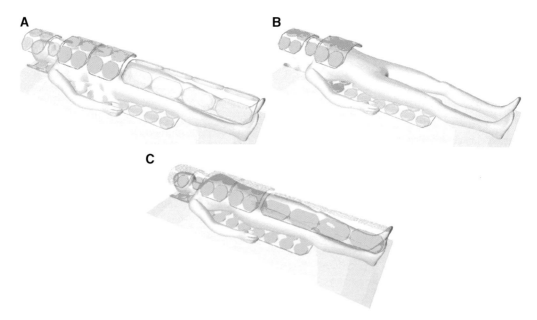

Fig. 3. The concept of TIM (total imaging matrix). Up to 76 coil elements can simultaneously be connected to the system. At any time, the signal from up to 32 coil elements can be fed into 32 independent parallel receive channels. (*A*) Coil system for imaging of thorax and abdomen. (*B*) Coil system for imaging of thorax, neck, and head. (*C*) Whole body imaging.

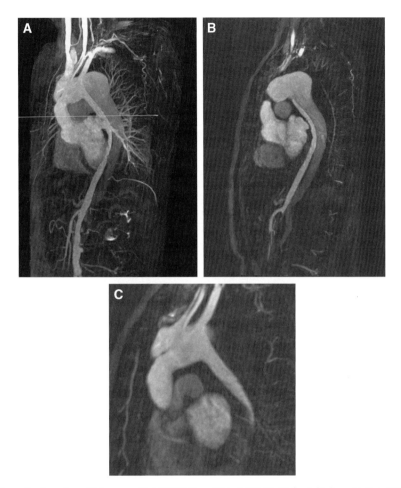

Fig. 4. Type A aortic dissection. Oblique sagittal MIP (*A*) and thin MIP (*B, C*) from high-resolution CEMRA showing true and false lumens that are separated by the intimal flap. (*B*) Extensive thrombus in the false lumen (*arrow*). (*C*) Dissection flap in the transverse aortic arch and extending in to the innominate artery (*arrows*).

projection (MIP) and volume-rendered (VR) display for improved segmentation and visualization of individual vascular segments.

Time-resolved contrast-enhanced MR angiography

Real-time visualization of the first pass of a contrast bolus has in the past been a unique feature of conventional x-ray angiography. Ultra-fast MR techniques can generate temporally resolved 3D MRA, which depicts the transit of the paramagnetic contrast agent through the vascular system [12,13].

In a first step, ultra-short TR sequences, in combination with sparse k-space sampling, generated complete 3D data sets in under 5 seconds. As

an example, with a TR of 1.8 milliseconds, 120 lines, and 16 partitions, the scan time is 3.5 seconds [14,15]. This is fast enough to clearly differentiate the arterial phase from the venous phase. Much faster scan times can be achieved with fewer partitions to produce quasi-projectional 3D MR angiograms [12]. The advantages to this approach are that high temporal frequency can be achieved and that each 3D data set is fully independent of its neighbors. The disadvantage of this approach is that if the MIP images are rotated off-axis, blurring may occur because the through-plane resolution is limited. Therefore, these data are best viewed on-axis where full spatial resolution is maintained.

Higher frame rates can be achieved only by reducing the size of k-space, which is regularly updated. The keyhole technique measures full

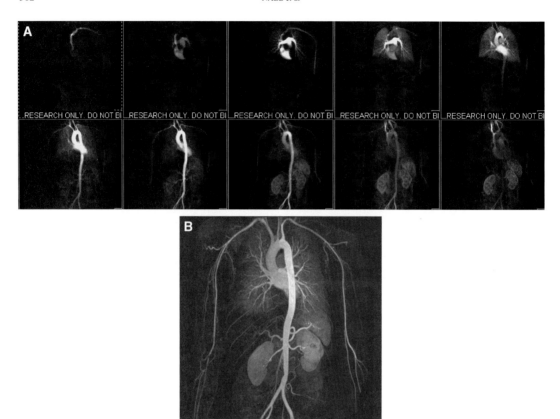

RESEARCH ONLY. DO NOT BI RESEARCH ONLY. DO NOT BI RESEARCH ONLY. DO NOT BI RESEARCH ONLY. DO NOT BI RESEARCH ONLY. DO NOT BI

Fig. 5. Coronal MIPs from time-resolved MRA (*A*) and coronal MIP from high-resolution CEMRA (*B*) showing the application of multi-coil in extended FOV imaging.

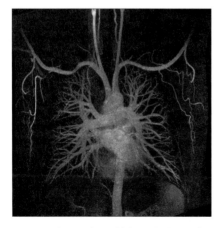

Fig. 6. Coronal MIP from high-resolution pulmonary CEMRA at 3T, acquired during a 20-second breath hold. Up to 5th order pulmonary arterial branches are visible.

k-space only once before the contrast injection, followed by a rapid, continuous update of only a small centerpiece of k-space [12]. Retrospectively, every center of k-space is filled with the peripheral k-space data that were measured before the contrast injection to create a series of data sets with good spatial resolution. The disadvantage of keyhole imaging is that small-detail resolution cannot be displayed because the corresponding k-space data are not updated during the contrast injection.

Korosec et al [13] described a k-space acquisition scheme whereby the low spatial frequency data were sampled more often than the high spatial frequency data. The high spatial frequency data were interpolated on a temporal basis to the time of corresponding central k-space data. The advantage of this approach is that the major contribution to image contrast lies in the data that are updated frequently, and interpolating the high spatial frequency data yields full 3D k-space

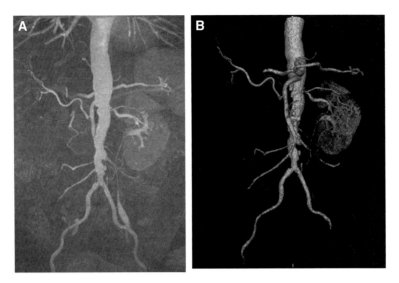

Fig. 7. Atherosclerosis. Coronal MIP (*A*) and 3D VR (*B*) from CEMRA at 3T shows atherosclerosis and tortuosity of abdominal aorta and irregularity at the common iliac bifurcation. The patient lost the right kidney as a consequence of severe atherosclerotic renal artery stenosis. A replaced hepatic artery from the superior mesenteric artery is noted as a normal variant.

data sets (ie, high spatial resolution). The disadvantage is that for rapidly changing processes, some edge artifact and blurring may occur due to the lower temporal resolution of the outer k-space segments.

In a similar approach, the time-resolved, echo-shared angiographic technique (TREAT) uses echo-sharing in which some k-space data are used for two subsequent frames (echo sharing). In 3D k-space, k_y and k_z are referred to as in-plane phase-encode direction and through-plane phase-encode direction, respectively. k-Space is divided into three segments in the k_y-k_z plane: A, B, and C (Fig. 1). In a standard acquisition, A, B, and C are acquired in a linear fashion, and this process is repeated until all frames are available. In the TREAT acquisition, the central segment, A, is acquired more frequently than the outer portions of k-space data, B and C. The reconstruction of 3D data is implemented as shown in

Table 1
Sequence parameters for thoraco-abdominal contrast-enhanced MR angiography at 1.5Tesla

Parameters	Conventional CEMRA	Time-resolved CEMRA
TR (ms)	2.78	1.97
TE (ms)	1.11	0.78
Flip angle	30	20
Bandwidth (Hz/pixel)	610	1090
Field of view (2 mm)	500 × 450	500 × 450
Matrix size	512 × 410	384 × 290
Voxel size (3 mm)	1.2 × 1 × 1.6	1.7 × 1.3 × 8
Parallel acquisition	GRAPPA × 2, R-L	GRAPPA × 2, R-L
Partial Fourier	7/8 along all logical axes	7/8 along all logical axes
Acquisition time (s)	20–24	1.6 per 3D slab; total: 20–24
Partition thickness (mm)	1.6	8
Contrast	30 mL at 2 mL/s	6 mL at 4 mL/s
Sequence	GRE	GRE-shared echo

Abbreviation: GRAPPA, generalized autocalibrating partially parallel acquisitions.

Table 2
Sequence parameters for thoraco-abdominal contrast-enhanced MR angiography at 3Tesla

Parameters	Conventional CEMRA	Time-resolved CEMRA
TR (ms)	2.84	1.99
TE (ms)	1.1	0.87
Flip angle	23	20
Bandwidth (Hz/pixel)	790	1300
Field of view (2 mm)	390 × 360	380 × 300
Matrix size	576 × 400	320 × 240
Voxel size (3 mm)	1 × 0.7 × 1.1	1.7 × 1.2 × 5
Parallel acquisition	GRAPPA × 3, R-L	GRAPPA × 3, R-L
Partial Fourier	7/8 along all logical axes	7/8 along all logical axes
Acquisition time (s)	20–24	1.1 per 3D slab; total: 20–24
Partition thickness (mm)	1.1	5
Contrast	25 mL at 1.5 mL/s	6 mL at 4 mL/s
Sequence	GRE	GRE-shared echo

Fig. 2. This reduces the time between each 3D volume-set and increases the frame rate of a multi-measurement acquisition. The time between 3D volumes is two thirds of what it would be in a standard acquisition without the echo-sharing.

A general limitation of all time-resolved MR angiography techniques is that the spatial resolution of the individual 3D data sets is limited when compared with single-phase MR angiography acquisitions. This limitation can be addressed with parallel imaging, using arrays of surface coils and receiver channels to reduce the number of phase-encode steps to be measured [16–19]. Parallel imaging is one of the most exciting recent advances in MR imaging. Implementations, such as simultaneous acquisition of spatial harmonics and sensitivity encoding, provide the framework for improved spatial and temporal resolution [20–23]. With parallel imaging, the individual signals from component coil elements in a radiofrequency coil array are used to substitute for some phase-encoding gradient steps, which can then be omitted. This allows a reduction of the acquisition time or an increase in the spatial resolution by the so-called "acceleration factor." The theoretical maximum attainable acceleration factor is equal to the number of coil elements along the phase-encoding direction. At the current state of development, SNR penalties limit the maximum acceleration factor to about four for most applications.

The SNR penalty of parallel imaging depends on the degree of k-space undersampling and the coil array geometry [22,24]. Fink et al [25] have reported time-resolved parallel 3D pulmonary MR angiography with parallel acquisition with promising results. As the acceleration factor increases, the noise amplification tends to be aggravated. The higher SNR available at 3.0T is potentially an advantage where higher acceleration factors are being considered.

Time-resolved MR angiography may provide supplemental functional information in several situations. Filling patterns in dissections,

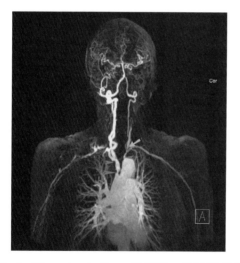

Fig. 8. Atherosclerosis. Coronal MIP from 3D CEMRA shows severe atherosclerosis of the supra-aortic vessels. Occlusion of right internal carotid, distal left common carotid (*arrow*), left internal carotid, left external carotid, proximal left subclavian (*arrowhead*), and a high-grade stenosis of brachiocephalic trunk (*arrowhead*), right subclavian, right proximal common carotid (*arrowhead*) is seen. A hypertrophic right vertebral artery is visible, which alone supplies the entire intracranial circulation and left arm. By using a 500 mm FOV, the head, neck, and chest vasculature is visualized in a single-station acquisition.

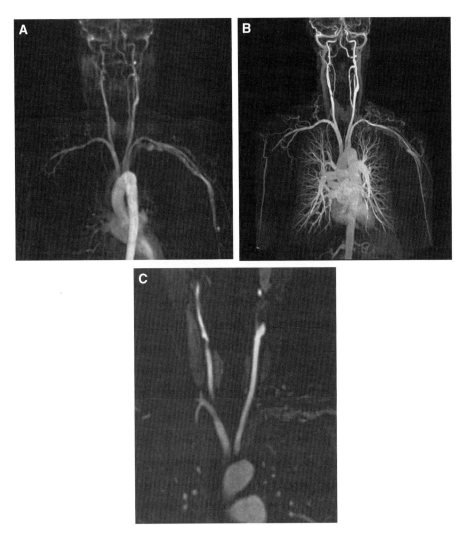

Fig. 9. Takayasu's arteritis. Coronal MIP from time-resolved MRA (*A*) and oblique sagittal MIP (*B*) and coronal thin MIP (*C*) image from CEMRA showing extensive irregularity of right subclavian artery (clinical history of Takayasu's arteritis) and a short focal area of critical stenosis in its distal course. There is a plaque presented at the right common carotid bifurcation with approximately 50% stenosis (*C*).

arteriovenous fistulae, or shunts are best appreciated with highly temporally resolved imaging. Other strengths of time-resolved MR angiography include relative insensitivity to motion and the requirement for only small doses of contrast [26].

Advances in multi-coil technology

Recent developments in MR scanner design and coil technology are relevant for CEMRA of the thorax and abdomen. Combining large arrays of surface coils with multiple independent

detectors [27,28] allows collection of signals from several object regions in parallel and extends the area from which high-sensitivity measurements can be obtained. As a result, improvements in SNR, field of view (FOV), or a combination of both are possible (Fig. 3) [19,27–29]. For best results, parallel imaging should include the use of multi-element arrays with a high sensitivity profile.

Commercial surface coil arrays can be interfaced with up to 32 independent wide-band receiver channels [30,31]. Extended FOV imaging may be useful where pathology extends beyond

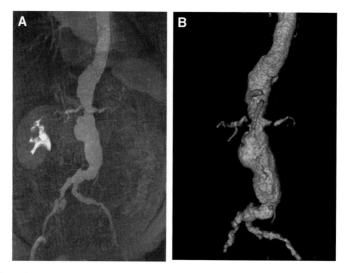

Fig. 10. Abdominal aortic aneurysm. Coronal MIP (*A*) and 3D VR (*B*) image from CEMRA at 3T showing an abdominal aortic aneurysm and severe atherosclerotic tortuosity of the abdominal aorta and bilateral renal artery segmental occlusion.

the coverage of a single-body array coil; for example, thoraco-abdominal aneurysms or aortic dissections may extend above and below the diaphragm (Fig. 4). By combining large FOV protocols with high spatial resolution matrices, extended coverage can be achieved with small voxels throughout the entire FOV (Fig. 5).

Higher magnetic field strength (3Tesla)

The main advantage of MR imaging at 3.0T is that the SNR is approximately doubled relative to 1.5T [32,33]. The theoretical SNR advantages at 3.0T are especially noticeable for MR angiography applications. The higher SNR gain at 3.0T can be used to reduce acquisition time, to improve spatial resolution, or both [32,34,35]. Also, because the longitudinal relaxation time (T1) of unenhanced blood increases with field strength [36], sensitivity to injected gadolinium agents for CEMRA is heightened. There are substantial technical challenges to large FOV imaging at 3.0T, particularly involving good RF field homogeneity. Also, the SAR at 3.0T is increased by a factor of four relative to 1.5T.

At our institution, we perform CEMRA at 3.0T over a wide spectrum of vascular territories, including carotids, chest, and abdomen, and the results have been uniformly positive (Figs. 6 and 7). It seems likely that the introduction of arrays of

more sensitive imaging coils and receiver channels at 3.0T will permit further improvement in imaging quality and performance, as it has at 1.5T [16–18].

Practical three-dimensional contrast-enhanced MR angiography

For thoraco-abdominal 3D CEMRA, we usually prescribe the imaging volume as a coronal or coronal-oblique acquisition aligned with the aorta. The imaging parameters are adjusted to provide the optimum balance between spatial resolution and anatomic coverage within a comfortable breath-hold. Tables 1 and 2 summarize typical sequence parameters used at our institution in clinical protocols for thoraco-abdominal CEMRA.

The acquisition of a precontrast data set is helpful to ensure proper anatomic coverage by the imaging volume and can be used for subtraction. Precontrast imaging also provides an opportunity for the patient and the operator to review breath-hold instructions. At least two postcontrast acquisitions should be performed because additional information can often be obtained with later acquisitions. Slowly filling structures, such as capacious aortic aneurysms or false channels, may not be optimally visualized with early-phase images.

For contrast administration, we use a bolus timing technique [2,37]. For most clinical applications, Gd-enhanced 3D MRA can be successfully

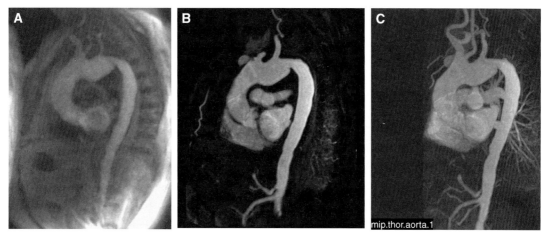

Fig. 11. Thoracic aortic aneurysm. (*A*) Sagittal MIP image from time-resolved MRA (800 millisecond acquisition). (*B*) Sagittal thin MIP image. (*C*) Sagittal oblique MIP images from high-resolution CEMRA showing an aneurysm of the ascending thoracic aorta involving the inferior wall of the transverse aortic arch.

performed using 20 to 30 mL of a Gd-based extracellular contrast agent, administered using a 20 or 22 G needle via an antecubital vein at 1 to 2 mL/s. A right-sided injection may reduce the tendency for signal loss at the origins of the great vessels, which sometimes occurs due to the high concentration of Gd within the left brachiocephalic vein [38]. It is also important that all contrast injections be followed by a 20 to 30 mL saline flush to prevent pooling within the tubing or peripheral veins. We generally supplement our thoraco-abdominal MRA protocols with a T1-weighted gradient echo fat sat sequence (T1 GRE-FS) after the contrast administration. This is often helpful for providing anatomic detail about the vessel wall and venous system.

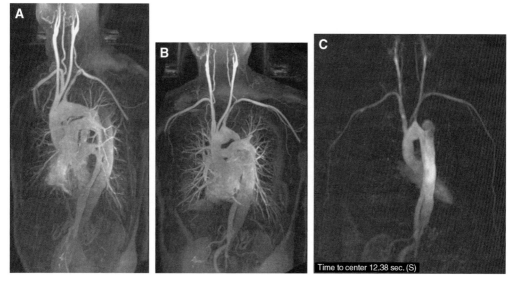

Fig. 12. Type B aortic dissection. Oblique sagittal MIP from high resolution CEMRA (*A, B*), showing true and false lumen of an aortic dissection, which are separated by the intimal flap. (*B*) Left renal artery arises from the false lumen (*arrow*). (*C*) Coronal MIP from time-resolved MRA shows delayed left renal parenchymal enhancement.

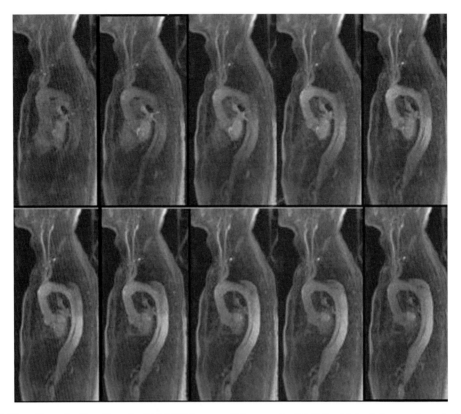

Fig. 13. Type B aortic dissection. Sagittal MIP images of time-resolved MRA obtained 1 second apart show the sequential filling of the true and false lumen of aortic dissection; retrograde filling of the false lumen is evident.

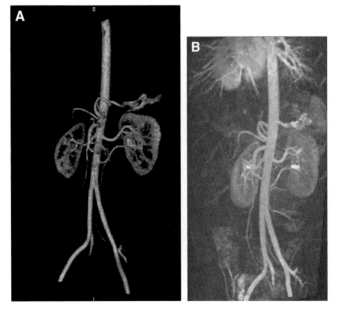

Fig. 14. Anomalous visceral arterial anatomy. Coronal oblique 3D VR (A) and coronal oblique MIP (B) from high-resolution CEMRA showing separate origins of the left gastric, splenic, and hepatic arteries directly from the aorta.

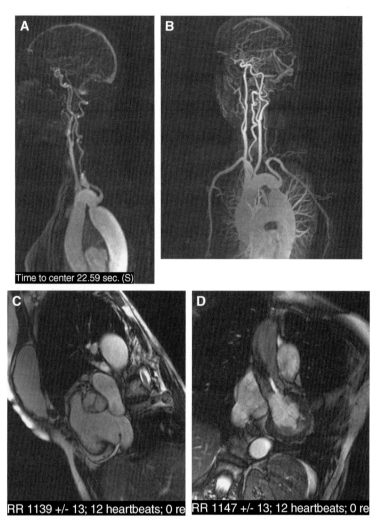

Fig. 15. Aortic coarctation. Sagittal MIP from time-resolved MRA (*A*) and oblique sagittal MIP from CEMRA (*B*) showing coarctation of the thoracic aorta. The presence of left PAPVR is noticeable (*arrow*). Cardiac cine (*C* and *D*) shows associated bicuspid aortic valve with moderate to severe stenosis.

Time-resolve MRA can be used as a complimentary study or in many instances can provide all the relevant diagnostic information required. At our institution, for time-resolved MRA, we use an ultrafast spoiled 3D GRE sequence with asymmetric k-space sampling and echo-sharing in all three axes to further shorten the acquisition time [12]. Other sequence parameters are shown in detail in Tables 1 and 2.

Clinical applications

Although MR imaging can be safely performed in certain emergency settings, it is more commonly used for nonacute clinical applications. Requiring only a peripheral intravenous catheter and administration of contrast agents characterized by an excellent safety profile [39,40], 3D CEMRA techniques have lowered the threshold for vascular imaging of the thorax and abdomen. The following discussion illustrates applications of CEMRA in several clinical scenarios.

Arterial occlusive disease

Atherosclerosis is a systemic process and is the most common cause of arterial occlusive disease. It commonly affects the aorta and its major branches, including the great supra aortic vessels,

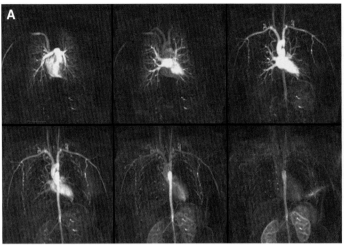
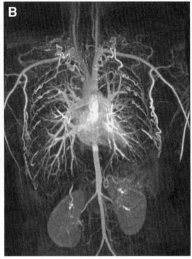

Fig. 16. Aortic coarctation. Coronal MIP from time-resolved MRA (*A*) and coronal MIP from high-resolution CEMRA (*B*) showing the significant stenosis of aorta distal to the left subclavian artery consistent with postductal aortic coarctation. Multiple dilated intercostal, internal mammary, and bronchial artery collaterals supply the descending aorta distal to the coarctation.

renal, mesenteric, iliac arteries, and their lower-extremity branches (Figs. 7 and 8). Manifestations of atherosclerosis include ulcers, vessel tortuosity, aneurysmal dilatation, stenosis, and occlusion. Atherosclerosis and its sequelae are leading causes of morbidity and mortality in the western world. The ability of MRA to provide reliable, non-invasive assessment of the arterial tree, even in patients with renal insufficiency, is a compelling argument for of its use in this population. Other causes of arterial occlusive disease include fibro-muscular dysplasia, which commonly affects the renal and mesenteric branches; vasculitic process-es such as Takayasu disease, which commonly affect the proximal portion of supra aortic vascu-lature (Fig. 9); inflammatory or neoplastic disor-ders; and postradiation arteritis. 3D CEMRA has been used effectively in these clinical settings.

Aorta

Although CT is more practical and available in acute, life-threatening conditions affecting the aorta, 3D CEMRA may have advantages in the more stable patient, even with advances in multi-detector CT.

Aortic aneurysm

Aortic aneurysm is a common clinical entity and may be classified according to its location, etiology, or shape. The predisposing factors typically include atherosclerosis, where aneurysms most commonly affect the descending aorta (Fig. 10); trauma; connective tissue disorders (eg, Erhlers-Danlos syndrome and Marfan syndrome); and rare infections (eg, syphilis) [41]. Close follow-up and consideration of elective surgery require accurate risk stratification. 3D CEMRA of an aortic aneurysm can demonstrate the site of aneurysm, its size and morphology, and relation-ship of the aneurysm to branch vessels and the presence of associated features such as thrombus or ulceration (Fig. 11). These findings can affect surgical decision making, and MR imaging is frequently used as a follow-up tool for monitoring the progression of disease.

3D CEMRA may be supplemented by the acquisition of a T1-weighted fat suppressed GRE sequence. This may be helpful for evalua-tion of the vessel wall and surrounding soft tissue. Where aneurysms involve the ascending aorta or sinuses of Valsalva, concomitant aortic valve disease can be readily evaluated using cardiac cine imaging.

Aortic dissection

Aortic dissection results from a spontaneous longitudinal separation of the aortic intima and adventitia and occurs due to the passage of blood to the tunica media of the aortic wall, causing it to split in two [42,43]. This results in the creation of

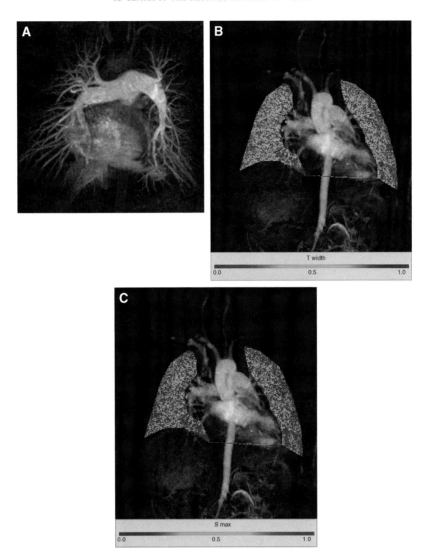

Fig. 17. Pulmonary hypertension. Coronal MIP image (*A*) from CEMRA at 3T shows significant dilatation of central pulmonary arteries and abnormal proximal-to-distal tapering. Color mapping of perfusion data from time-resolved MRA shows prolonged mean transit time (*B*) and decreased maximum signal intensity (*C*) in the lung periphery in this patient.

a true and false lumen separated by an intimal flap, which is the typical imaging finding of aortic dissection. Systemic hypertension is the underlying cause in the majority of aortic dissections. Other predisposing factors are aortic coarctation, iatrogenic injury, cystic media necrosis, Marfan syndrome, Ehler-Danlos syndrome, Turner syndrome, and Behcet disease.

Aortic dissections are classified as Stanford Type A (involving the ascending thoracic aorta ± aortic arch) (see Fig. 4) or Stanford Type B (in which dissection flap begins beyond the origin of

the left subclavian artery) (Fig. 12). Type A dissections are surgical emergencies due to the risk of myocardial infarction from involvement of the coronary arteries and of pericardial tamponade secondary to aortic rupture into the pericardium. Type B dissections are usually managed medically.

MR imaging has high sensitivity and specificity for detection of dissection [44,45]. The diagnosis can be made on the localizer images in many instances, and Single-shot TrueFISP has recently been shown to be highly accurate for the diagnosis and classification of aortic dissection [46]. 3D

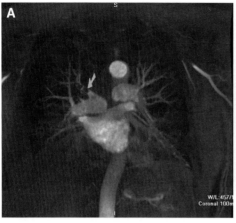
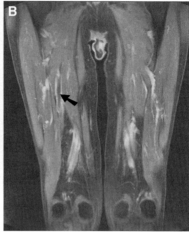

Fig. 18. Pulmonary embolism. Coronal MPR from high-resolution CEMRA (*A*) showing extensive thromboemboli in the right superior pulmonary artery (*arrow*). (*B*) Coronal T1-fatsat image of the thighs shows the presence of extensive thrombosis in the right femoral vein (*arrow*).

CEMRA of dissection can provide dynamic functional and cross-sectional information and can show the extent of dissection, involvement of branch vessels, and the location of re-entry sites.

A separate CE-MRA study of the abdomen may be required to assess distal dissections extending into the abdominal aorta, renal, and mesenteric arteries. Large FOV imaging can display the entire aorta in a single acquisition in most instances (Figs. 4 and 12). With T1 GRE-FS imaging, intramural hematomas or thrombosed false lumens may be highlighted. Dark blood techniques may help to differentiate intramural hematoma from a thrombosed false lumen in aortic dissection [11,47].

Time-resolved MRA is especially useful in dissection. Sequential filling of the true and false lumen, the entry and exit points of the dissection, pseudo aneurysms, or intramural hematomas may have characteristic appearances (Fig. 13). Another advantage of MR in aortic dissection is the ability to perform cine and velocity-encoded phase imaging. Flow velocity and direction, cardiac function, aortic valve involvement, and the severity of regurgitation can be obtained and used for close clinical follow-up of these patients [48,49].

Congenital abnormalities

Double aortic arch, right-sided aortic arch, coarctation, and anomalies affecting the position or the number of branches of the aorta can be readily shown with CEMRA. Aberrant subclavian artery origins, bovine arch, and visceral artery anatomic anomalies can be easily demonstrated, and 3D postprocessing can be used effectively when 3D vascular anatomy is complex (Figs. 7 and 14) [50,51].

Coarctation of the aorta is the most common aortic congenital abnormality, typically caused by a stenosis at the junction of the aortic arch and descending aorta. It is classified as postductal, which is a discrete focal narrowing of the aortic isthmus distal to the origin of the left subclavian artery (usually incidental finding in adults), or preductal, which is a hypoplasia of a longer segment of aortic arch after the origin of the innominate artery (usually symptomatic in infants).

In the evaluation of aortic coarctation, 3D CEMRA allows depiction of the involved segment, determination of the length and diameter of the aorta, and depiction of collateral supplies (Figs. 15 and 16). Considering the low risk profile of MR imaging, it has a strong role in long-term follow-up and pre- and postoperation evaluation of these patients. Cine imaging of the heart should accompany an assessment for aortic coarctation because these patients may have associated congenital heart disease, such as bicuspid aortic valve (Fig. 15). In the evaluation of aortic coarctation, time-resolved MRA may show sequential filling of chest wall collaterals (Fig. 16). Velocity-encoded cine can be used for quantitative measurements of velocity and flow proximal and distal to the stenosis and helps assess the severity of stenosis [52]. It is helpful for long-term monitoring of disease progression and for follow-up of patients with previous repair

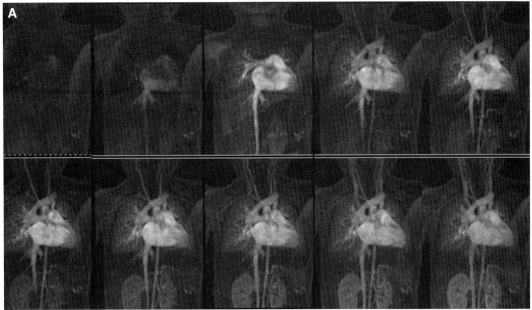

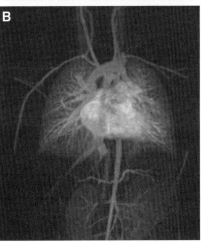

Fig. 19. PAPVR in a 2-year-old child. Coronal MIP images from time-resolved MRA (*A*) and coronal MIP image from CEMRA (*B*) showing PAPVR with a prominent left vertical vein draining in to the left brachiocephalic vein.

because residual coarctation can present later in life even after a repair [53]. Pseudocoarctation is an important differential diagnosis; it resembles a co-arctation but is caused by aortic kinking just distal to the origin of the left subclavian artery. It is not hemodynamically flow limiting and therefore is not associated with collaterals.

Pulmonary vasculature

In the lungs, x-ray computed tomography (CT) is widely regarded as the technique of choice for the workup of acute and chronic pulmonary vascular disease. The success of CT in the thorax is due in part to the high spatial resolution and advances in multi-slice technology, which have dramatically increased the speed and simplicity of CT. There remains a subset of patients who are not candidates for CT and in whom CEMRA in the lungs may be pivotal. MR imaging of pulmonary vasculature has been challenging for a variety of reasons, most importantly due to respiratory motion and suscep-tibility artifact at air–tissue interfaces.

The advent of faster imaging protocols has overcome most of these limitations, and high-resolution pulmonary MRA can now resolve up

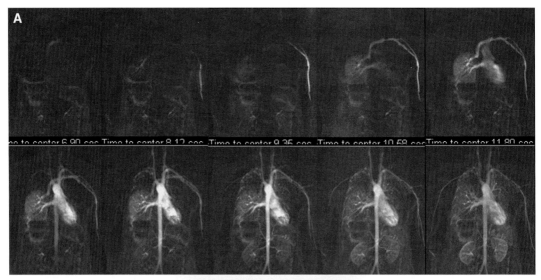

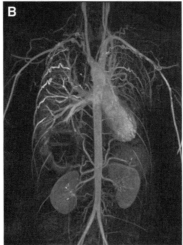

Fig. 20. Pulmonary atresia with Glenn shunt. (*A*) Coronal MIP images from time-resolved MRA show the absence of main and left pulmonary arteries and a patent Glenn shunt to the right pulmonary artery. Occlusion of right vertebral and subclavian artery is noted from a previous Mustard procedure. Early venous enhancement of the right lower lobe indicates arteriovenous shunting. A metallic artifact is seen in the right upper and lower lobe secondary to embolization coils. Delayed perfusion of the left lung is via an IVC-right pulmonary artery Glenn shunt. (*B*) Coronal MIP image from CEMRA shows large tortuous right intercostal collaterals reconstituting flow to the right axillary artery and tortuous left intercostal and bronchial arteries.

to 5th order pulmonary branches in a comfortable breath hold. In the clinical setting, the need for fast image acquisition during a short breath hold has opened up new applications for dynamic pulmonary time-resolved MRA [12,15,54]. Time-resolved MRA can combine dynamic and morphologic information and provide insight into cardiopulmonary hemodynamics and lung perfusion. 3.0T imaging provides SNR at a higher

baseline level and is more tolerant of parallel acquisition schemes and short readout times. At our institution, preliminary results with pulmonary CEMRA and time-resolved MRA at 3T have been positive (see Fig. 6).

Analysis of perfusion data provides several parameters of physiologic relevance, including the time to peak, mean transit time, and maximum signal intensity. These can be presented as

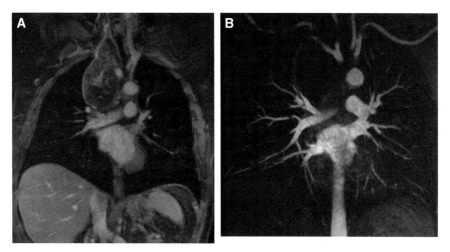

Fig. 21. Intrathoracic thyroid mass. Coronal Flash 2D T1 Fatsat postcontrast (*A*) and Coronal thin MIP from CEMRA (*B*) at 3T reveals an encapsulated, well-defined heterogeneous mass in right paratracheal region that enhances centrally and inhomogeneously. Adjacent vascular structures are mildly displaced but are not invaded.

color-coded maps that permit visual assessment of regional perfusion (Fig. 17).

Pulmonary embolism

CTA is rapidly gaining acceptance as the imaging test of choice in acute pulmonary embolism (PE). There are several studies that have described the use of pulmonary MRA for PE, documenting high sensitivity and specificity in large lobar and segmental vessels [55–58]. The sensitivity decreased for emboli in the subsegmental vessels [58,59]. Dynamic MRA provides functional and perfusion information that offers supplemental information to pulmonary MRA, and pulmonary perfusion quantification has been shown to be feasible and sensitive in the detection of perfusion defects [60,61]. Another positive attribute of MRA in suspected thromboembolic disease is that it can be complemented by MR venography of the pelvic and femoral veins (Fig. 18).

MRA may have a role in the follow-up of patients treated for acute PE and for the diagnosis of chronic PE. The signs of chronic PE on MRA include vascular webs, wall thickening, distal arterial tapering, and multiple distal perfusion defects [62].

Pulmonary arterial hypertension

Pulmonary arterial hypertension is diagnosed when pulmonary arterial pressure is > 30 mm Hg by cardiac catheterization and can be primary or secondary to congenital heart disease, chronic lung disease, or chronic thromboembolism. A

decreased number of segmental or subsegmental pulmonary arteries and abnormal tapering of segmental vessels (pruning) are the most common characteristic findings (see Fig. 17) [62–64]. Time-resolved MRA may demonstrate right to left shunts, and cine MR imaging with velocity encoding can provide information regarding cardiac function and chamber size and can provide quantitative measurements of blood velocity and flow in the pulmonary artery [65,66].

Anomalous pulmonary venous return

Typically, there are two superior (right and left) and two inferior (right and left) pulmonary veins. Altered development of the pulmonary venous system typically results from persistent communication with the systemic system, causing anomalous pulmonary venous drainage. These abnormalities can be complete or partial and are often associated with intracardiac congenital heart diseases, such as atrial septal defect. Several studies have shown the feasibility and accuracy of 3D CEMRA in the depiction of anomalous veins and the location of drainage (Fig. 19) [67–69].

Pulmonary arteriovenous malformations

Pulmonary arteriovenous malformations (AVMs) are seen mainly in the periphery and bases of the lungs and can be acquired (iatrogenic) or congenitally associated with diseases such as hereditary hemorrhagic telangiectasia (Osler-Weber disease). 3D CEMRA can accurately demonstrate pulmonary AVM, in most instances

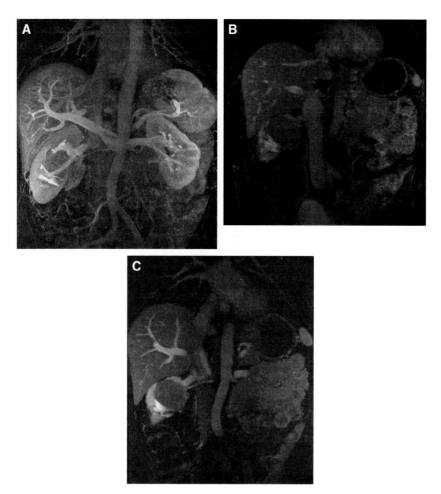

Fig. 22. Renal mass. (*A*) Coronal MIP from the venous-phase 3D CEMRA. (*B* and *C*) T1-FS post-contrast at 3T showing a cystic right renal mass and its association to the right renal vein and IVC. Also shown in (*B*) is a hemangioma in the caudate lobe.

as contrast pooling in the dilated vessel segment of the shunt. Time-resolved MRA can demonstrate sequential filling of the AVM. The value of pulmonary MRA for the pre- and post-treatment management of patients with AVMs has been demonstrated in several studies (Fig. 20) [70–72].

Tumors

Infiltration of vessels in cases of mediastinal, lung, or renal tumors can be assessed with CEMRA [73]. Acquisition of venous phases should be performed because a major complication of these tumors is the obstruction of the veins due to compressive effect or direct invasion. The combination of CEMRA and a T1-weighted (T1 GRE-

FS) pre- and postcontrast imaging of the tumor in coronal and axial planes is useful in visualizing tumor extension and involvement of the vasculature, for evaluating surrounding soft tissue, and for presurgical planning (Figs. 21 and 22).

Venography

Central thoracic vein

Thrombosis of systemic chest veins is an important cause of morbidity in patients with malignancy, hematologic disease, or long-term indwelling catheters. Several reports have proposed the use of contrast-enhanced 3D MR venography (CEMRV) techniques for the evaluation of thrombo-occlusive disease of the chest

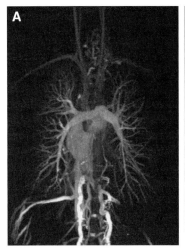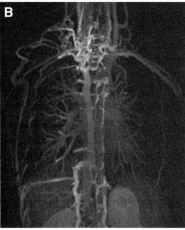

Fig. 23. Venous obstruction in a subject with lupus anticoagulant syndrome. Coronal MIP images from the arterial (*A*) are venous phase (*B*) of high-resolution CEMRA: The right subclavian vein is occluded proximally, the SVC is occluded, and the azygous vein is significantly dilated. Multiple large tortuous collaterals are seen in the neck and anterior mediastinum. The hemiazygous, paravertebral, intercostal, and abdominal wall are extensively dilated, and large esophageal and gastric varices are seen.

veins [74,75]. 3D CEMR venography, timed for venous imaging, has been shown to be a reliable tool for the evaluation of thoracic veins and identification of venous thrombosis [76–78]. 3D CEMRV can also be used for the evaluation of patients with known poor venous access who require central venous catheters, such as patients receiving intravenous chemotherapy regimens. Steady-state free precession (SSFP) pulse sequences provide a high venous SNR, especially after the administration of a Gd contrast agent, and SSFP should be considered as an adjunct or alternative method for venous imaging [79].

Using time-resolved MRA obviates the need for contrast bolus timing and has been shown to be reliable for the display of central veins. This type of dynamic imaging allows for the assessment of thoracic veins in different arm positions (Fig. 23) [80].

Pulmonary venous mapping

In patients with atrial fibrillation, radiofrequency ablation often has curative potential. CEMRA is used for pulmonary venous mapping before catheter-guided radiofrequency ablation and for postprocedural follow-up [81,82].

Summary

With the strategies presented in this article, relevant disease involving the thoraco-abdominal vessels can be well depicted by 3D CEMRA. Aneurysms, dissections, occlusions, congenital lesions, and anatomic anomalies are readily assessed. Time-resolved MRA provides supplemental information in shunts, dissections, aneurysms, and AVMs. Velocity-encoded imaging may help further characterize lesions and may provide useful functional information to grade and monitor the progression of stenotic disease. 3.0T imaging and recent development in multicoil RF technology will further improve the performance of 3D CEMRA in terms of temporal and spatial resolution.

References

[1] Prince MR, Yucel EK, Kaufman JA, et al. Dynamic gadolinium-enhanced three-dimensional abdominal MR arteriography. J Magn Reson Imaging 1993;3: 877–81.

[2] Earls JP, Rofsky NM, DeCorato DR, et al. Breath-hold single-dose gadolinium-enhanced three-dimensional MR aortography: usefulness of a timing examination and MR power injector. Radiology 1996;201:705–10.

[3] Kreitner KF, Kunz RP, Kalden P, et al. Contrast-enhanced three-dimensional MR angiography of the thoracic aorta: experiences after 118 examinations with a standard dose contrast administration and different injection protocols. Eur Radiol 2001; 11:1355–63.

[4] Maki JH, Prince MR, Londy FJ, et al. The effects of time varying intravascular signal intensity and

k-space acquisition order on three-dimensional MR angiography image quality. J Magn Reson Imaging 1996;6:642–51.

[5] Wilman AH, Riederer SJ, King BF, et al. Fluoroscopically triggered contrast-enhanced three-dimensional MR angiography with elliptical centric view order: application to the renal arteries. Radiology 1997;205:137–46.

[6] Goyen M, Herborn CU, Lauenstein TC, et al. Optimization of contrast dosage for gadobenate dimeglumine-enhanced high-resolution whole-body 3D magnetic resonance angiography. Invest Radiol 2002;37:263–8.

[7] Hany TF, Schmidt M, Hilfiker PR, et al. Optimization of contrast dosage for gadolinium-enhanced 3D MRA of the pulmonary and renal arteries. Magn Reson Imaging 1998;16:901–6.

[8] Leung DA, McKinnon GC, Davis CP, et al. Breathhold, contrast-enhanced, three-dimensional MR angiography. Radiology 1996;200:569–71.

[9] Prince MR, Narasimham DL, Stanley JC, et al. Breath-hold gadolinium-enhanced MR angiography of the abdominal aorta and its major branches. Radiology 1995;197:785–92.

[10] Hartnell GG, Finn JP, Zenni M, et al. MR imaging of the thoracic aorta: comparison of spin-echo, angiographic, and breath-hold techniques. Radiology 1994;191:697–704.

[11] Krinsky GA, Rofsky NM, DeCorato DR, et al. Thoracic aorta: comparison of gadolinium-enhanced three-dimensional MR angiography with conventional MR imaging. Radiology 1997;202:183–93.

[12] Finn JP, Baskaran V, Carr JC, et al. Thorax: low-dose contrast-enhanced three-dimensional MR angiography with subsecond temporal resolution—initial results. Radiology 2002;224:896–904.

[13] Korosec FR, Frayne R, Grist TM, et al. Time-resolved contrast-enhanced 3D MR angiography. Magn Reson Med 1996;36:345–51.

[14] Carr JC, Laub G, Zheng J, et al. Time-resolved three-dimensional pulmonary MR angiography and perfusion imaging with ultrashort repetition time. Acad Radiol 2002;9:1407–18.

[15] Goyen M, Laub G, Ladd ME, et al. Dynamic 3D MR angiography of the pulmonary arteries in under four seconds. J Magn Reson Imaging 2001;13: 372–7.

[16] de Zwart JA, Ledden PJ, van Gelderen P, et al. Signal-to-noise ratio and parallel imaging performance of a 16-channel receive-only brain coil array at 3.0 Tesla. Magn Reson Med 2004;51:22–6.

[17] King SB, Peterson DG, Varosi S, et al. A comparison of 1, 4, and 8 channel phased array head coils at 1.5 T. Presented at the 9th Annual Meeting of the International Society for Magnetic Resonance in Medicine. Glasgow (Scotland), April 21–27, 2001.

[18] Bodurka J, Ledden PJ, van Gelderen P, et al. Scalable multichannel MRI data acquisition system. Magn Reson Med 2004;51:165–71.

[19] Hayes CE, Roemer PB. Noise correlations in data simultaneously acquired from multiple surface coil arrays. Magn Reson Med 1990;16:181–91.

[20] Sodickson DK, McKenzie CA, Li W, et al. Contrast-enhanced 3D MR angiography with simultaneous acquisition of spatial harmonics: a pilot study. Radiology 2000;217:284–9.

[21] Weiger M, Pruessmann KP, Kassner A, et al. Contrast-enhanced 3D MRA using SENSE. J Magn Reson Imaging 2000;12:671–7.

[22] Pruessmann KP, Weiger M, Scheidegger MB, et al. SENSE: sensitivity encoding for fast MRI. Magn Reson Med 1999;42:952–62.

[23] Griswold MA, Jakob PM, Heidemann RM, et al. Generalized autocalibrating partially parallel acquisitions (GRAPPA). Magn Reson Med 2002; 47:1202–10.

[24] Sodickson DK, Manning WJ. Simultaneous acquisition of spatial harmonics (SMASH): fast imaging with radiofrequency coil arrays. Magn Reson Med 1997;38:591–603.

[25] Fink C, Bock M, Puderbach M, et al. Partially parallel three-dimensional magnetic resonance imaging for the assessment of lung perfusion: initial results. Invest Radiol 2003;38:482–8.

[26] Frayne R, Grist TM, Swan JS, et al. 3D MR DSA: effects of injection protocol and image masking. J Magn Reson Imaging 2000;12:476–87.

[27] Hayes CE, Hattes N, Roemer PB. Volume imaging with MR phased arrays. Magn Reson Med 1991; 18:309–19.

[28] Roemer PB, Edelstein WA, Hayes CE, et al. The NMR phased array. Magn Reson Med 1990;16:192–225.

[29] Constantinides CD, Westgate CR, O'Dell WG, et al. A phased array coil for human cardiac imaging. Magn Reson Med 1995;34:92–8.

[30] Hardy CJ, Darrow RD, Saranathan M, et al. Large field-of-view real-time MRI with a 32-channel system. Magn Reson Med 2004;52:878–84.

[31] Zhu Y, Hardy CJ, Sodickson DK, et al. Highly parallel volumetric imaging with a 32-element RF coil array. Magn Reson Med 2004;52:869–77.

[32] Campeau NG, Huston J III, Bernstein MA, et al. Magnetic resonance angiography at 3.0 Tesla: initial clinical experience. Top Magn Reson Imaging 2001; 12:183–204.

[33] Willinek WA, Born M, Simon B, et al. Time-of-flight MR angiography: comparison of 3.0-T imaging and 1.5-T imaging–initial experience. Radiology 2003; 229:913–20.

[34] Thulborn KR. Clinical rationale for very-high-field (3.0 Tesla) functional magnetic resonance imaging. Top Magn Reson Imaging 1999;10:37–50.

[35] Robitaille PM, Abduljalil AM, Kangarlu A. Ultra high resolution imaging of the human head at 8 tesla: 2K x 2K for Y2K. J Comput Assist Tomogr 2000;24:2–8.

[36] Rinck PA, Muller RN. Field strength and dose dependence of contrast enhancement by gadolinium-based MR contrast agents. Eur Radiol 1999;9:998–1004.

[37] Hany TF, McKinnon GC, Leung DA, et al. Optimization of contrast timing for breath-hold three-dimensional MR angiography. J Magn Reson Imaging 1997;7:551–6.

[38] Lee VS, Martin DJ, Krinsky GA, et al. Gadolinium-enhanced MR angiography: artifacts and pitfalls. AJR Am J Roentgenol 2000;175:197–205.

[39] Shellock FG, Kanal E. Safety of magnetic resonance imaging contrast agents. J Magn Reson Imaging 1999;10:477–84.

[40] Shehadi WH. Contrast media adverse reactions: occurrence, recurrence, and distribution patterns. Radiology 1982;143:11–7.

[41] Joyce JW, Fairbairn JF Jr, Kincaid OW, et al. Aneurysms of the thoracic aorta: a clinical study with special reference to prognosis. Circulation 1964;29:176–81.

[42] Nienaber CA, von Kodolitsch Y, Nicolas V, et al. The diagnosis of thoracic aortic dissection by non-invasive imaging procedures. N Engl J Med 1993; 328:1–9.

[43] DeSanctis RW, Doroghazi RM, Austen WG, et al. Aortic dissection. N Engl J Med 1987;317:1060–7.

[44] Summers RM, Sostman HD, Spritzer CE, et al. Fast spoiled gradient-recalled MR imaging of thoracic aortic dissection: preliminary clinical experience at 1.5 T. Magn Reson Imaging 1996;14:1–9.

[45] Prince MR, Narasimham DL, Jacoby WT, et al. Three-dimensional gadolinium-enhanced MR angiography of the thoracic aorta. AJR Am J Roentgenol 1996;166:1387–97.

[46] Pereles FS, McCarthy RM, Baskaran V, et al. Thoracic aortic dissection and aneurysm: evaluation with nonenhanced true FISP MR angiography in less than 4 minutes. Radiology 2002;223:270–4.

[47] Wolff KA, Herold CJ, Tempany CM, et al. Aortic dissection: atypical patterns seen at MR imaging. Radiology 1991;181:489–95.

[48] Didier D, Ratib O, Lerch R, et al. Detection and quantification of valvular heart disease with dynamic cardiac MR imaging. Radiographics 2000;20: 1279–99 [discussion: 1299–301].

[49] Barkhausen J, Goyen M, Ruhm SG, et al. Assessment of ventricular function with single breath-hold real-time steady-state free precession cine MR imaging. AJR Am J Roentgenol 2002;178:731–5.

[50] Soler R, Rodriguez E, Requejo I, et al. Magnetic resonance imaging of congenital abnormalities of the thoracic aorta. Eur Radiol 1998;8:540–6.

[51] Roche KJ, Krinsky G, Lee VS, et al. Interrupted aortic arch: diagnosis with gadolinium-enhanced 3D MRA. J Comput Assist Tomogr 1999;23: 197–202.

[52] Mohiaddin RH, Kilner PJ, Rees S, et al. Magnetic resonance volume flow and jet velocity mapping in aortic coarctation. J Am Coll Cardiol 1993;22: 1515–21.

[53] Bogaert J, Kuzo R, Dymarkowski S, et al. Follow-up of patients with previous treatment for coarcta-tion of the thoracic aorta: comparison between contrast-enhanced MR angiography and fast spin-echo MR imaging. Eur Radiol 2000;10:1847–54.

[54] Hatabu H, Tadamura E, Levin DL, et al. Quantitative assessment of pulmonary perfusion with dynamic contrast-enhanced MRI. Magn Reson Med 1999;42:1033–8.

[55] Meaney JF, Weg JG, Chenevert TL, et al. Diagnosis of pulmonary embolism with magnetic resonance angiography. N Engl J Med 1997;336:1422–7.

[56] Steiner P, McKinnon GC, Romanowski B, et al. Contrast-enhanced, ultrafast 3D pulmonary MR angiography in a single breath-hold: initial assessment of imaging performance. J Magn Reson Imaging 1997;7:177–82.

[57] van Beek EJ, Wild JM, Fink C, et al. MRI for the diagnosis of pulmonary embolism. J Magn Reson Imaging 2003;18:627–40.

[58] Gupta A, Frazer CK, Ferguson JM, et al. Acute pulmonary embolism: diagnosis with MR angiography. Radiology 1999;210:353–9.

[59] Meaney JF, Ridgway JP, Chakraverty S, et al. Stepping-table gadolinium-enhanced digital subtraction MR angiography of the aorta and lower extremity arteries: preliminary experience. Radiology 1999; 211:59–67.

[60] Fink C, Risse F, Buhmann R, et al. Quantitative analysis of pulmonary perfusion using time-resolved parallel 3D MRI: initial results. Rofo Fortschr Geb Rontgenstr Neuen Bildgeb Verfahr 2004;176:170–4.

[61] Kluge A, Dill T, Ekinci O, et al. Decreased pulmonary perfusion in pulmonary vein stenosis after radiofrequency ablation: assessment with dynamic magnetic resonance perfusion imaging. Chest 2004; 126:428–37.

[62] Ley S, Kauczor HU, Heussel CP, et al. Value of contrast-enhanced MR angiography and helical CT angiography in chronic thromboembolic pulmonary hypertension. Eur Radiol 2003;13:2365–71.

[63] Laffon E, Laurent F, Bernard V, et al. Noninvasive assessment of pulmonary arterial hypertension by MR phase-mapping method. J Appl Physiol 2001; 90:2197–202.

[64] Kreitner KF, Ley S, Kauczor HU, et al. Chronic thromboembolic pulmonary hypertension: pre- and postoperative assessment with breath-hold MR imaging techniques. Radiology 2004;232:535–43.

[65] Hoeper MM, Tongers J, Leppert A, et al. Evaluation of right ventricular performance with a right ventricular ejection fraction thermodilution catheter and MRI in patients with pulmonary hypertension. Chest 2001;120:502–7.

[66] Saba TS, Foster J, Cockburn M, et al. Ventricular mass index using magnetic resonance imaging accurately estimates pulmonary artery pressure. Eur Respir J 2002;20:1519–24.

[67] Prasad SK, Soukias N, Hornung T, et al. Role of magnetic resonance angiography in the diagnosis of major aortopulmonary collateral arteries and partial

anomalous pulmonary venous drainage. Circulation 2004;109:207–14.

[68] Puvaneswary M, Leitch J, Chard RB. MRI of partial anomalous pulmonary venous return (scimitar syndrome). Australas Radiol 2003;47:92–3.

[69] Balci NC, Yalcin Y, Tunaci A, et al. Assessment of the anomalous pulmonary circulation by dynamic contrast-enhanced MR angiography in under four seconds. Magn Reson Imaging 2003;21:1–7.

[70] Dinsmore BJ, Gefter WB, Hatabu H, et al. Pulmonary arteriovenous malformations: diagnosis by gradient-refocused MR imaging. J Comput Assist Tomogr 1990;14:918–23.

[71] Goyen M, Ruehm SG, Jagenburg A, et al. Pulmonary arteriovenous malformation: characterization with time-resolved ultrafast 3D MR angiography. J Magn Reson Imaging 2001;13:458–60.

[72] Ohno Y, Hatabu H, Takenaka D, et al. Contrast-enhanced MR perfusion imaging and MR angiography: utility for management of pulmonary arteriovenous malformations for embolotherapy. Eur J Radiol 2002;41:136–46.

[73] Kauczor HU, Gamroth AH, Tuengerthal SJ, et al. [MR angiography: its use in pulmonary and mediastinal space-occupying lesions.] Rofo 1992;157:15–20 [in German].

[74] Li W, David V, Kaplan R, et al. Three-dimensional low dose gadolinium-enhanced peripheral MR venography. J Magn Reson Imaging 1998;8:630–3.

[75] Lebowitz JA, Rofsky NM, Krinsky GA, et al. Gadolinium-enhanced body MR venography with subtraction technique. AJR Am J Roentgenol 1997; 169:755–8.

[76] Thornton MJ, Ryan R, Varghese JC, et al. A three-dimensional gadolinium-enhanced MR venography technique for imaging central veins. AJR Am J Roentgenol 1999;173:999–1003.

[77] Shinde TS, Lee VS, Rofsky NM, et al. Three-dimensional gadolinium-enhanced MR venographic evaluation of patency of central veins in the thorax: initial experience. Radiology 1999;213:555–60.

[78] Kroencke TJ, Taupitz M, Arnold R, et al. Three-dimensional gadolinium-enhanced magnetic resonance venography in suspected thrombo-occlusive disease of the central chest veins. Chest 2001;120: 1570–6.

[79] Foo TK, Ho VB, Marcos HB, et al. MR angiography using steady-state free precession. Magn Reson Med 2002;48:699–706.

[80] Goyen M, Barkhausen J, Kuehl H, et al. [Contrast-enhanced 3D MR venography of central thoracic veins: preliminary experience.] Rofo 2001;173:356–61 [in German].

[81] Tsao HM, Chen SA. Evaluation of pulmonary vein stenosis after catheter ablation of atrial fibrillation. Card Electrophysiol Rev 2002;6:397–400.

[82] Collins JD, Song GK, Bello D, et al. Pre-ablative pulmonary venous mapping by high-resolution MR angiography facilitates electrophysiologic pulmonary vein ablation and reduces fluoroscopic time in patients with paroxysmal atrial fibrillation [abstract]. Presented at the North American Society for Cardiac Imaging 30th Annual Meeting and Scientific Session in conjunction with the Third International Workshop on Coronary MR and CT Angiography. Dallas (TX), September 21–24, 2002.

ELSEVIER
SAUNDERS

Magn Reson Imaging Clin N Am
13 (2005) 381–395

**MAGNETIC
RESONANCE
IMAGING CLINICS
of North America**

Female Pelvis

Michèle A. Brown, MD*, Claude B. Sirlin, MD

*Department of Radiology, UCSD Medical Center, 200 West Arbor Drive,
San Diego, CA 92103-8756, USA*

The anatomy of the female pelvis is shown in exquisite detail by MR imaging. MR imaging has become the imaging modality of choice for the diagnosis of congenital uterine anomalies and benign acquired gynecologic disease. MR imaging also has clear indications for pretreatment assessment of uterine malignancies and characterization of adnexal masses. This article reviews current MR imaging techniques, normal anatomy, and commonly encountered benign and malignant diseases of the female pelvis.

MR imaging technique

Patients are imaged best with an empty bladder after fasting for at least 4 hours. Antispasmodics, such as glucagon, may be used to decrease motion artifact that is related to bowel peristalsis. Some centers also use intravaginal gel to distend the vaginal fornices. Imaging is performed with the patient supine unless she is in late pregnancy, in which case a decubitus position is preferred to decrease pressure on the inferior vena cava. A phased-array coil should be used in most instances. Endoluminal coils or small surface coils may provide improved resolution for specific indications.

There are many MR sequence protocol options for imaging the female pelvis. The appropriate choice depends on the specific clinical question, available equipment, and expertise. The following general protocol suggestions use sequences that

are widely available. First, a large field of view coronal T2-weighted (T2w) single shot echo train spin-echo image is obtained, such as half-Fourier single shot turbo spin-echo. Subsequent images are obtained with a small field of view (20–24 cm) to maximize spatial resolution; these include axial and sagittal T2w echo train spin-echo and axial T1-weighted (T1w) spoiled gradient echo in- and out-of-phase. Sequence planes are angled to the uterus or cervix to provide true long- and short-axis views of these structures. This can be accomplished by first obtaining T2w echo train spin-echo or T2w/T1w steady-state free precession images axial to the patient. These sequences delineate the endometrial and endocervical canals and are used to prescribe oblique sagittal T2w images that are oriented parallel to the endometrial or endocervical canal. From the oblique sagittal images, oblique axial T2w and dual echo T1w images are prescribed in a plane that is perpendicular to the endometrial or endocervical canal (short-axis view). In cases of uterine anomalies, oblique coronal T2w images also are obtained. Fat-saturation is not applied routinely to T2w sequences in the female pelvis; however a fat-suppressed T1w image is helpful in cases of suspected endometriosis to detect small endometrial deposits.

For benign disease, exclusive use of breath-hold sequences usually is sufficient and serves to minimize examination time and increase through put. For evaluation of cancer, longer duration high-resolution T2w echo train spin-echo and postgadolinium fat-suppressed T1w images are needed. Sequential postgadolinium breath-hold three-dimensional fast gradient echo images are

* Corresponding author.
   E-mail address: m9brown@ucsd.edu (M.A. Brown).

used for dynamic imaging. For evaluation of fetal anomalies, MR imaging relies almost exclusively on ultrafast sequences, such as T2w single-shot echo train spin-echo and T2/T1w steady-state free precession gradient echo.

Normal

The uterus has three distinct zones on T2w images in women of reproductive age [1]. The central high-signal intensity represents the endometrium. The low signal intensity middle layer is the junctional zone, which corresponds to the inner myometrium. The outer intermediate signal intensity corresponds to the outer myometrium (Fig. 1). The endometrial thickness varies depending on hormonal status. Reports that describe the normal thickness of the junctional zone differ, with an average of 2 mm to 8 mm [2]. High temporal resolution MR imaging reveals that the appearance of the junctional zone is in constant flux, which is believed to be due to inner myometrial uterine peristalsis [3]. In postmenopausal women the uterus typically is small and the zonal anatomy is indistinct.

On unenhanced T1w images, the uterus has homogenous signal intensity that is similar to that of muscle; the zonal anatomy usually is not apparent. Occasionally, the endometrium can be identified by subtly higher signal intensity than the myometrium. The appearance of uterus on

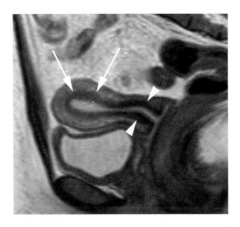

Fig. 1. Normal uterus and cervix. Sagittal T2-weighted image shows central hyperintense endometrium, middle hypointense junctional zone (*arrows*), and outer intermediate signal intensity myometrium. The junctional zone is continuous with the fibrous stroma of the cervix (*arrowheads*).

gadolinium-enhanced T1w images depends on the phase in which images are acquired. On arterial and venous phases, the myometrium tends to be homogeneously hyperintense, in contrast to the slowly enhancing endometrium, which appears distinctly hypointense. On more delayed images, however, the endometrium becomes slightly hyperintense relative to the outer myometrium, whereas the junctional zone becomes slightly hypointense. Thus, on delayed phase T1w images, the relative signal intensity of the three uterine zones is similar to unenhanced T2w images, although the contrast between the zones is subtler.

The cervix has four layers on T2w images [4]. Hyperintense mucus is seen centrally, surrounded by high signal intensity endocervix that contains mucosal folds (plica palmatae). The endocervix is surrounded by the hypointense fibrous stroma, which is continuous with the junctional zone. The endocervical fibrous stroma usually is differentiated easily from the uterine junctional zone because it tends to be thicker and more hypointense. The peripheral intermediate signal intensity corresponds to smooth muscle and is continuous with the outer myometrium. The cervix tends to enhance more slowly and less homogeneously than the adjacent myometrium. The mildly heterogeneous and hypointense appearance of the normal cervix on delayed images should not be misinterpreted as cancer or other pathology.

The vagina has three layers on T2w images: central high signal intensity mucosa and fluid, middle low signal intensity submucosa and muscularis, and outer high signal intensity vaginal venous plexus that contains slow venous flow [5]. After gadolinium administration, the vaginal wall enhances intensely.

The female urethra has a target or bulls-eye appearance on axial T2w and enhanced T1w images and is best seen using high-resolution techniques [6]. There is a low signal intensity outer muscular ring, a high signal intensity middle vascular submucosal ring, and a low signal intensity central mucosal dot (Fig. 2). At the center, a tiny central hyperintense dot of urine or mucus is sometimes seen on T2w images. After gadolinium administration, the middle submucosal layer enhances brightly relative to the rest of the urethra and appears as a continuous ring.

The ovaries are nearly always visible in premenopausal women but may not be seen after menopause. If not obvious on initial inspection of

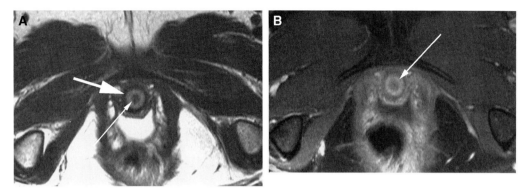

Fig. 2. Normal urethra. (*A*) Axial T2-weighted image shows a low signal intensity outer muscular ring (*large arrow*), a high signal intensity middle vascular submucosal ring, and a low signal intensity central mucosal dot (*small arrow*). (*B*) Axial postgadolinium fat-suppressed T1-weighted image shows that the middle submucosal layer (*arrow*) enhances more than the inner and outer layers.

images, the ovaries often can be identified by following the course of the gonadal vessels or round ligaments. On T2w images, the ovaries contain low signal intensity central stroma and high signal intensity follicles and functional cysts of varied sizes. Cysts are common in ovaries, regardless of patient age and hormonal status. Corpus luteal cysts have thick irregular walls that enhance intensely. Hemorrhagic cysts are bright on T1w images [7].

Benign disease

Müllerian duct anomalies

Müllerian duct anomalies occur in less than 1% of women; however, the incidence is much higher in women who are undergoing fertility assessment. In addition to impaired fertility, these anomalies may lead to primary amenorrhea, menstrual disorders, recurrent miscarriage, premature labor, or intrauterine growth retardation. Accurate diagnosis is important to guide treatment. Although transvaginal ultrasound and hysterosalpingography are helpful and used widely, each has limitations. MR imaging is the imaging test of choice [8]. The widely used modified Buttram and Gibbons classification and corresponding MR imaging features are described below [8,9]. Despite the classification scheme, these anomalies represent a spectrum of disease, and complex anomalies may show characteristics of multiple classes. In the case of a complex anomaly, it is important to describe the individual

components rather than the class it most resembles [8].

- Class I: Segmental agenesis or hypoplasia. MR imaging reveals an absent or small uterus, cervix, or vagina, depending on the affected segment. Typically, uterovaginal agenesis is seen best on sagittal T2w sequences.
- Class II: Unicornuate uterus. MR imaging shows an elongated uterus with or without a rudimentary horn. The rudimentary horn may contain endometrium and may communicate with the main endometrium. The presence of endometrium is seen best on T2w images.
- Class III: Uterus didelphys. MR imaging shows two uteri and cervices, often separated widely. Vaginal septa are associated with uterus didelphys more often than the other anomalies, and these septa may obstruct and result in hematocolpometria.
- Class IV: Bicornuate uterus. MR imaging reveals divergent uterine horns more than 4 cm apart that are divided by a muscular and fibrous septum. An indentation in the fundus of more than 1 cm in depth suggests bicornuate over septate uterus, and this is seen best on a true coronal image oriented to the uterus.
- Class V: Septate uterus. This is the most common Müllerian duct anomaly and has high association with infertility. MR imaging shows a convex or minimally indented (<1 cm) fundus and a fibrous septum and normal distance between the uterine horns

(2–4 cm). To differentiate from bicornuate, it is helpful to obtain a true coronal image oriented to the uterus (Fig. 3).

Class VI: Arcuate uterus. Considered a mild septate uterus in the original classification and a normal variant by some, an arcuate uterus has questionable impact on fertility. MR imaging shows a short, broad septum.

Class VII: Diethylstilbestrol (DES) exposure. This category includes various anomalies that are associated with DES, such as hypoplasia, T-shaped uterus, constrictions, polypoid defects, synechiae, and marginal irregularities. These patients also are at risk for developing clear cell carcinoma of the vagina. On MR imaging, a T-shaped endometrium is seen best on oblique coronal images parallel to the endometrium, and constrictions are seen as focal thickening of the junctional zone.

Leiomyomas

Leiomyomas are common benign smooth muscle tumors that may cause bleeding, pain, infertility, second trimester abortions, or dystocia. Degeneration is common, and painful hemorrhagic degeneration is especially common during pregnancy. Other complications, such as torsion, infection, and sarcomatous degeneration are rare

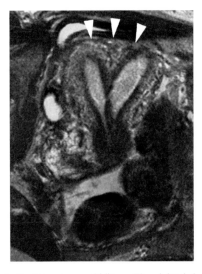

Fig. 3. Septate uterus. Oblique T2-weighted imaged obtained coronal to the uterus shows a central muscular and fibrous septum with a normal convex fundal margin (*arrowheads*).

[10–12]. MR imaging is highly accurate for detecting, localizing, and characterizing leiomyomas. MR imaging is particularly helpful to distinguish between a pedunculated subserosal leiomyoma and an ovarian mass, to demonstrate the exact size and location before myomectomy, to distinguish leiomyomas from adenomyosis, and to identify complications.

On MR imaging, typical leiomyomas are sharply marginated lesions of low signal intensity on T2w sequences (Fig. 4). Degenerative changes may lead to heterogeneous increased signal intensity on T2w images, or increased signal intensity on T1w images in the case of hemorrhagic degeneration. No criteria exist to exclude sarcomatous degeneration with certainty; however it should be suspected if a large lesion is seen in a postmenopausal woman, especially if there has been rapid growth or if indistinct margins are present [10,11].

Treatment options for patients who have symptomatic leiomyomas include gonadotropin-releasing hormone analogs, hysterectomy, myomectomy, or uterine artery embolization (UAE). Investigation is ongoing into other minimally invasive methods of treatment, such as MR imaging–guided focused ultrasound therapy [12,13]. Pretreatment MR imaging is helpful for choosing initial therapy and monitoring outcome in patients who undergo uterine-sparing treatment. Fibroids that do not enhance are unlikely to respond to UAE, so administration of gadolinium chelates is helpful for patient selection. Additionally, contrast-enhanced images allow documentation of devascularization after UAE [11,14] and may identify ovarian artery collaterals that feed refractory fibroids in patients who do not respond.

Adenomyosis

Adenomyosis is a common condition which is defined as endometrial stroma and glands within the myometrium. Similar to fibroids, adenomyosis can lead to dysmenorrhea and menorrhagia. Unlike fibroids, adenomyosis is treated with hysterectomy; no other treatment options have proved to be consistently efficacious, although there are reports of success with UAE. On MR imaging, thickening of the hypointense junctional zone is seen on T2w images (Fig. 5). Characteristically, the thickening has ill-defined or lobulated borders. Although reported threshold values vary, thickening of 12 mm or more suggests the diagnosis.

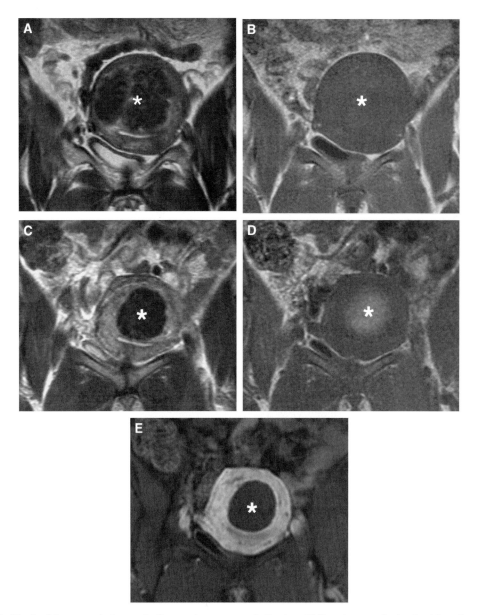

Fig. 4. Uterine leiomyoma before and after uterine artery embolization. Oblique images obtained axial to the uterus before embolization demonstrate a typical leiomyoma (*), which is hypointense on T2-weighted images (*A*) and of intermediate signal intensity on T1-weighted images (*B*). After embolization, the leiomyoma (*) is smaller and slightly more hyperintense on T2-weighted images (*C*) and hyperintense on T1-weighted images (*D*), with no enhancement on postgadolinium fat-suppressed T1-weighted images (*E*). These changes reflect hemorrhagic infarction.

Multiple punctate foci of hyperintensity are seen frequently on T2w images. Bright foci on T1w images are seen much less frequently, but when present, support the diagnosis. Cystic adenomyosis that results from extensive hemorrhage may appear as well-circumscribed, cystic myometrial lesions which contain blood products of different ages. The focal form, adenomyoma, may mimic leiomyoma, and the distinction is important for proper management. On T2w images, features that suggest adenomyosis include poorly defined borders; elliptical or lobulated, rather than round shape; contact with the junctional zone; minimal mass effect on the endometrium; and high signal

386   BROWN & SIRLIN

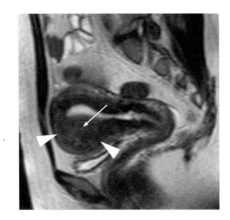

Fig. 5. Adenomyosis. Sagittal T2-weighted images shows focal thickening of the junctional zone (*arrowheads*). Scattered punctate hyperintense foci (*arrow*) can be seen which represent islands of endometrium within the myometrium.

intensity foci or linear striations that radiate out from the endometrium into the myometrium [11].

Endometriosis

Endometriosis may present with pain or infertility. The most commonly involved structures are the ovaries, the cul-de-sac and posterior uterine wall, the uterosacral ligaments, the anterior uterine wall, and the bladder dome. On T1w images, endometriomas are of high signal intensity and often are homogeneously "lightbulb" bright; this signal intensity is more conspicuous on fat-suppressed images [15]. If gadolinium chelates are administered, smooth uniform ring

enhancement on delayed images is characteristic; the central portion of the lesion does not enhance. On T2w images, endometriomas may demonstrate low signal intensity ("shading") that presumably is due to repeated bleeding and the build-up of blood products that shorten T2 (Fig. 6). This profound T2 shortening is a helpful finding because it is uncommon in functional or hemorrhagic cysts [7]. When using all of these signal characteristics, the sensitivity of MR imaging for detecting endometriomas is high. MR imaging may not detect small superficial lesions that are seen at laparoscopy; however MR imaging may surpass laparoscopy at detecting deep pelvic endometriosis, which is symptomatic more frequently [16].

Dermoid

Dermoid cysts are the most common ovarian neoplasm. Symptoms, when present, are related to mass effect, or rarely, torsion, infection, or rupture. Malignant transformation is rare and usually occurs in postmenopausal women [17]. Characteristic MR imaging features include fat, fluid-fluid levels, and Rokitansky nodules. Standard T1w and T2w imaging sequences can support the diagnosis of a teratoma; however, fat-saturated or out-of-phase T1w images will improve diagnostic confidence (Fig. 7) [18]. Calcifications, if present, may be difficult to identify on MR images.

Polycystic ovary syndrome

Polycystic ovary syndrome represents a spectrum of disease that may manifest clinically with

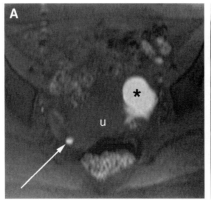
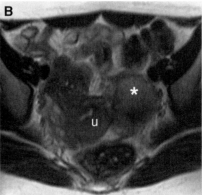

Fig. 6. Endometriosis. Axial images shows a mass (*) to the left of the uterus (*u*) that demonstrates homogeneous high signal intensity on fat-suppressed T1-weighted images (*A*) and graded intermediate to low signal intensity on T2-weighted images (*B*). Fat-suppressed T1-weighted images are helpful to demonstrate small endometrial deposits (*arrow, A*) that cannot be distinguished on other sequences.

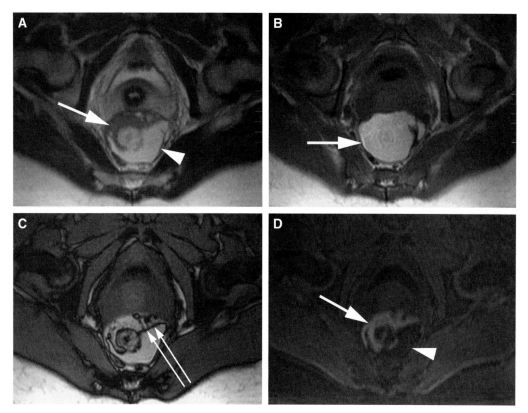

Fig. 7. Dermoid. Oblique axial images demonstrate a mass that is heterogeneous on T2-weighted images with intermediate signal intensity components (*arrow, A*) and high signal intensity components (*arrowhead, A*). The mass is entirely high signal intensity on in-phase T1-weighted images (*arrow, B*). On out-of-phase T1-weighted images, low signal "India ink" artifact (*arrows, C*) demonstrates that the lesion contains fat and water-based tissue. (*D*) Fat-suppressed T1-weighted images confirm the presence of gross fat (*arrowhead*) in addition to other components that are not completely suppressed (*arrow*).

hirsutism, irregular bleeding, or infertility. Obesity is an associated characteristic but does not define the disease [19]. On MR imaging, the ovaries are normal to large in size with multiple small peripheral follicles of uniform size. Occasionally, a dark capsule and central stroma are seen on T2w images (Fig. 8). Unlike normal ovaries, the small uniform follicles do not become hemorrhagic and are consistently bright on T2w images and dark on T1w images. There is overlap between the MR imaging appearance of normal and polycystic ovaries, and diagnosis requires the proper clinical setting [20].

Pelvic congestion syndrome

Pelvic congestion syndrome can be suggested in patients who have pelvic varices if the appropriate clinical syndrome of chronic pelvic pain exists. The syndrome typically affects multiparous women. Patients report a dull, deep ache that is made worse by standing. The clinical diagnosis is challenging; patients who are suspected of having this condition often undergo venography, which is invasive and frequently negative. MR imaging provides a noninvasive venogram, and the addition of routine sequences for evaluation of pelvic anatomy permits diagnosis of other possible causes of pain, such as adenomyosis. On T1w and T2w images, serpentine parauterine and para-ovarian vessels are noted. With dynamic gadolinium-enhanced imaging, reflux can be seen down enlarged gonadal veins on early images, and the pelvic varices enhance intensely [21].

Pelvic floor relaxation

Pelvic floor relaxation is common in parous women; symptoms include urinary or fecal incontinence and prolapse of the cervix or uterus.

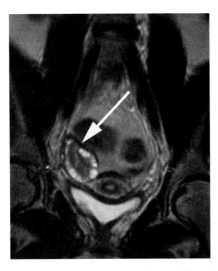

Fig. 8. Polycystic ovary syndrome. Coronal T2-weighted image shows a slightly enlarged right ovary (*arrow*) with peripheral follicles of equal size and low signal intensity central stroma.

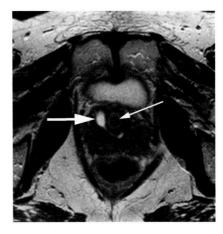

Fig. 9. Urethral diverticulum. Axial T2-weighted image demonstrates a small hyperintense fluid collection (*large arrow*) peripheral to the central mucosa (*small arrow*) and partially surrounding the urethra. The connection to the central mucosal layer is not seen.

MR imaging is helpful for patients who have symptoms that involve more than one compartment and patients who are undergoing repeat operations. The MR imaging technique relies on sagittal midline images during rest and during strain, typically with a fast cine T2w or T2/T1w sequence. The descent of all three compartments can be quantified, and none should descend more than 2 cm below the pubococcygeal line. High-resolution axial T2w images also are used to identify pelvic floor musculature in detail [22].

Urethral diverticulum

Urethral diverticula are difficult to diagnose clinically because symptoms can be varied and nonspecific [23]. MR imaging is highly accurate for evaluation of suspected urethral diverticula and depicts the relationships with surrounding structures, which aids surgical planning [24]. On MR imaging, a focus or foci of signal intensity that is consistent with urine is seen peripheral to the urethral mucosal layer (Fig. 9). Diverticula often assume a C-shape surrounding the urethra, in which case they sometimes are called "saddle-bag diverticula" [25]. High-resolution T2w images axial to the urethra are especially useful. If a lesion is detected on the noncontrast images, high-resolution gadolinium-enhanced T1w fat-suppressed images are helpful to delineate the point of communication with the urethral lumen

and exclude solid enhancing components that would suggest carcinoma.

Malignant disease

Cervical carcinoma

Approximately 85% of cervical carcinomas are squamous cell carcinomas, whereas the remainder consists of adenocarcinomas, adenosquamous carcinomas, and undifferentiated carcinomas. Widespread use of the Papanicolaou smear has led to a decreased incidence of squamous cell carcinoma, and an increased relative incidence of adenocarcinomas [26]. Cervical cancer spreads by direct extension or through lymphatics. Hematogenous spread is rare. Cervical carcinoma is staged clinically according to the International Federation of Gynecology and Obstetrics (FIGO) staging system, which is an important determinant of prognosis and choice of treatment. The treatment of stage Ib and IIa disease may vary; however, traditionally, FIGO stage IIa or lower stage tumors are treated surgically, whereas higher stage tumors are treated with radiation therapy. FIGO staging has a high error rate compared with surgical staging; an important role of MR imaging is to increase pretreatment staging accuracy in patients who have low-stage disease [27]. MR imaging also detects lymphadenopathy, which affects prognosis and management, but is not part of FIGO staging. MR imaging also is helpful for lesions that are endocervical or suspected of extension to the parametrium. MR imaging is the modality of choice for staging cervical cancer when the diagnosis is made during pregnancy. It was reported that overall, MR imaging is more cost effective than the traditional evaluation with tests such as cystoscopy, barium enema, and intravenous urography [28].

Sagittal and axial T2w sequences provide good contrast between the tumor and normal cervix. Oblique axial images that are oriented perpendicular to the cervical canal may improve staging accuracy over straight axial images [29]. Cervical cancer has high signal intensity compared with the cervical stroma (Fig. 10). An intact low signal intensity rim that surrounds the tumor indicates it is limited to the cervix and was shown to be highly accurate for excluding parametrial invasion [26]. Dynamic imaging with gadolinium was reported to help determine the extent of invasion [30]. Parametrial extension indicates stage IIb disease and is diagnosed by disruption of the dark cervical stroma and abnormal soft tissue or stranding of the parametrial fat.

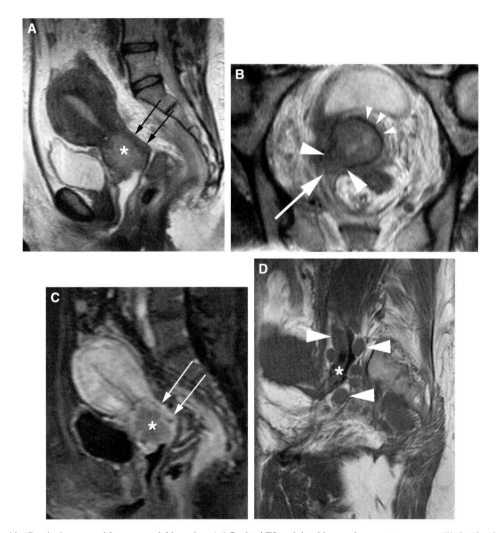

Fig. 10. Cervical cancer with parametrial invasion. (*A*) Sagittal T2-weighted image demonstrates a mass (*) that has high signal intensity compared with the cervical stroma (*arrows*). (*B*) Oblique T2-weighted image axial to the cervix demonstrates disruption of the dark cervical stroma (*large arrowheads*) and abnormal soft tissue extending into the parametrial fat (*arrow*), indicating parametrial invasion. On the opposite side, the dark line of the fibrous cervical stroma is intact (*small arrowheads*). (*C*) Sagittal postgadolinium fat-suppressed T1-weighted image shows that the mass (*) enhances less than cervical stroma (*arrows*). (*D*) Sagittal T1-weighted image shows enlarged lymph nodes (*arrowheads*) along the iliac vessels (*). Lymphadenopathy affects prognosis but is not part of FIGO staging.

T1w sequences are used to detect the presence of lymphadenopathy. Para-aortic, obturator, and iliac nodes should be no larger than 1 cm, whereas parametrial nodes should be no larger than 5 mm; however, central necrosis of a lymph node may be more specific than size criteria [31]. Sensitivity for malignant lymphadenopathy is low. This may improve with increasing availability of ultrasmall paramagnetic iron oxide particle contrast agents [32].

Endometrial carcinoma

Nearly 90% of all endometrial carcinomas are adenocarcinomas. Endometrial carcinoma first invades the myometrium, and lymphatic and hematogenous spread of endometrial carcinoma occurs later than in cervical carcinoma. The FIGO classification is used for tumor staging. MR imaging is indicated for patients who have advanced disease or high histologic grade tumors. MR imaging also is helpful to determine if an adenocarcinoma that is diagnosed by cervical biopsy is endometrial or cervical in origin (Fig. 11) [26–28]. In addition, MR imaging can be performed if endovaginal ultrasound is technically limited because of body habitus or fibroids. The depth of myometrial invasion can be estimated on MR imaging and predicts the likelihood of lymph node metastasis and overall prognosis. Lymph node metastasis is seen in 3% of patients who have superficial myometrial invasion and in 40% of patients who have deep myometrial invasion [33].

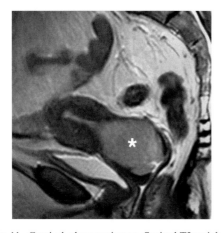

Fig. 11. Cervical adenocarcinoma. Sagittal T2-weighted image in a patient who has adenocarcinoma that was diagnosed by biopsy shows a mass (*) centered at the cervix. Distinguishing cervical from endometrial origin is important for proper treatment.

Endometrial abnormality and myometrial invasion can be seen on T2w images that are oriented sagittal and axial to the uterus, rather than to the patient. Endometrial carcinoma is similar in signal intensity to normal endometrium, and small or superficial cancers may not be seen. If the tumor becomes large enough, the endometrial canal is widened, and a heterogeneous mass with areas of high and low signal intensity is visualized. This finding is not specific for cancer, however; endometrial hyperplasia or endometrial polyps may have a similar appearance. Disruption of the normal junctional zone suggests myometrial invasion, and abnormal signal that extends to the outer half of the myometrium suggests deep myometrial invasion, with its associated increased probability of lymph node metastases (Fig. 12). Irregularity of the serosal surface suggests extension beyond the uterus. It is important to consider that the junctional zone is not seen in all postmenopausal women; nonvisualization of the junctional zone should not be interpreted, in the absence of other findings, as evidence of myometrial invasion. Gadolinium-enhanced T1w images are helpful for evaluating the local extent of disease, whether or not the junctional zone is well-seen on T2w images. Endometrial cancer enhances less than the surrounding myometrium on delayed images, whereas normal endometrium enhances more than myometrium. Pregadolinium T1w and postgadolinium fat-suppressed T1w images allow detection of lymphadenopathy. Detection relies on the criterion of size that is greater than 1 cm; signal intensity is not helpful in smaller lymph nodes [34].

Ovarian carcinoma

Ovarian cancer typically presents with advanced disease and is staged surgically. MR imaging has a limited role in the preoperative assessment of patients who have advanced disease but may be helpful to characterize adnexal masses as suspicious or benign. Studies have reported high accuracy [35,36]. Ovarian dermoids, most endometriomas, and pedunculated subserosal fibroids can be diagnosed definitively with MR imaging. For other masses, MR imaging features that favor malignancy include size larger than 4 cm, large solid component, wall or septal thickness of greater than 3mm, nodularity, and necrosis. A study of 163 lesions found that vegetations within a cystic lesion and ascites were the two best predictors of malignancy [36]. Most ovarian

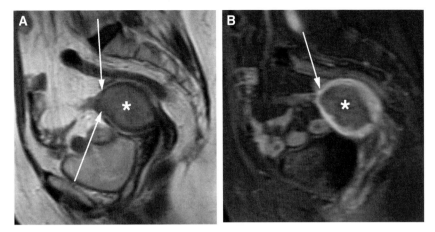

Fig. 12. Endometrial carcinoma. (*A*) Sagittal T2-weighted image shows a large mass (*) distending the endometrial cavity. The mass is lower in signal intensity than normal endometrium. Disruption of the junctional zone (*arrows*) indicates myometrial invasion. (*B*) Sagittal postgadolinium fat-suppressed T1-weighted image shows a thin rim of intact myometrium (*arrow*) not seen on T2-weighted images because of adjacent bowel. The mass (*) enhances less than the surrounding myometrium.

cancers are epithelial, most commonly serous or mucinous cystadenocarcinoma. Depending on cell type, up to 50% of ovarian neoplasms are bilateral. The typical pattern of spread is peritoneal, although lymphatic spread also occurs. The MR imaging appearance of primary epithelial neoplasms is a variable combination of cystic and solid components (Fig. 13). Gadolinium administration aids in the detection of solid and necrotic components, thick septations or vegetations, and peritoneal implants. Other cell types, such as sex cord stromal tumors and germ cell tumors, tend to be more solid and heterogeneous. Although some of these are associated with hemorrhage, distinction from endometriomas is usually possible because endometriomas tend to be homogeneously lightbulb bright on T1w images and demonstrate smooth peripheral enhancement after administration of gadolinium chelates, whereas hemorrhagic cancers tend to be

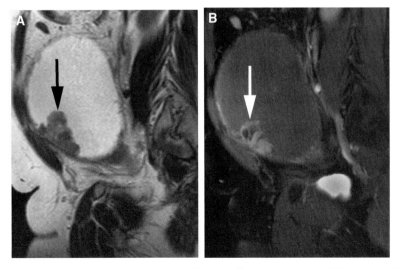

Fig. 13. Ovarian carcinoma. Sagittal T2-weighted (*A*) and postgadolinium fat-suppressed T1-weighted (*B*) images show a large cystic mass with enhancing solid mural nodules (*arrow*).

heterogeneously bright and demonstrate central, nodular, or irregular enhancement. Ovarian metastases may contain low signal on T2w images as a result of intense stromal reaction that occurs in the ovary as a response to the tumor [37]. Although MR imaging has a high accuracy for differentiating benign from malignant masses, the overlap in imaging appearance among cell types makes it difficult to predict histology based on MR imaging appearance.

Obstetric MR imaging

Ultrafast MR imaging techniques, such as single shot echo train spin-echo and steady-state gradient echo, provide excellent resolution for imaging the fetus and mother without radiation or sedation [38]. Late in pregnancy, patients should be imaged in a decubitus position to relieve pressure on the inferior vena cava. The use of MR imaging in obstetric patients is increasing, and there are no reports of adverse effects on the fetus from routine MR imaging sequences [39,40]. Until there is extensive experience in humans, MR imaging should be used only when ultrasound is inconclusive and should be avoided in the first trimester because of increased theoretic risk in the setting of rapid organogenesis. It also was suggested that gadolinium chelates be avoided during pregnancy. These agents cross the placenta, are excreted by the fetal urinary tract, and are swallowed by the fetus. If the benefit of contrast is believed to outweigh the theoretic risks, it is suggested that informed consent be obtained before contrast administration [41].

Fetal and placental imaging

The MR imaging appearances of many fetal anomalies have been described. The diagnostic accuracy of MR imaging is reported to be superior to sonography in some central nervous system anomalies and in complex malformations [42–44]. The fetal MR imaging examination typically is tailored to the specific question and may require multiple oblique planes of imaging. The fetal brain is usually seen well on T2w single shot echo train spin-echo images that are obtained coronal, axial, and sagittal to the fetal head (Fig. 14) [43]. T2w/T1w steady-state free precession images may be helpful if flow-related dephasing artifacts degrade the single shot echo train spin-echo images. For evaluation of congenital diaphragmatic hernia or cystic adenomatous

malformation, sagittal and coronal images of the fetus at the level of the diaphragm allow distinction of the thorax and abdomen. Many fetal anomalies can be evaluated with MR imaging, and it should be considered an adjunct to ultrasound in the evaluation of fetal anatomy.

Because of the large field of view possible, the entire placenta can be imaged by MR imaging. In cases that prove difficult for sonographic evaluation, MR images can diagnose placenta previa with high accuracy. Placenta accreta is an important cause of perinatal maternal mortality and often is a challenging diagnosis with ultrasound. MR imaging may be diagnostic and provide an estimation of the extent of invasion that greatly aids surgical planning. The normal placenta is homogenously bright on T2w images and intermediate on T1w images in the second trimester. In the third trimester, the internal architecture becomes apparent. In placenta accreta, the architecture is distorted, dark bands are seen on T2w images, and a convex bulge beyond the expected smooth margin of the uterus may be noted (Fig. 15) [45]. Some investigators have found gadolinium to be helpful; because of the potentially deadly consequences of placenta accreta, its use would be justified if needed for accurate diagnosis.

Maternal imaging

MR imaging has been used successfully to evaluate pregnant patients who have acute abdominal or pelvic pain without ionizing radiation. In patients who have indeterminate ultrasound, MR imaging has a high accuracy for detecting the cause of pain and usually requires no contrast

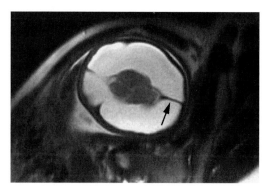

Fig. 14. Hydranencephaly. T2-weighted single shot echo train spin-echo image axial to the fetal head shows severe hydranencephaly with a partially intact falx (*arrow*), but no residual cortical tissue.

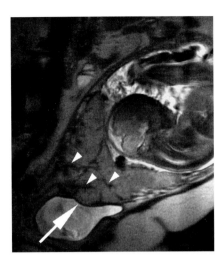

Fig. 15. Invasive placenta. Sagittal T2-weighted image shows an abnormal placenta with multiple dark bands (*arrowheads*), myometrial thinning, and an abnormal bulge in the outer uterine contour (*arrow*) indenting the bladder. Pathologic evaluation revealed invasion through uterine serosa indicating placenta percreta.

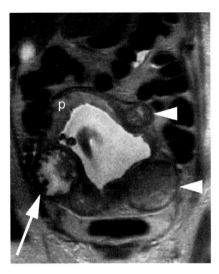

Fig. 16. Painful degenerating leiomyoma in pregnancy. Coronal T2-weighted image shows extensive degeneration of a right-sided leiomyoma (*arrow*) corresponding to the area of pain and exquisite tenderness. Several other leiomyomas (*arrowheads*) are seen with varying degrees of degeneration. The patient's clinical presentation mimicked appendicitis. p, placenta.

material (Fig. 16) [46–48]. Acute conditions that may be diagnosed on MR imaging include appendicitis, obstructing ureteral stone, degenerating fibroids, ovarian torsion, and small bowel obstruction. Single shot echo train spin-echo typically is used; other sequences may be added, depending on the specific clinical question. Such sequences may include heavily T2w single shot echo train spin-echo for MR cholangiopancreatography or MR urography, fat-suppressed T2w images for detection of inflammation, and time of flight or phase contrast for imaging vascular structures without contrast [46,48].

MR imaging is excellent for characterizing adnexal masses during pregnancy, whether they are symptomatic or discovered incidentally. If surgery is necessary, it is best performed in the second trimester [49]. MR imaging also is helpful for patients who are diagnosed with cervical cancer during pregnancy. Depending on the stage of disease, the patient may be encouraged strongly to terminate and undergo immediate treatment. MR is the imaging modality of choice because of its accuracy for staging and safety in pregnancy. T2w images may provide adequate visualization without contrast; however, if necessary, the use of contrast may be warranted because of the importance of accurate staging for proper management.

Lower stage cancers may be monitored closely with delay of therapy until delivery [50].

Summary

MR is the diagnostic imaging modality of choice for many disorders of the female pelvis. Benign uterine disease is well-demonstrated using rapid sequences and minimal examination time, whereas evaluation of malignancy is best performed with high-resolution techniques. Widespread availability of ultrafast sequences has expanded MR imaging applications to include evaluation of pelvic floor relaxation and fetal anomalies. Promising developments, such as new contrast agents, MR-guided focused ultrasound, and 3 tesla imaging, suggest continued advancement of MR imaging in the care of patients who have gynecologic disease.

References

[1] Hricak H, Alpers C, Crooks LE, et al. Magnetic resonance imaging of the female pelvis: initial experience. AJR Am J Roentgenol 1983;141(6):1119–28.
[2] Brown HK, Stoll BS, Nicosia SV, et al. Uterine junctional zone: correlation between histologic findings and MR imaging. Radiology 1991;179(2):409–13.

[3] Togashi K, Nakai A, Sugimura K. Anatomy and physiology of the female pelvis: MR imaging revisited. J Magn Reson Imaging 2001;13(6): 842–9.

[4] Scoutt LM, McCauley TR, Flynn SD, et al. Zonal anatomy of the cervix: correlation of MR imaging and histologic examination of hysterectomy specimens. Radiology 1993;186(1):159–62.

[5] Hricak H, Chang YC, Thurnher S. Vagina: evaluation with MR imaging. Part I. Normal anatomy and congenital anomalies. Radiology 1988;169: 169–74.

[6] Hricak H, Secaf E, Buckley DW, et al. Female urethra: MR imaging. Radiology 1991;178:527–35.

[7] Outwater EK, Dunton CJ. Imaging of the ovary and adnexa: clinical issues and applications of MR imaging. Radiology 1995;194:1–18.

[8] Troiano RN, McCarthy SM. Mullerian duct anomalies: imaging and clinical issues. Radiology 2004; 233(1):19–34.

[9] The American Fertility Society classifications of adnexal adhesions, distal tubal obstruction, tubal occlusion secondary to tubal ligation, tubal pregnancies, mullerian anomalies and intrauterine adhesions. Fertil Steril 1988;49:944–55.

[10] Murase E, Siegelman ES, Outwater EK, et al. Uterine leiomyomas: histopathologic features, MR imaging findings, differential diagnosis, and treatment. Radiographics 1999;19(5):1179–97.

[11] Ascher SM, Jha RC, Reinhold C. Benign myometrial conditions: leiomyomas and adenomyosis. Top Magn Reson Imaging 2003;14(4):281–304.

[12] Wallach EE, Vlahos NF. Uterine myomas: an overview of development, clinical features, and management. Obstet Gynecol 2004;104(2):393–406.

[13] Hindley J, Gedroyc WM, Regan L, et al. MRI guidance of focused ultrasound therapy of uterine fibroids: early results. AJR Am J Roentgenol 2004; 183(6):1713–9.

[14] Pelage JP, Guaou NG, Jha RC, et al. Uterine fibroid tumors: long-term MR imaging outcome after embolization. Radiology 2004;230(3):803–9.

[15] Ha HK, Lim YT, Kim HS, et al. Diagnosis of pelvic endometriosis: fat supressedT1-weighted vs. conventional MR images. AJR Am J Roentgenol 1994;163: 127–31.

[16] Bazot M, Darai E, Hourani R, et al. Deep pelvic endometriosis: MR imaging for diagnosis and prediction of extension of disease. Radiology 2004; 232(2):379–89.

[17] Kido A, Togashi K, Konishi I, et al. Dermoid cysts of the ovary with malignant transformation: MR appearance. AJR 1999;172:445–9.

[18] Kier R, Smith RC, McCarthy SM. Value of lipid- and water-suppression MR images in distinguishing between blood and lipid within ovarian masses. AJR Am J Roentgenol 1992;158:321–5.

[19] Guzick DS. Polycystic ovary syndrome. Obstet Gynecol 2004;103(1):181–93.

[20] Kimura I, Togashi K, Kawakami S, et al. Polycystic ovaries: implications of diagnosis with MR imaging. Radiology 1996;201:549–52.

[21] Gupta A, McCarthy S. Pelvic varices as a cause for pelvic pain: MRI appearance. Magn Reson Imaging 1994;12:679–81.

[22] Fielding JR. MR imaging of pelvic floor relaxation. Radiol Clin N Am 2003;41(4):747–56.

[23] Romanzi LJ, Groutz A, Blaivas JG. Urethral diverticulum in women: diverse presentations resulting in diagnostic delay and mismanagement. J Urol 2000; 164:428–33.

[24] Khati NJ, Javitt MC, Schwartz AM, et al. MR imaging diagnosis of a urethral diverticulum. Radiographics 1998;18:517–22.

[25] Blander DS, Broderick GA, Rovner ES. Images in clinical urology. Magnetic resonance imaging of a "saddle bag" urethral diverticulum. Urology 1999;53:818–9.

[26] Kaur H, Silverman PM, Iyer RB, et al. Diagnosis, staging, and surveillance of cervical carcinoma. AJR Am J Roentgenol 2003;180(6):1621–31.

[27] Peppercorn PD, Jeyarajah AR, Woolas R, et al. Role of MR imaging in the selection of patients with early cervical carcinoma for fertility-preserving surgery: initial experience. Radiology 1999;212(2):395–9.

[28] Hricak H, Powell CB, Yu KK, et al. Invasive cervical carcinoma: role of MR imaging in pretreatment work-up–cost minimization and diagnostic efficacy analysis. Radiology 1996;198(2):403–9.

[29] Shiraiwa M, Joja I, Asakawa T, et al. Cervical carcinoma: efficacy of thin-section oblique axial T2-weighted images for evaluating parametrial invasion. Abdom Imaging 1999;24(5):514–9.

[30] Seki H, Azumi R, Kimura M, et al. Stromal invasion by carcinoma of the cervix: assessment with dynamic MR imaging. AJR Am J Roentgenol 1997;168(6): 1579–85.

[31] Yang WT, Lam WW, Yu MY, et al. Comparison of dynamic helical CT and dynamic MR imaging in the evaluation of pelvic lymph nodes in cervical carcinoma. AJR Am J Roentgenol 2000;175(3):759–66.

[32] Harisinghani MG, Saini S, Weissleder R, et al. MR lymphangiography using ultrasmall superparamagnetic iron oxide in patients with primary abdominal and pelvic malignancies: radiographic-pathologic correlation. AJR Am J Roentgenol 1999;172(5): 1347–51.

[33] Chen SS, Lee L. Retroperitoneal lymph node metastases in stage I carcinoma of the endometrium: correlation with risk factors. Gynecol Oncol 1983; 16(3):319–25.

[34] Chaudhry S, Reinhold C, Guermazi A, et al. Benign and malignant diseases of the endometrium. Top Magn Reson Imaging 2003;14(4):339–57.

[35] Komatsu T, Konishi I, Mondai M, et al. Adnexal masses: transvaginal US and gadolinium-enhanced MR imaging assessment of intratumoral structure. Radiology 1996;198:109–15.

[36] Sohaib SA, Sahdev A, Van Trappen P, et al. Characterization of adnexal mass lesions on MR imaging. AJR Am J Roentgenol 2003;180(5):1297–304.

[37] Ha HK, Baek SY, Kim SH, et al. Kruckenberg's tumor of the ovary: MR imaging features. AJR 1995; 164:1435–9.

[38] Levine D, Barnes PD, Sher S, et al. Fetal Fast MR imaging: reproducibility, technical quality, and conspicuity of anatomy. Radiology 1998;206:549–54.

[39] Kanal E. Pregnancy and the safety of magnetic resonance imaging. Magn Reson Imag Clin N Am 1994;2:309–17.

[40] Dempsey MF, Condon B, Hadley DM. MRI safety review. Semin Ultrasound CT MR 2002;23:392–401.

[41] Shellock FG, Kanal E. Safety of magnetic resonance imaging contrast agents. J Magn Reson Imaging 1999;10(3):477–84.

[42] Nagayama M, Watanabe Y, Okumura A, et al. Fast MR imaging in obstetrics. Radiographics 2002;22: 563–80.

[43] Levine D, Barnes PD, Madsen JR, et al. Central nervous system abnormalities assessed with prenatal magnetic resonance imaging. Obstet Gynecol 1999; 94(6):1011–9.

[44] Kubik-Huch RA, Huisman TA, Wisser J, et al. Prenatal diagnosis of fetal malformations by ultrafast magnetic resonance imaging. Prenat Diagn 1998; 11:1205–8.

[45] Maldjian C, Adam R, Pelosi M, et al. MRI appearance of placenta percreta and placenta accreta. Magn Reson Imaging 1999;17(7):965–71.

[46] Leyendecker JR, Gorengaut V, Brown JJ. MR imaging of maternal diseases of the abdomen and pelvis during pregnancy and the immediate postpartum period. Radiographics 2004;24: 1301–16.

[47] Cobben LP, Groot I, Haans L, et al. MRI for clinically suspected appendicitis during pregnancy. AJR Am J Roentgenol 2004;183:671–5.

[48] Eyvazzadeh AD, Pedrosa I, Rofsky NM, et al. MRI of right-sided abdominal pain in pregnancy. AJR Am J Roentgenol 2004;183:907–14.

[49] Curtis M, Hopkins MP, Zarlingo T, et al. Magnetic resonance imaging to avoid laparotomy in pregnancy. Obstet Gynecol 1993;82(5):833–6.

[50] Nguyen C, Montz FJ, Bristow RE. Management of stage I cervical cancer in pregnancy. Obstet Gynecol Surv 2000;55(10):633–43.

ELSEVIER
SAUNDERS

Magn Reson Imaging Clin N Am
13 (2005) 397–400

MAGNETIC
RESONANCE
IMAGING CLINICS
of North America

Index

Note: Page numbers of article titles are in **boldface** type.

A

Abdomen, and pelvis, fundamentals of MR imaging techniques applied to, 241–242, 243
echo-train spin-echo sequences of, 246–247
fat-suppressed spoiled gradient-echo sequences of, 245
imaging of, at 1.5 Tesla, and optimization at 3 Tesla, **241–254**
optimization at 3 Tesla in, 247–254
balanced-echo sequences in, 250–251
dielectric effect at 3 Tesla in, 250
echo time in, 249
echo-train refocusing flip angle in, 250
potential limitation of, 252
single shot turbo spin-echo echo-train length in, 249–250
single shot turbo spin-echo sequences in, 248–250
summary of, 253
three-dimensional gradient-echo THRIVE in, 253
two-dimensional gradient-echo sequences in, 251–252
MR imaging of, general approach to, 247
out-of-phase spoiled gradient-echo sequences of, 244–245
spoiled gradient-echo sequences of, 244
standard spin-echo and fast spin-echo sequences of, 245–246
T1-weighted sequences of, 242
T2-weighted sequences of, 245–247
three-dimensional spoiled gradient-echo sequences of, 245

Adenocarcinoma, pancreatic, 317–321

Adenomyomatosis, MR imaging in, 301–302

Adenomyosis, 384–386

Aortic aneurysm, abdominal, 366, 370
thoracic, 367, 370

Aortic dissection, 370–371
type B, 367, 368, 371

Arterial occlusive disease, 369–370

Arteriovenous malformations, pulmonary, 375–376

Atherosclerosis, 369–370
MR imaging at 3.0T in, 363, 364, 366

B

Biliary system, anatomic variants of, 298–299
benign tumors of, 305
biliary calculi and, 303–304
congenital defects of, 303
gallbladder and, MR imaging of, **295–311**
malignant tumors of, 306
normal anatomy of, 297
obstruction of, 305
postoperative complications of, 306–308
primary sclerosing cholangitis of, 304
secondary cholangitis of, 305

Bowel, large, and small, combined imaging of, 356–357
inflammation of, MR colonography for detection of, 355
MR imaging of, **349–358**
small, **331–348**
coils of, 334
distension of, MR imaging of, 334
MR enteroclysis, technique of, 337–338, 339
MR follow through technique, 337
MR imaging of, clinical indications for, 338–344
oral contrast agents for, 334–337
protocols for, 331–338
sequences for, 331–334

Breast cancer, pancreatic metastasis from, 327, 328

Budd-Chiari syndrome, 288, 289

C

Calculi, of biliary system, 303–304

Cancer, acquired capabilities of, 228

Changing Your Address?

Make sure your subscription changes too! When you notify us of your new address, you can help make our job easier by including an exact copy of your Clinics label number with your old address (see illustration below.) This number identifies you to our computer system and will speed the processing of your address change. Please be sure this label number accompanies your old address and your corrected address—you can send an old Clinics label with your number on it or just copy it exactly and send it to the address listed below.

We appreciate your help in our attempt to give you continuous coverage. Thank you.

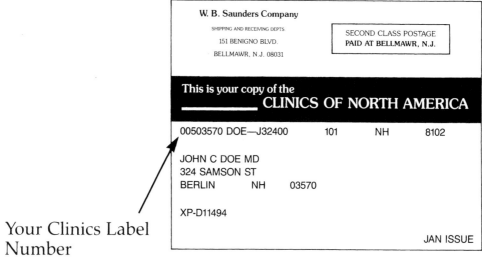

W. B. Saunders Company

SHIPPING AND RECEIVING DEPTS.

151 BENIGNO BLVD.

BELLMAWR, N.J. 08031

SECOND CLASS POSTAGE
PAID AT BELLMAWR, N.J.

This is your copy of the
_____ **CLINICS OF NORTH AMERICA**

00503570 DOE—J32400   101   NH   8102

JOHN C DOE MD
324 SAMSON ST
BERLIN   NH   03570

XP-D11494

JAN ISSUE

Your Clinics Label Number

Copy it exactly or send your label
along with your address to:
W.B. Saunders Company, Customer Service
Orlando, FL 32887-4800
Call Toll Free 1-800-654-2452

Please allow four to six weeks for delivery of new subscriptions and for processing address changes.

Practice, Current, Hardbound:
SATISFACTION GUARANTEED

YES! Please start my subscription to the **CLINICS** checked below with the ❑ first issue of the calendar year or ❑ current issues. If not completely satisfied with my first issue, I may write "cancel" on the invoice and return it within 30 days at no further obligation.

Please Print:

Name _____

Address_____

City_____ State _____ ZIP _____

Method of Payment

❑ Check (payable to **Elsevier**; add the applicable sales tax for your area)

❑ VISA   ❑ MasterCard   ❑ AmEx   ❑ Bill me

Card number _____ Exp. date _____

Signature _____

Staple this to your purchase order to expedite delivery

❑ **Adolescent Medicine Clinics**
  ❑ Individual $95
  ❑ Institutions $133
  ❑ *In-training $48

❑ **Anesthesiology**
  ❑ Individual $175
  ❑ Institutions $270
  ❑ *In-training $88

❑ **Cardiology**
  ❑ Individual $170
  ❑ Institutions $266
  ❑ *In-training $85

❑ **Chest Medicine**
  ❑ Individual $185
  ❑ Institutions $285

❑ **Child and Adolescent Psychiatry**
  ❑ Individual $175
  ❑ Institutions $265
  ❑ *In-training $88

❑ **Critical Care**
  ❑ Individual $165
  ❑ Institutions $266
  ❑ *In-training $83

❑ **Dental**
  ❑ Individual $150
  ❑ Institutions $242

❑ **Emergency Medicine**
  ❑ Individual $170
  ❑ Institutions $263
  ❑ *In-training $85
    ❑ Send CME info

❑ **Facial Plastic Surgery**
  ❑ Individual $199
  ❑ Institutions $300

❑ **Foot and Ankle**
  Individual $160
  Institutions $232

❑ **Gastroenterology**
  ❑ Individual $190
  ❑ Institutions $276

❑ **Gastrointestinal Endoscopy**
  ❑ Individual $190
  ❑ Institutions $276

❑ **Hand**
  ❑ Individual $205
  ❑ Institutions $319

❑ **Heart Failure (NEW in 2005!)**
  ❑ Individual $99
  ❑ Institutions $149
  ❑ *In-training $49

❑ **Hematology/ Oncology**
  ❑ Individual $210
  ❑ Institutions $315

❑ **Immunology & Allergy**
  ❑ Individual $165
  ❑ Institutions $266

❑ **Infectious Disease**
  ❑ Individual $165
  ❑ Institutions $272

❑ **Clinics in Liver Disease**
  ❑ Individual $165
  ❑ Institutions $234

❑ **Medical**
  ❑ Individual $140
  ❑ Institutions $244
  ❑ *In-training $70
    ❑ Send CME info

❑ **MRI**
  ❑ Individual $190
  ❑ Institutions $290
  ❑ *In-training $95
    ❑ Send CME info

❑ **Neuroimaging**
  ❑ Individual $190
  ❑ Institutions $290
  ❑ *In-training $95
    ❑ Send CME inf0

❑ **Neurologic**
  ❑ Individual $175
  ❑ Institutions $275

❑ **Obstetrics & Gynecology**
  ❑ Individual $175
  ❑ Institutions $288

❑ **Occupational and Environmental Medicine**
  ❑ Individual $120
  ❑ Institutions $166
  ❑ *In-training $60

❑ **Ophthalmology**
  ❑ Individual $190
  ❑ Institutions $325

❑ **Oral & Maxillofacial Surgery**
  ❑ Individual $180
  ❑ Institutions $280
  ❑ *In-training $90

❑ **Orthopedic**
  ❑ Individual $180
  ❑ Institutions $295
  ❑ *In-training $90

❑ **Otolaryngologic**
  ❑ Individual $199
  ❑ Institutions $350

❑ **Pediatric**
  ❑ Individual $135
  ❑ Institutions $246
  ❑ *In-training $68
    ❑ Send CME info

❑ **Perinatology**
  ❑ Individual $155
  ❑ Institutions $237
  ❑ *In-training $78
    ❑ Send CME inf0

❑ **Plastic Surgery**
  ❑ Individual $245
  ❑ Institutions $370

❑ **Podiatric Medicine & Surgery**
  ❑ Individual $170
  ❑ Institutions $266

❑ **Primary Care**
  ❑ Individual $135
  ❑ Institutions $223

❑ **Psychiatric**
  ❑ Individual $170
  ❑ Institutions $288

❑ **Radiologic**
  ❑ Individual $220
  ❑ Institutions $331
  ❑ *In-training $110
    ❑ Send CME info

❑ **Sports Medicine**
  ❑ Individual $180
  ❑ Institutions $277

❑ **Surgical**
  ❑ Individual $190
  ❑ Institutions $299
  ❑ *In-training $95

❑ **Thoracic Surgery (formerly Chest Surgery)**
  ❑ Individual $175
  ❑ Institutions $255
  ❑ *In-training $88

❑ **Urologic**
  ❑ Individual $195
  ❑ Institutions $307
  ❑ *In-training $98
    ❑ Send CME info

---

*To receive in-training rate, orders must be accompanied by the name of affiliated institution, dates of residency and signature of coordinator on institution letterhead. Orders will be billed at the individual rate until proof of resident status is received.

© **Elsevier 2005.** Offer valid in U.S. only. Prices subject to change without notice. **MO 10807 DF4176**

BUSINESS REPLY MAIL

FIRST-CLASS MAIL   PERMIT NO 7135   ORLANDO FL

POSTAGE WILL BE PAID BY ADDRESSEE

PERIODICALS ORDER FULFILLMENT DEPT
ELSEVIER
6277 SEA HARBOR DR
ORLANDO FL 32821-9816